CBT for Adult

A Practical Gu

for Clinicians

CBT for Adults:
A Practical Guide
for Clinicians

Lynne M. Drummond

RCPsych Publications

© The Royal College of Psychiatrists 2014

RCPsych Publications is an imprint of the Royal College of Psychiatrists,
21 Prescot Street, London E1 8BB
http://www.rcpsych.ac.uk

British Library Cataloguing-in-Publication Data.
A catalogue record for this book is available from the British Library.
ISBN 978 1 909726 27 7

Distributed in North America by Publishers Storage and Shipping Company.

The views presented in this book do not necessarily reflect those of the Royal College of Psychiatrists, and the publishers are not responsible for any error of omission or fact.

The Royal College of Psychiatrists is a charity registered in England and Wales (228636) and in Scotland (SC038369).

Printed by Bell & Bain Limited, Glasgow, UK.

To Laura, Neal and Hugh

Contents

Tables, boxes, figures and case examples

Foreword

In recent years effective cognitive–behavioural therapies have become widely used. They can help many individuals to overcome a broad range of problems in order to live normal lives. As there are few easy guides to such therapies for would-be therapists, this new book is most welcome. Clinicians wishing to apply behavioural and cognitive procedures can learn more from how-to-do-it guidance than from theoretical disquisitions. In this easy-to-read book therapists can find a wide variety of case histories of therapy in sufficient detail to use similar methods in their own work. The book contains many examples of careful treatment applications that will allow practitioners to skilfully meet the needs of their own patients. An important advance concerns self-help for anxiety disorders. Self-exposure can be so successful that, as this book notes, in most individuals with anxiety disorder clinician-accompanied exposure is unnecessary. The therapist's main task is to encourage the patient to work out and complete suitable exposure targets and to monitor progress towards their achievement. Lynne Drummond gives clear guidance on this topic.

Also mentioned is a National Institute of Mental Health (NIMH) multicentre controlled study of the treatment of depression. In that study interpersonal therapy was at least as effective as cognitive therapy. The cognitive part of cognitive therapy may be redundant, the core element to the various successful brief psychotherapies for depression being task-oriented problem-solving. However, cognitive therapy on its own can, too, be therapeutic.

Other relatively recent knowledge concerns medication combined with exposure in some individuals with anxiety disorders. In a large controlled study of agoraphobia with panic in London and Toronto, high doses of benzodiazepines interfered with exposure in the long term and should therefore be avoided. In contrast, in additional work, antidepressants did not interfere with exposure and indeed could enhance it when depression complicated the phobia/panic or obsessive–compulsive problem. Moreover, a variety of antidepressant drugs can be used in such cases as no particular class is yet known to be specific to any given anxiety syndrome.

It is encouraging that clinicians can quickly learn to guide patients to complete behavioural and cognitive treatments for a large number of clinical problems that help many people improve within a few weeks, and in more difficult cases within a few months. This volume by Dr Drummond is an excellent guide for clinicians who want to learn how to do this.

Emeritus Professor Isaac M. Marks
Institute of Psychiatry, King's College London

Preface

This book is designed for clinicians as a practical guide to treating adults with psychological and psychiatric disorders using cognitive and behavioural interventions. I firmly believe that clinicians learn best from patients, and so I have included illustrative case history material throughout. The book is similar in format to an earlier book I co-authored with Richard Stern, *The Practice of Behavioural and Cognitive Psychotherapy*, published in 1991. Indeed, a few of the case histories originally appeared in the earlier book but are still relevant and I am extremely grateful to Richard Stern and Cambridge University Press for allowing me to reuse them here.

The whole subject of cognitive–behavioural psychotherapy has developed significantly since that first volume. In 1991, the 'cognitive revolution' was taking hold and cognitive therapy was being hailed as a panacea for a whole range of psychiatric and psychological conditions. Sadly and inevitably, it did not live up to all the claims that were then being made. More recently the role of cognitive interventions has been identified in a number of conditions, including depression and anxiety disorders. Cognitive therapy is a useful and often necessary adjunct for the treatment of other conditions, including body dysmorphic disorder, health anxiety, hypochondriasis and social anxiety. The development of the so-called 'third generation' or 'third wave' therapies has seen a move back to behavioural treatments with less emphasis on the cognitive elements. All these more recent interventions are described but with a note of caution that there is still a relative lack of good-quality, robust research on many of these.

The aim of this book is to be a practical guide to interventions using clinical examples. It is not full of theory. A theoretical overview is presented in each chapter and is developed as different approaches are discussed. This is designed to ensure a clinician understands why different techniques may be applied to different patients. Key references are presented so that anyone who is interested in looking into this further can easily do so, and I have also listed books for further reading.

No one should ever think any book will equip them to be able to apply all the therapies. Anyone embarking on these treatments is best advised to obtain supervision from a fully accredited cognitive–behavioural therapy (CBT) supervisor. Some of the simpler techniques, however (such as 'cleaning up a patient's lifestyle' in Chapter 9), could be applied with little or no supervision. Hopefully, I will give readers new therapeutic ideas and encourage them to develop further skills.

I hope you enjoy this book and find it useful. My hope is that it will have a place in your office used for clinical work with patients and will be referred to when making clinical decisions about care.

L.M.D.

Structure of the book

The order of the chapters is based on the introduction of the various theories and techniques to be used. It is intended that the more straightforward theories and techniques are presented first, before moving on to more complex paradigms and methods. In other words, after exploring assessment for CBT, the book starts with behavioural treatments such as exposure-based therapies and then examines reinforcement and skill acquisition. Subsequent chapters introduce cognitive theory and practice and also start to look at the third wave treatments. Later chapters in the book cover more complex applications of CBT in conditions including personality disorder and psychoses. Finally, the possibility of integrating CBT with other treatments is discussed before starting to look at what the future may hold for CBT.

Chapter 1

This chapter starts by looking at the history of CBT. Starting at the beginning of the 20th century with the behaviourist movement, it follows the development of pragmatic treatments based on observation of clinical situations and the behaviour of the individual rather than on theory. Indeed, usually the theories were developed to describe the clinical findings rather than *vice versa*. Exposure-based treatments, reinforcement schedules and skills training are mentioned. The theories and treatments that comprise the so-called cognitive revolution are examined and the reversion back to more behavioural methods is explored. Finally, the chapter considers where CBT has come in the past 50 years and postulates some of what the future may hold.

Chapter 2

This chapter examines the pivotal importance of measurement and its role in CBT. Being a pragmatic approach to psychological and psychiatric distress and disorders, the idea that each patient was their own 'single-case' experiment was the hallmark of CBT. Although there are strong theoretical concepts which underpin CBT treatments, the use of the single-case design, whereby improvement or deterioration is objectively measured, shaped the development of treatments. Indeed, sometimes it was observations about the effect of different interventions which led to the theory rather than the traditional approach of theory leading to treatments. It is thus vital that anyone embarking on CBT has a firm understanding of an approach to measurement that is both reliable and valid.

Chapters 3, 4 and 5

These chapters focus mainly on the role of reinforcement and how it can be used effectively in skill acquisition. The different types of reinforcers are described and the potential role they may have in the treatment as well as the genesis of psychological and behavioural disorders. The way that complex skills can be divided into their component behaviours and taught using reinforcement is then discussed in the application in social skills, relationship, communications and sexual skills training. The recently developed treatment of integrative couple therapy is also briefly mentioned.

Chapters 6 and 7

The next two chapters examine the role of exposure treatments and their role in the management of phobic anxiety and OCD. They are deliberately at the start of the book as they describe one of the most straightforward treatment paradigms in CBT, which is still the good standard treatment for these conditions.

Chapters 8 and 9

Chapter 8 introduces the basic theories of cognitive therapy expanded on in Chapter 9. These chapters demonstrate the practical application of cognitive interventions in depression and generalised anxiety and how these treatments are combined with some of the behavioural treatments already discussed. The concept of CBT involving both cognitive and behavioural components is then further developed in the succeeding chapters.

In addition, some of the so-called third generation treatments involving mindfulness are introduced and described.

Chapters 10 and 11

The importance of combining firm behavioural principles and treatment in combination with cognitive interventions is emphasised in these chapters which look at health anxiety and body dysmorphic and eating disorders.

Chapter 12

The principles and application of motivational interviewing are discussed in detail. Treating addictions using complex integration of cognitive reattribution combined with behavioural coping skills is described. Relapse prevention strategies are important for all conditions but are particularly vital when dealing with addictive behaviour. These are tackled fully in this chapter.

Chapter 13

The application of CBT in the treatment of psychoses is studied. Effective medication and early treatment has meant many more people with psychoses are potentially amenable to CBT. However, it is still necessary to proceed slowly and with care in applying these techniques to people with severe, enduring psychotic disorders. There is demonstration of how CBT techniques can be used to engage the patient in therapy and to start to examine some of the thoughts underpinning the symptoms of psychoses.

Chapter 14

This chapter describes the development of the CBT model to derive schema-based CBT for people with personality disorders.

The third generation treatment of dialectical behaviour therapy is then explored along with its application in people with borderline personality disorder. There is a discussion about the shortfalls in current research in these methods.

Chapter 15

Cognitive–behavioural therapy is usually not delivered in isolation but in combination with other therapies. This chapter examines which combinations are helpful and which can be a hindrance to progress. The most frequent combination is CBT and psychopharmacological interventions and these are explored in detail. The combination of different types of psychological treatment is then discussed, starting with eye movement desensitisation and reprocessing in combination with CBT. The potential negative effect that delivering two models of psychotherapy can have will also be examined. Finally, more 'hybrid' models of therapy such a cognitive analytical therapy and systemic therapy are explored.

Abbreviations

ACT   acceptance and commitment therapy

A&E   accident and emergency

BDD   body dysmorphic disorder

BDI   Beck Depression Inventory

BMI   body mass index

BPD   borderline personality disorder

CAT   cognitive analytical therapy

CBT   cognitive–behavioural therapy

DBT   dialectical behaviour therapy

DIRT   danger ideation reduction therapy

ECT   electroconvulsive therapy

EDNOS   eating disorders not otherwise specified

EMDR   eye movement desensitisation and reprocessing

ERP   graded exposure and self-imposed response prevention

FAP   functional analytic psychotherapy

GP   general practitioner

IAPT   Improving Access to Psychological Therapies

ICT   integrative couple therapy

MBCT   mindfulness-based cognitive therapy

NAT   negative automatic thought

NHS   National Health Service

NICE   National Institute for Health and Care Excellence (until May 2013 the National Institute for Health and Clinical Excellence)

NIMH   National Institute of Mental Health

OCD	obsessive–compulsive disorder
PTSD	post-traumatic stress disorder
RCT	randomised controlled trial
REBT	rational emotive behavioural therapy
SLOF	Specific Level of Functioning Assessment
SNRI	serotonin-noradrenaline reuptake inhibitor
SRI	serotonin reuptake inhibitor
SSRI	selective serotonin reuptake inhibitor
YBOCS	Yale–Brown Obsessive Compulsive Scale

Introduction

Overview

This chapter will examine the development and future of cognitive–behavioural therapy (CBT). Starting with the ideas of behaviourism and the development of conditioning theory, it moves to examine the exposure theory and its application in clinical practice. This sets the groundwork for the concept of pragmatic treatments based on direct clinical observations rather than being guided purely by theoretical models. Mention will be made of other third wave treatments such as mindfulness, behavioural activation, dialectical behaviour therapy (DBT), acceptance and commitment therapy and integrative couple therapy, the cognitive–behavioural analysis system of psychotherapy and functional analytic psychotherapy. Finally, there is a summary concerning research and CBT and a look towards possible future developments.

The development of CBT: history, theory and practice

First generation therapies

Behaviourism arose at the beginning of the 20th century. Its central tenet is that all organisms react to the external environment with a variety of behaviours. These behaviours are learnt and are in response to reinforcement, and so it follows that psychological and psychiatric conditions are seen largely as being due to maladaptive learnt behaviour in response to the environment.

Key people who developed the theories of behaviourism were:

- Ivan Pavlov (classical conditioning; Pavlov, 1927)
- Edward Lee Thorndike (pioneer of using animals in psychological experiments; Thorndike, 1933)
- John Broadus Watson (animal studies and also genesis of phobias in humans – the 'Little Albert' experiment; Watson, 1925)
- Burrhus Frederic Skinner (operant conditioning; Skinner 1950).

It was not until mid-20th century that the potential for using behavioural methods to treat patients with psychological conditions was realised. Joseph Wolpe developed a technique called systematic desensitisation for the treatment of phobic anxiety (Wolpe, 1958). In this technique, the patient is taught deep muscle relaxation and a very detailed hierarchy of fears is produced. The patient is very gradually exposed to the fear while inducing relaxation. This treatment worked at reducing anxiety but was painstakingly slow and any therapeutic gains tended to be lost if the patient subsequently became anxious. Thus the treatment was rendered virtually obsolete in the 1970s with the development of graded *in vivo* exposure.

Real-life exposure methods were pioneered by James Watson and Isaac Marks (1971) in the treatment of phobic disorder. Following on from this, a range of conditions were added to those that could be treated using behavioural psychotherapy. These behavioural approaches remain the treatments of choice for most phobic anxiety, obsessive–compulsive disorders, skill-deficit disorders (e.g. social and sexual) and mild to moderate depression (behavioural activation). They are also a major component of the treatment of many conditions, including health anxiety and hypochondriasis, body dysmorphic disorder, eating disorders, addictive problems, and schizophrenia.

Second generation therapies

Simultaneously with the development of behavioural psychotherapy Albert Ellis, an American psychologist who had trained as a psychoanalyst, broke away from the psychoanalytic school and established the basis of rational emotive behavioural therapy (REBT; Ellis 1962). In REBT (also known as rational emotive therapy and rational therapy) the basic theory is that, in the main, people are not disturbed by negative events but by their beliefs about these events. These beliefs involve the world, themselves and others. The ABC model states that 'A' – the activating event (or adversity) contributes to 'C' – the behavioural and emotional consequences. However, the 'B' – beliefs about the activating event – moderates this response. The activating event can either be an external event or a thought about the past, present or future. In therapy, patients are asked to confront these beliefs with rational responses.

Aaron Temkin Beck was also trained as a psychoanalyst and worked as a psychiatrist in Pennsylvania. He started by experimentally investigating psychoanalytical concepts and through this developed his model for depression (Beck *et al*, 1979) and, subsequently, anxiety disorder (Beck *et al*, 1985) and personality disorder (Beck *et al*, 2003). It is this form of cognitive intervention which is the most widely used with patients and it is referred to in this book. Beck described the negative automatic thoughts (NATs) and how these could be challenged to alter mood. The approach is described in full in Chapters 8, 9 and 10.

Introduction to third generation (third wave) CBT

At the turn of the 20th century, many therapists and researchers began to question the shortcomings of CBT. There developed a group of loosely connected therapies which have been called 'third wave' or 'third generation' CBT therapies. These therapies have several things in common:

- all are empirically based and subjected to scientific evaluation
- all move to being more behavioural in orientation and less concerned with cognitions *per se*
- rather than examining the content of cognitions, these therapies concentrate on how the patient responds to these cognitions (i.e. looks at the direct behaviour resulting from these).

Therapies that are included under this heading are:

- mindfulness
- behavioural activation
- acceptance and commitment therapy (ACT)
- dialectical behaviour therapy (DBT)
- integrative couple therapy (ICT)
- other therapies (e.g. functional analytic psychotherapy).

To practise some of these therapies, such as DBT and the cognitive–behavioural analysis system of psychotherapy, requires therapists to attend a separate course as well as receive supervision.

The issue with many of these third generation CBT methods is currently the lack of empirical evidence of their efficacy in treating disorders. A recent Cochrane review of treatments for depression found two studies examining ACT and one examining behavioural activation which met the criteria for analysis. The final conclusion was that both treatments appeared as effective as CBT in acute depression (Hunot *et al*, 2013).

Current position regarding CBT

Over the past 50 years, behavioural psychotherapy treatments have been developed for a variety of conditions. These treatments are simple, effective and have a strong evidence base for a range of psychological conditions. Although they require the therapist to have the ability to form a good relationship with the patient and to be empathic and sensitive to the patient's emotions, they do not require a high level of specialised training beyond that. All that is needed is a core mental health professional experience, some background knowledge and clinical supervision to enable most people to conduct exposure therapies and devise skills acquisition and reinforcement regimes. Owing to this, the key advantages of behavioural psychotherapy are that it is effective (see list of conditions which can be treated earlier in this chapter), it is cheap (highly specialised therapists are not necessary) and it produces rapid results.

The development of CBT meant that the range of conditions which could be treated using a pragmatic evidence-based method widened and included, for example, generalised anxiety and panic, depression as well as health anxiety, body dysmorphic disorder and social anxiety. Very soon CBT was being hailed as a panacea that could solve a range of psychiatric conditions. Inevitably this meant it would not live up to all the extreme expectations. Some of the treatments are less evidence-based than others. Also there has been a tendency to 'throw out the baby with the bath water' as many therapists now only use CBT for conditions where an evidence-based treatment was established. For example, cognitive approaches were often applied in simple phobias and obsessive–compulsive disorder (OCD) where there is no evidence to suggest these are preferable to the simpler methods of exposure. As will be suggested in Chapter 7, it may be preferable to focus the cognitive approaches in these conditions on people who have specific problems in performing exposure methods.

Overall, CBT is:

- intellectually more attractive to therapists (and some patients) than behavioural psychotherapy
- more expensive than behavioural psychotherapy (therapists need more training and treatment tends to take longer)
- known to be effective in certain conditions such as depression, generalised anxiety, health anxiety and social anxiety
- being used for some conditions with little evidence base to demonstrate its efficacy, where caution is needed in claiming its superiority to other methods
- well established with a large number of CBT-trained therapists available across the high-income countries.

The third generation therapies have recognised some of the shortfalls of concentrating on cognitions and represent a move back to more strictly behavioural methods. Many of the treatments remain quite complex and involved, and yet there is considerable overlap between many of them. There is a need for detailed, good-quality research to examine not only their true effectiveness but also which components of the packages are the most valuable. In general, third generation therapies:

- represent a move back to more behavioural methods
- often are contained in complex packages (with the exception of behavioural activation)
- often require therapists to attend dedicated courses, training only in one particular therapy, making them expensive and, some being patented, exclusive; they are thus, in general, more expensive to deliver
- are not as well researched as the rest of CBT
- need to have the effective components of these complex packages isolated.

Human nature means that even if we have good, effective, reliable treatments available, we will tend to be attracted to the newer, more exciting treatments that are developed and forget the advantages of some of the older methods. As will be shown throughout the book, often treatments change with fashion, whereas existing treatments may work as well or better than the ones which have replaced them. One example is in the use of long-term schema-focused CBT for personality disorder and DBT for personality disorder. There is research to suggest that these approaches are superior to waiting-list controls (Stoffers *et al*, 2012), but there is difficulty in claiming with confidence that they are preferable to more traditional psychodynamic psychotherapy or the more recently introduced psychoanalytically oriented day-patient mentalisation-based treatment. Given these provisos, it is difficult to know the value of the new treatments in the long term.

New developments and the future

New developments which have proven useful include computerised treatment packages. These computerised treatments were first introduced in the 1980s (e.g. Carr *et al*, 1988). They became more widespread with the greater availability of computers in the home as well as at specialist centres. The evidence base for this type of approach is growing in the area of anxiety disorders and depression (Andrews *et al*, 2010; Christensen *et al*, 2014). Increasing availability of mobile technology has led to the development of mobile phone and tablet applications which mean the patient can access therapy wherever they wish (Watts *et al*, 2013). There is huge potential for technology to deliver more therapy in more sophisticated ways in the future. However, there should be a note of caution as already there is a plethora of programmes purporting to treat common psychological conditions. These vary in their quality and the evidence behind their advice. Whereas some individuals with milder conditions may be able to access these programmes and complete them unaided to good effect, many more will also require some advice and guidance from trained professionals to assist them in the choice and application of the treatment. The use of such applications is thus often best thought of as a way of delivering therapy to more people but still requiring some trained interventions from a professional.

Another development in the UK was the launch in 2007 of the government initiative Improving Access to Psychological Therapies (IAPT). This scheme aimed to introduce into primary care widespread services providing CBT treatment to people with depression and anxiety disorders (Clark *et al*, 2009). This initiative has resulted in thousands more people receiving appropriate and effective treatment at an early stage. Treatment is delivered by specially trained graduate workers and supervised by trained psychologists. However, the sheer volume of patients accessing these services has led to a tendency for a 'one-size-fits-all' approach in some cases. Whereas overall excellent outcomes have been obtained, some patients slip through the net. There are now fewer trained CBT therapists in secondary care services and most secondary care services specialise in the psychoses and bipolar disorders. Some more severely ill patients with anxiety and obsessive–compulsive disorders require more specialist interventions, which are frequently unavailable. We need to continue to monitor the outcome with the IAPT services and ensure that those with more complex conditions are signposted appropriately to experts in the field. For example, a recent meeting of OCD Action (a national UK charity supporting people with OCD) highlighted that some individuals with OCD are receiving generic anxiety management training rather than the graded exposure they require (J. Rose, 2014, personal communication).

The future is always difficult to predict and undoubtedly will involve 'forgetting' some of the old effective treatments as people try to invent newer, more 'fashionable' ways of treating patients. It is to be hoped, however, that with increasing reliance on treatment protocols and reviews of the literature, we can maintain the older reliable and effective treatments while fully scientifically investigating newer treatments and developing newer, more cost-efficient treatments for a wider number of patients.

Key learning points

- First wave behavioural treatments are still valid, useful, cost-efficient treatments for a variety of psychological disorders, including obsessive–compulsive disorders, phobic anxiety, social skills deficits and habit disorders.
- Second wave treatments include CBT for depression, generalised anxiety, social anxiety and health anxiety.
- Third wave treatments involve a mixed bag of treatments, generally with a move away from cognitive therapy and back to more behavioural methods. Many of these treatments also involve mindfulness.
- There is, so far, less robust evidence for third wave treatments than for behavioural or cognitive interventions.
- Third generation treatments include:
  - mindfulness, a form of meditation where the individual is encouraged to concentrate on the 'here and now'
  - behavioural activation
  - acceptance and commitment therapy
  - dialectical behaviour therapy
  - integrative couple therapy
  - other therapies (e.g. functional analytic psychotherapy and the cognitive–behavioural analysis system of psychotherapy)
- The development of IAPT services in the UK has vastly increased the number of patients with anxiety and depressive disorders who can receive treatment.
- Computerised CBT is now realistically available to most of the population and is developing rapidly.

References

Andrews G, Cuiipers P, Craske MG, *et al* (2010) Computer therapy for the anxiety and depressive disorders is effective, acceptable and practical health care: a meta-analysis. *PLoS One*, **5**: e13196.

Beck AT, Rush AJ, Shaw BF, *et al* (1979) *Cognitive Therapy of Depression*. Guilford Press.

Beck AT, Emery G, Greenberg RL (1985) *Anxiety Disorders and Phobias: A Cognitive Perspective*. Basic Books.

Beck AT, Freeman A, Davis DD (2003) *Cognitive Therapy of Personality Disorders*. Guilford Press.

Carr AC, Ghosh A, Marks IM (1988) Computer-supervised exposure treatment for phobias. *Canadian Journal of Psychiatry*, **33**: 112–17.

Christensen H, Batterham B, Calear A (2014) Online interventions for anxiety disorders. *Current Opinion in Psychiatry*, **27**: 7–13.

Clark DM, Layard R, Smithies R, *et al* (2009) Improving Access to Psychological Therapies: initial evaluation of two UK demonstration sites. *Behaviour Research and Therapy*, **47**: 910–20.

Ellis A (1962) *Reason and Emotion in Psychotherapy*. Lyle Stuart.

Hunot V, Moore TH, Caldwell DM, *et al* (2013) Third wave cognitive and behavioural therapies versus other psychological therapies for depression. *Cochrane Database of Systematic Reviews*, **10**: CD008704.

Pavlov IP (1927) *Conditioned Reflexes: An Investigation of the Physiological Activity of the Cerebral Cortex* (transl GV Anrep). Oxford University Press.

Skinner BF (1950) Are theories of learning necessary? *Psychology Reviews*, **57**: 193–216.

Stoffers JM, Vollm BA, Rucker G, *et al* (2012) Psychological therapies for people with borderline personality disorder. *Cochrane Database of Systematic Reviews*, **15**: CD005652.

Thorndike EL (1933) *An Experimental Study of Rewards*. Teachers College, Columbia University.

Watson JB (1925) *Behaviorism*. WW Norton.

Watson JP, Marks IM (1971) Relevant and irrelevant fear in flooding – a crossover study of phobic patients. *Behavior Therapy*, **2**: 275–93.

Watts S, Mackenzie A, Thomas C, *et al* (2013) CBT for depression: a pilot RCT comparing mobile phone vs computer. *BMC Psychiatry*, **13**: 409.

Wolpe J (1958) *Psychotherapy by Reciprocal Inhibition*. Stanford University Press.

Further reading

Beck AT, Rush AJ, Shaw BF, *et al* (1979) *Cognitive Therapy of Depression*. Guilford Press.

Beck AT, Emery G, Greenberg RL (1985) *Anxiety Disorders and Phobias: A Cognitive Perspective*. Basic Books.

Buckley KW (1989) *Mechanical Man: John Broadus Watson and the Beginnings of Behaviorism*. Guilford Press.

Crane R (2009) *Mindfulness-Based Cognitive Therapy*. Routledge.

Ellis A (1962) *Reason and Emotion in Psychotherapy*. Lyle Stuart.

Flaxman PE, Blackledge JT, Bond PW (2011) *Acceptance and Commitment Therapy*. Routledge.

Linehan MM (1993) *Cognitive Behavioural Treatment of Borderline Personality Disorder*. Guilford Press.

Marks IM (1987) *Fears, Phobias and Rituals*. Oxford University Press.

Marks IM (1988) *Cure and Care of Neuroses*. Wiley.

Skinner BF (1953) *Science and Human Behaviour*. Free Press.

Skinner BF (1974) *About Behaviorism*. Random House.

Assessment

> Overview
>
> This chapter gives a full description of assessment of the patient for CBT and the development of the cognitive–behavioural formulation. The assessment starts with a full description of a thorough psychiatric history and looks at various *aides-memoires* and models of symptom development before demonstrating how a full cognitive–behavioural formulation can be derived. There is full description of the measurement of problems, the identification of goals and the roles of behavioural tests and questionnaire assessment.

Many people assume that there is a great mystery to the art of performing a good cognitive–behavioural assessment. In fact, this is far from the truth and any thorough clinician should elicit sufficient information to enable an adequate formulation to be made, and to implement a treatment regime. Following this procedure, measures of the problem are used to gauge the severity and to enable both the therapist and the patient to monitor progress, success or failure of the treatment.

To obtain a CBT assessment does, of course, require that the therapist is a skilled interviewer who is familiar with putting people at ease and dealing with patients. As the skills of psychiatric and general psychological interviewing are beyond the scope of this book, any reader who is unsure about this should not attempt CBT assessment until they have undergone a refresher course.

The chapter is divided into four main sections. The first concentrates on CBT history-taking and assessment, the second on the CBT formulation, the third on the education of the patient and planning treatment, and finally, the fourth section discusses the use of baseline and successive measures of the problem. As CBT psychotherapists come from a whole range of mental healthcare professions, it is important that these assessment procedures are used as an adjunct to rather than a replacement for general assessment procedures. All therapists should have a protocol in their mind for obtaining general information and assessing psychiatric patients. Just because a patient arrives at a clinic referred for CBT does not exclude the possibility of other major mental health problems, or even serious physical disorder. For example, a patient was referred to me with 'agoraphobia', subsequently diagnosed as chronic fatigue due to chronic lymphatic leukaemia; another patient was referred with 'generalised anxiety and depersonalisation' but was found to have temporal lobe epilepsy; and many patients are referred with various anxiety syndromes whereas in fact they are severely depressed and need the depression treated first.

The first section of this chapter is aimed at a medical audience who will normally combine a diagnostic psychiatric interview with the initial CBT assessment. Non-medical readers may still find this helpful, though they may wish to concentrate on the subsection on checklists and mnemonics (pp. 10–13) and add this to the normal assessment procedures as appropriate to their mental health discipline.

From medical assessment to CBT assessment

In most specialties of medicine, the doctor takes a full history from the patient and then assesses the symptoms and signs to arrive at a diagnosis. If a patient was seen by a surgeon and said they had 'appendicitis', it is unlikely that the doctor would write this down as a diagnosis unquestioned. Unfortunately, this is not always the case in psychiatry. Patients may say they have 'panic attacks' or 'generalised anxiety' and the psychiatrist may not fully investigate the statement. They may obtain exhaustive details of the patient's family and early history but fail to gain precise descriptions of current symptomatology. With any symptom it is worth looking at ten main questions which make the unlikely mnemonic of 'Dad's car fad' (Box 2.1).

After obtaining details of the symptoms in this way, it is important then to trace the progress from their onset, with any variations in symptomatology and details of the circumstances and life events which may have occurred at various times throughout the history. This information is vital as it may radically alter the formulation and resultant treatment. For example, a 25-year-old woman presented with a 2-year history of fear of dirt and germs as she worried that she might catch a fatal disease. This fear was accompanied by avoidance of touching anything that had been touched by other people unless using tissues or rubber gloves and extensive hand-washing and cleaning rituals. Whereas at first this may have appeared to be a straightforward obsessive–compulsive history which would be best treated by graduated exposure to the feared situation in real life and self-imposed response prevention (see Chapter 7), it transpired that these started following a vicious rape attack. Treatment therefore needed to start by addressing her post-traumatic stress disorder (PTSD; see Chapter 15) before proceeding to treatment of the residual OCD.

Box 2.1 Ten questions instrumental in obtaining accurate psychiatric diagnosis – the 'Dad's car fad' mnemonic

Description. Full description of what the patient means by the symptom. What does it feel like? What happens?

Associated phenomena. Description of the thoughts, fears and emotions of the patient at the time of experiencing their symptoms.

Duration. Duration of all the symptoms.

Severity. Severity of all the symptoms.

Course. A chronological description of what happens from the very first symptom to resolution of the symptom.

Aggravating factors. Does anything make the symptoms worse or more likely to occur?

Relieving factors. Does anything make the symptoms better or less likely to occur?

Frequency and periodicity. How often do these symptoms occur and do they vary in severity?

Associated phenomena. Any other symptoms that have occurred? If the answer is affirmative, then repeat the same questions with each of these symptoms.

Diurnal variation. What time of day, when, where and with whom do the symptoms occur?

Once the full history of presenting complaints has been obtained in this way, the rest of the details of the patient's life history, family history, past medical and psychiatric problems and their treatments, drug history and social circumstances is obtained in the usual way. Whereas in a CBT assessment much less emphasis is placed on this information than on the presenting complaints, it is foolhardy to miss out these major areas. To exclude these enquiries could mean that important information which may alter the formulation and recommended treatment regime is missed.

The next stage is the mental state examination, which is followed by sharing the formulation with the patient, educating them about their problem and the suggested treatment before moving on to obtaining baseline measures and planning treatment in more detail with the patient.

Such an assessment may sound daunting at first sight, however, there are a number of mnemonics and checklists that can be used by the therapist to ensure all the vital information is obtained.

Checklists and mnemonics

When assessing a psychiatric symptom or problem behaviour, it is initially useful to think of two mnemonics, both remembered by the letters ABC: 'antecedents, behaviours and beliefs, and consequences'; 'affect, behaviour and cognition'.

Antecedents, behaviours and beliefs, and consequences

This mnemonic, coined by O'Leary & Wilson (1975), serves to remind the therapist that the antecedents and consequences of a behaviour, as well as the patient's beliefs about it, can modify the frequency of the behaviour. Clearly these factors should be examined and form part of the formulation as treatment will usually be geared towards modifying them.

For example, in the case of June, a patient with agoraphobia whose full history is given in Chapter 6 (Case example 6.1, pp. 77–80), the problem could be presented graphically (Fig 2.1).

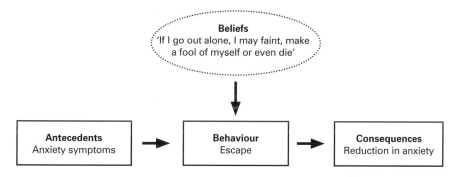

Fig 2.1 Relationship between antecedents, beliefs, behaviour and consequences (Case example 6.1).

Although similar analysis could be applied to all the case histories given in this book, the case of Flora (Case example 2.1, continued in Chapter 3, p. 32) also demonstrates the model (Fig. 2.2).

Case example 2.1: Incontinence treated with CBT

Flora, an 82-year-old woman, had a cerebrovascular accident 2 years earlier that had resulted in moderate intellectual impairment. She had spent the past 2 years living in a care home, where incontinence was a problem to the staff, who had to change her pad 8 or 9 times daily. This was not felt to be organic in origin, but attempts to regularly 'toilet' Flora had not produced any obvious success. Despite this, it was noted with interest that Flora was rarely incontinent overnight. The staff found her difficult because of her problem and requested she be moved to a more intensive nursing facility. Her GP referred her to the clinic for CBT.

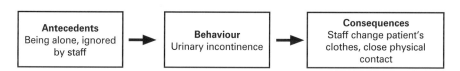

Fig. 2.2 Relationship between antecedents, behaviour and consequences (beliefs unknown); Case example 2.1.

Affect, behaviour and cognition

This mnemonic can not only be used to describe symptoms in a cognitive and behavioural formulation but also act as a useful model to describe how various treatments alter symptoms (Fig. 2.3).

This model demonstrates how affect, behaviour and cognition are all interdependent and how physical symptoms can alter all three. For example, if we move clockwise around the diagram, and start with affect, it is immediately obvious that how an individual feels affects the way that person thinks. Similarly, how someone thinks affects what they do and what someone does has an effect on how they feel. The same interrelationships can be seen by moving anticlockwise round the diagram. Physical symptoms can also affect an individual's thoughts, emotions and behaviour, and *vice versa*. Some drugs directly relate to physical symptoms, such as beta-blockers for anxiety, which may reduce symptoms without directly treating the problem.

If this model is applied to June (Case example 6.1), Fig 2.4 is obtained. From this example, it will be seen that the therapist decided to treat June purely by the behavioural technique of graduated exposure. This is because of the interdependent relationship of the various facets of psychiatric symptomatology. Altering June's behaviour was sufficient to alter her negative cognitions, disturbed affect and physical symptoms. This fact is important, as therapists can become prematurely seduced into cognitive therapy with a patient with catastrophic cognitions, instead of using the

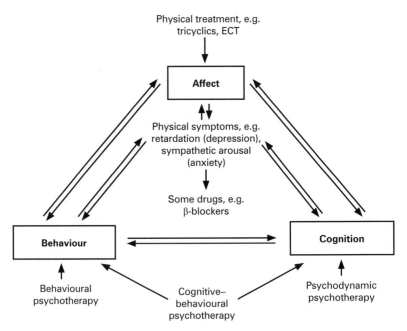

Fig 2.3 Relationship between different types of symptoms and therapeutic strategies.

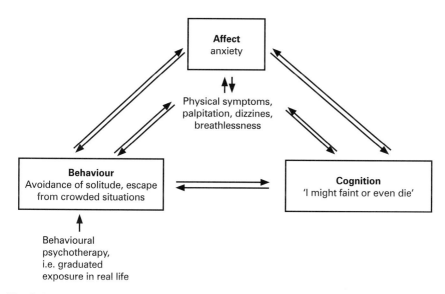

Fig. 2.4 Application of ABC model for June (Case example 6.1).

easier and less time-consuming behavioural methods, which are often the most powerful way of altering cognitions.

Predisposing, precipitating and perpetuating factors (the three Ps)

Assessment of these factors is a vital part of any CBT assessment and is fundamental in formulation and treatment planning. The case history of Lorraine and Michael (Case example 5.3, pp. 62–67) demonstrates some of these factors (Table 2.1).

In this example, it is clearly important for the therapist to be sensitive to and address many of the predisposing and precipitating factors as well as those which are perpetuating the problem.

Table 2.1 Factors affecting sexual dysfunction (Lorraine, Case example 5.3)[a]

Predisposing factors	Inadequate sexual information Parental attitude to sex School attitude to sex Belief that sex was 'dirty'
Precipitating factors	No clear precipitant as lifelong problem but perhaps parental disapproval when Lorraine moved in with Michael
Perpetuating factors	Guilt Continued parental disapproval Fear of pregnancy Michael's attitudes and beliefs

a. Lorraine had received very little sexual education at school or at home and found her first discussions about sex traumatic and unpleasant. She had been taught to consider sex as a sin and dirty. Michael had had early loss of confidence during sex as was told his penis was small.

Abbreviated assessment or screening

It is sometimes necessary to carry out an abbreviated form of assessment owing to lack of time. In these cases it is often useful to remember the plan of behavioural assessment described by Lazarus (1973) as necessary information to devise a behavioural programme. A brief CBT assessment can also be performed in this way, provided a full diagnostic and psychiatric assessment has been carried out.

Lazarus' scheme can be remembered by the mnemonic BASIC ID. This represents the major headings in history-taking: behaviour, affect, sensations, imagery, cognition, interpersonal relationships, drugs (Box 2.2 presents this schema based on Case example 8.3).

Box 2.2 BASIC ID history-taking

Behaviour Freda described how she felt she lacked energy and was thus less able to go out with friends. Although she had had a difficult few years initially caring for her elderly father and then her mother, she still had a large number of friends with whom she could socialise and had managed to ensure she had gone out at least once a week while caring for her parents. Since her mother had been admitted to a care home, Freda found she had withdrawn much more from her previous social life. She had increasingly stopped going out and instead concentrated wholly on her work and visiting her mother in the care home. At assessment, she said 'I think I've forgotten how to have fun!'.

Affect Her mood was low and flat. It was difficult for her to experience enjoyment any more. Even her favourite foods did not taste as good as they had in the past. While at work, Freda often felt agitated and dissatisfied with her performance. She was frequently anxious as she felt she was not performing to her full potential. Freda also admitted that she regularly felt guilty for not caring for her mother herself. Expressing her hopelessness, she said 'I feel I am a failure at everything...I am no good at work; I failed my father as I couldn't keep him alive; I've abandoned my mother to a care home and now I can't even be bothered to be a good wife to my husband or a good friend to anyone.'

Sensations Freda said she spent much of her time feeling extremely tired and exhausted. She had experienced a number of physical problems recently including more frequent headaches, muscle pains as well as general lethargy. If she did make an effort to engage in a pleasurable activity, she found she enjoyed it much less that she had done in the past. In her words, 'everything is flat and dull now'.

Imagery Freda admitted that she frequently had images of bad events befalling herself, for instance losing her job owing to her worsened performance. She also had frequent images of bad things happening, for example her mother falling out of bed in the care home and not getting the help she required, her children being involved in a catastrophic accident. These images made her anxious as well as deeply concerned about her own perceived lack of energy as she felt she 'should be able to cope and just get on with things'.

Cognition   Freda had multiple beliefs concerning her perceived failure and inadequacy as a daughter, a wife, a mother, a work colleague; and a friend. She felt she was a total failure in everything. At times she had felt it would be better if she died but she had no intention to harm herself as she realised this would greatly upset her family and friends. Freda also had high standards to which she felt she should always aspire. Extremely critical of herself, she found it hard to take any credit for her previous successes in life.

Interpersonal relationships   Although very close to her mother, Freda tearfully admitted that she had not always had such a close relationship with her father. She found him overbearing and had frequently rebelled against him when she was younger. This thought did worry her and she wondered if she had partially caused the stress leading to his demise. She married her husband at the age of 25 and he had been her first and only sexual partner. She described him as a 'good man, a good father and a caring husband'. Often she worried that he would become bored with her and her depression and leave her. Although he was caring, supportive and would help her whenever he could, he was 'not a man who would handle emotion' and so she had been unable to confide all her worries in him. Whereas she had been close to both her daughter and son when they were growing up, they had moved to different parts of the UK due to their jobs. Her daughter telephoned her regularly every week but her son was more sporadic about when he called. Freda worried that her son did not call owing to her failure as a mother, despite being reassured by her friends that this was unlikely to be the case and that he was just busy with his own life. She had good close friends whom she had known since school days. Before her depression, she would go out with friends once a week and she would also go out for a meal or to the theatre or cinema with her husband every 2–3 weeks.

Drugs   Freda was a social drinker who, prior to her mother going into a home, would go out with friends once a week and drink a glass or two of wine (175 ml) on each occasion. She did not drink alone but only in social situations. Thus she had not drunk anything for the previous 4 months as her husband never drank at home with her. She did not smoke and had never used any illicit drugs. Her GP had prescribed sertraline 50 mg a day for her but she had refused to take this as she felt taking drugs was 'a sign of weakness'. She also was on calcium and vitamin D_3 supplement but no other medications.

Cognitive–behavioural formulation

Examples of cognitive–behavioural formulations will be given throughout this book. However, it is worthwhile asking what a cognitive–behavioural formulation is and how it differs from any other type of formulation. Generally, it could be said that it is a hypothesis about a disorder, behaviour or symptom which attempts to identify any possible predisposing, precipitating and perpetuating factors or mechanisms. A formulation may be presented in a few sentences or as a diagram. It is not carved in tablets of stone and thus the formulation may alter as treatment progresses and other factors come to light. Usually it is helpful to share the formulation with the patient. It is often beneficial for them to see that their problem, which may have previously seemed insurmountable, can be summarised in a few short sentences and become more manageable. Discussing the formulation with the patient also presents an opportunity for the therapist to ensure that they have understood the problem fully, as well as helping patients to feel that the therapist has taken note of them. An example of a CBT formulation is given in Box 2.3 (based on Case example 6.3, pp. 82–84) and presented in a diagram (Fig. 2.5).

Box 2.3 A CBT formulation

'Gwen, although you do not describe any problems with hospital and dental procedures before the age of 14, the history of your mother and maternal aunt having similar problems suggests that there may well be some genetic predisposing factors, as well as the fact that you may have learned that these procedures might be accompanied by anxiety and fainting.

After your routine medical examination, you experienced minor symptoms of light-headedness and nausea when told you would need to have a blood sample taken. The fact that the doctor was unsympathetic and the nurse held on to you tightly and roughly would have increased your unpleasant sensations as well as being aversive in their own right. After the procedure, you fainted. You therefore learned to associate visiting doctors with feeling ill and frequently fainting.

Because of your unpleasant experiences, you started to reduce the number of visits to the doctor and dentist. Also, you told me that on several occasions you had walked out of a doctor's or dentist's surgery because you had catastrophic thoughts that you were going to be ill. These thoughts led to you having symptoms of feeling nauseous and unwell. Avoiding those visits and walking out of the doctor's is likely to make your fear of the situation worse. High anxiety is horrible and therefore a reduction in anxiety is like a reward. In your case, escaping from the situation or avoiding the situation reduced your anxiety. These behaviours were then 'rewarded' by a reduction in anxiety. If you reward any behaviour, you increase the chances of it recurring. Therefore, every time you escaped from or avoided contact with doctors and dentists, you served to increase your fear and strengthen your belief that avoidance and escape were the only way to avoid unpleasant sensations. You, therefore, became increasingly phobic of these situations until the present time'.

Education and planning treatment

Cognitive–behavioural therapy differs from most other types of psychiatric treatment, as the aim is nearly always to train the patient to become their own therapist. The advantages of this approach are in the cost-efficiency of therapist time, as well as enabling the patient to monitor and implement appropriate action if there are any early signs of relapse. However, this type of approach does mean that more time needs to be spent in the early stages of treatment, in explaining the exact reasons for any suggested remedy.

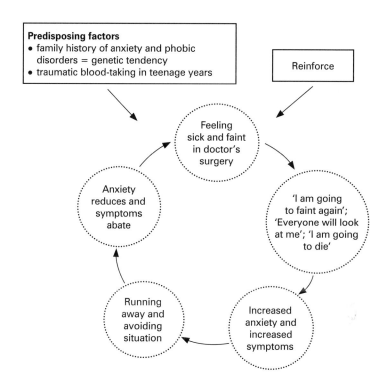

Predisposing factors
- family history of anxiety and phobic disorders = genetic tendency
- traumatic blood-taking in teenage years

Reinforce

Feeling sick and faint in doctor's surgery

Anxiety reduces and symptoms abate

'I am going to faint again'; 'Everyone will look at me'; 'I am going to die'

Running away and avoiding situation

Increased anxiety and increased symptoms

Fig. 2.5 Diagram of formulation for severe blood and injury phobia.

The case histories described in this book will also demonstrate that a high level of motivation and adherence to therapy is needed, as the patient is often asked to do things that are frightening or aversive to them. Adherence can often be dramatically improved by the therapist ensuring that the information given to the patient is honest, accurate and not overly optimistic or pessimistic. Treatment is usually designed by the patient and therapist together, and not in a (traditionally) prescriptive manner. The term 'collaborative empiricism' has been used to describe the way in which patient and therapist work together to find an answer to the patient's problems (Beck *et al*, 1979).

Examples of patient education and treatment planning will be seen throughout the book. An example is given here in Box 2.4, again based on the story of Gwen (Case example 6.3, pp. 82–84).

Once the therapist had answered the patient's questions about anxiety and treatment, the next stage is to establish the overall targets which the patient wishes to achieve by treatment and then work out a hierarchy of situations of varying difficulty. To judge the difficulty of each situation, the therapist may ask the patient to rate their anxiety on a 9-point scale (Fig. 2.6), which will be used frequently throughout this book and is described fully by Marks (1986).

Box 2.4 Patient education and treatment planning

'The first thing I want to explain to you is about anxiety. Anxiety is an extremely unpleasant experience but it is important to remember that it does no harm to you. People do not die or go mad from anxiety. Second, anxiety does reduce if you remain in situations for long enough.

In your case, when in a fear-provoking situation such as visiting a doctor, you initially experience typical symptoms of anxiety such as a pounding heart and feeling shaky. If possible you will try to escape at this time. However, as I have already explained to you, although escaping seems a good idea at the time as it reduces your anxiety, you are teaching yourself that the only way to deal with the situation is to escape from it or to avoid it completely and therefore, each time you escape from a situation, you make the problem worse.

If you do not manage to escape from the situation, another physical mechanism comes into operation and you feel nauseous, dizzy and frequently faint. This is also a part of the anxiety reaction. In the majority of fear-provoking situations, we react with what is known as the 'fight or flight' reaction, which we recognise by a rapid heartbeat and increased rate of breathing. This reaction is inbuilt and instinctive and prepares our bodies for the physical exertion of either running away or fighting the threat. However, in situations where injury is inevitable many animals, including ourselves, have an inbuilt reaction which in many ways is opposite to the fight or flight reaction. In this case, the heart slows down, breathing becomes shallow and nausea and vomiting may occur. This reduction in blood flow means that, if injury occurs, you are less likely to bleed to death than if your heart was pumping away at full rate. This is all very well in the wild, but your body is oversensitive to non-life-threatening situations such as a visit to a doctor or dentist.

The way to help is by asking yourself to gradually face up to the things that you fear, and to remain there long enough until your anxiety symptoms subside. This often takes between 1 and 2 hours. We will now work out together a series of situations which are increasingly difficult, and which you will need to master for treatment.

For the early exposure sessions at each stage of difficulty, we may have to start with you lying flat to reduce the risk of fainting. Your anxiety will reduce as you practise each stage, and we will move you gradually into a more upright position.

I should also emphasise that, although the treatment sounds difficult, the majority of patients who have this treatment improve. Do you have any questions about anything I have said?'

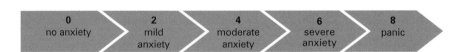

Fig 2.6 Nine-point scale for anxiety.

It is important not to swamp the patient with too much information and to ensure that it has been understood. Information and vocabulary need to be tailored to the educational and intellectual level appropriate for each patient. In addition, the patient's social circumstances and preferences must be taken into consideration. This does not mean that treatments without an evidence base should be offered based on patient preference but that all options that have been shown to be useful should be discussed along with the advantages and disadvantages of each. It is then acceptable to present the treatment package the therapist feels will be the most useful. Patients may wish to debate this care plan and the overall package may need modification as a result.

Finally, patients often forget what has been discussed in the clinic and it is useful to provide them with some form of written information to be taken away. This may be in the form of information sheets or by recommending a particular self-help book. (At the end of most chapters I have listed workbooks for therapists and appropriate self-help texts that can be suggested to patients to read.) Please always remember to first read any book you recommend to ensure it is in keeping with your advice. Also remember that some patients may not wish to read a whole book and so shorter texts and individualised material may be more appropriate.

However, it is also important to give some tailor-made written material of what was discussed in the session and how the patient's problem is viewed. It is often useful to jot down the main points of the formulation on a piece of paper and give this along with the diagram of how the problem is maintained. This can be written during the interview with the patient and initially used to illustrate the information given about anxiety (Box 2.5; full patient history is given in Case example 8.3, pp. 121–124).

Box 2.5   Information given to patient about anxiety

In the example of Freda, a 50-year-old office supervisor treated for depression by cognitive therapy whose case history is described in Chapter 8, the following was said:

'I understand how very low you have been feeling and you have explained fully to me how recent events have contributed to these feelings. However, it is often the case that it is not events themselves that lead us to feel low but some thoughts that rush into our mind and make us feel miserable.

If I can demonstrate this, I want you to imagine that on my next appointment with you, you did not arrive and did not telephone to cancel. Now, imagine that I am prone to get depressed, my thoughts might be something like this: "She's not arrived, she must think I am a hopeless therapist. Everyone will soon learn about this and realise how useless a therapist I am. I must be a complete failure, no one could possibly love me. It is pointless continuing to live like this." Now what do you think I would feel like after having thoughts like that?'

Freda replied with a laugh, 'Very low and desperate, but that really is not logical because if I had not arrived I might have forgotten the appointment, or written it down wrongly in my diary, or been caught in traffic, or many other things. Also just because one patient missed an appointment does not mean you are a hopeless therapist, and even if you did believe you were a hopeless therapist, it would not mean you were a total failure and no one could love you.'

The therapist answered, 'That is right, it does sound silly when stated in this way, but I think we will discover that it is no more irrational than many of the thoughts which run through all of our minds from time to time, and are now contributing to you feeling depressed. These thoughts are called negative automatic thoughts, and to illustrate what I mean I would like you to describe to me the last time you had a bout of feeling really low and what was happening at that time.'

Freda then described an incident in which she had been having a cup of coffee with a friend. The friend had casually mentioned that her daughter had passed a piano examination recently. Freda found that she felt miserable. The therapist asked her to imagine herself back in that situation, and to repeat out loud the thoughts which went through her mind at that time. The following sequence was obtained:

'My daughter did not have the chance to learn the piano. I must be such a hopeless mother that I did not encourage her sufficiently. This pattern will continue throughout her life and she will be a failure. Once she is unemployed she will blame and hate me. I am no good as a mother, she would be better off living without me.'

The therapist then encouraged Freda to examine the evidence which supported and refuted the first of these thoughts: her daughter not learning the piano meant that she was a hopeless mother, who did not encourage her sufficiently. A more rational response was produced, namely that her daughter had showed no interest in learning a musical instrument and that she had been more interested in gymnastics, which she kept up until leaving for university.

Following this, the therapist explained the major thinking errors which people commonly make. These thinking errors are listed fully in Freda's case history in Chapter 8 (p. 121). Examples from Freda's own history were used to illustrate these where possible or the therapist gave another example. These thinking errors were then written down for Freda to read at home. She was also asked to fill in a diary over the next week:

1 Write down each negative thought you have and record the time and place when you had the thought. Put this in the left-hand column on a sheet of paper.
2 In the right-hand column on the sheet of paper, put down any evidence you can think of to contradict the negative thought. If you cannot think of any contradictory evidence at this stage, just leave the right-hand column blank.'

Later in Chapter 8 the reader will find a description of how this diary recording develops into the 'two-column technique', which is integral to cognitive therapy of depression.

Thes two examples (Boxes 2.4 & 2.5) should give the reader an idea of the level of information needed to gain a patient's cooperation with treatment. It is often useful to perform at least some basic measures of the problem at the same time, as these may help the patient to focus on areas of difficulty when planning treatment with the therapist.

Measures and rating scales

Are measures really necessary?

Measurement of the problem is taken very seriously in CBT. Each patient may be considered as their own single-case experiment. There are several advantages to this type of approach. In initial stages it can encourage the patient to express their own targets and goals of treatment, which may prevent the therapist fruitlessly trying to pursue a line without the patient's interest.

I experienced an example of this recently, when supervising a trainee psychiatrist in the treatment of a patient with agoraphobic and social phobic problems. Progress was very slow, despite the trainee spending 2–3 h in the supermarket with the patient twice a week. Further questioning of the trainee revealed that the programme had been almost entirely suggested by the doctor, with little input from the patient. Also no measures had been taken as the trainee felt they were superfluous and irrelevant. The trainee was instructed to have another session with the patient in which a full list of measures were completed. This session revealed that the patient had little interest in being able to travel to a supermarket, as she was quite happy for her sister to do the shopping. Thus she had never performed any of the between-session homework self-exposure suggested by the trainee. Her only target of treatment at the time was to be able to travel on a bus to visit her elderly, frail parents who lived some miles away and who she had not seen for a year. Changing the treatment programme to tackle this goal greatly improved her motivation, and she achieved her target within three sessions.

Measurement allows the patient and the therapist to monitor progress and to ensure the treatment programme is working. Failure to progress is therefore recognised early and the treatment can either be changed or any sticking points dealt with. In the example cited earlier, if the trainee had monitored his patient's progress, he would have realised much sooner that she was failing to make progress, and could thus have saved himself several fruitless hours of standing in a supermarket. Also, he would have been able to question the patient sooner and may have discovered her failure to comply with homework tasks and her lack of interest in the target of treatment.

The patient may suffer from amnesia about the original problem and overestimate or, more commonly, underestimate the progress or lack of it. This is illustrated by the case example of Mrs B, a 35-year-old housewife who had a 10-year history of fear of contamination by grease, leading to excessive washing and cleaning rituals. At initial assessment, she was housebound, spending her day cleaning the house. Family members were required to strip down to their underwear standing on newspaper at the door before entering the house and changing into non-contaminated clothes. Non-family visitors were not admitted to the house. Treatment was on an out-patient and domiciliary basis, and consisted of graduated exposure in real life to the feared situation and self-imposed response prevention. However, the patient's high anxiety meant that progress was inevitably slow. After 4 weeks of therapy she announced, 'Really, you are wasting your time. I am no better and, in fact, I think I am even more anxious than before treatment now'. The therapist was able to demonstrate to her how many more things she was doing since the beginning of treatment, and how her anxiety ratings as well as her score on the Yale–Brown Obsessive Compulsive Scale (YBOCS; Goodman *et al*, 1989) and the Sheehan Disability Scale (Sheehan *et al*, 1996) showed a steady improvement. This greatly cheered Mrs B, who was able to continue treatment, feeling encouraged.

The therapist may also under-appreciate the severity of the patient's presenting problem, and underestimate or, more commonly, overestimate the patient's progress. This is shown by the case history of Mrs L, a 45-year-old woman who had experienced recurrent bouts of depression over the previous 25 years and had received a range of medication. A recent episode of depression had commenced 2 months earlier, and for the previous 6 weeks she had been attending a consultant psychiatrist, who had prescribed a new antidepressant drug for her. He felt sure that this had been of some benefit to her, though Mrs L denied this.

Whereas some patients do present with a full range of biological features of depression which resolve completely after a few weeks of appropriate treatment, in the majority it is far more equivocal. A more objective measure such as the quickly completed 13-item short form of the Beck Depression Inventory (BDI; Beck *et al*, 1974) would have only taken a few minutes at each appointment, and would have provided another and more reliable source of information.

Objectivity and types of measurement

Some forms of measurement are obviously more objective that others. For most clinical cases, the use of self-report or therapist-report questionnaires combined with the patient's, their relatives' and the therapist's observations should suffice, but it is useful to consider all types of measure. The major categories of measure used are listed below in approximate order of increasing objectivity.

Self-report

This could just be asking the patient a question like, 'How often do you experience your tic in a day?', which is likely to result in an inaccurate answer but will provide a rough guide to frequency of behaviours. Self-report can be made of more use by asking the patient to fill in a questionnaire containing a number of standard items or by the use of visual analogue scales. Once the patient has completed the questionnaire, an element of self-observation in relation to the rated items often operates and subsequent ratings are often more reliable than initial self-report ratings.

Relatives' reports

Reports from relatives can be useful but are dependent on the relationship between the patient and the family member and can occasionally result in friction between them. They mainly serve as a confirmation of the patient's report.

Self-observation

This requires the patient to monitor their own behaviour over a period of time. This is done most frequently with the use of a diary.

Relatives' observation

A relative can also be asked to monitor the patient's behaviour and record it in a diary, as can anyone living in the situation of 'pseudo relative', for instance nursing staff on a ward.

Impartial professional interview and rating

These measures are frequently used in research and involve a professional person who is not involved with, or is masked to, the patient's treatment rating their progress. Frequently, questionnaires are used for this.

Direct observation by role-play (impartial professional rater)

For some problems, such as anger management training, social skills training and marital communication skills training, role-play can be used to assess the patient's mastery of specific techniques. Objectivity in the use of role-play as a measure can only be achieved by asking a non-involved suitable professional to rate performance. This could be done either with the use of a one-way screen or, more commonly, by recording the role-play on camera.

Direct observation *in vivo*

With certain behaviours the therapist can directly observe a patient's progress in real life, for example a patient with obsessive–compulsive contamination fears may have initially been unable to touch a rubbish bin, but during treatment achieves this.

The reliability of these types of measures can be increased by setting up a standard 'behavioural avoidance test' or 'behavioural experiment' which can be performed by the patient repeatedly during treatment and used to monitor progress. An example of this would be a journey for a patient with agoraphobia which might follow a set route, starting with a walk, continuing with a visit to a small shop and buying an item such as a newspaper, then moving on to a bus journey, to large, busy shops and eventually to a train journey. The patient could be asked to return with certain items to prove that they were reporting their actual success accurately. Once again, a 'neutral' professional may be used to assess progress in a behavioural experiment.

Direct observation of result of behaviour

The most obvious (and most objective) example of this type of measure is that success or otherwise of a CBT treatment of obesity is judged by weight change. Unfortunately, such objective criteria are rarely available in clinical practice.

Measures and questionnaires

The actual use of different measures and questionnaires is obviously a matter which is subject to a great deal of individual variation, personal preference and personal prejudice. Every psychiatric or psychological journal contains examples of research in which a wide variety of questionnaires have been used to measure a range of parameters.

For someone new to the discipline of CBT, it is best to keep ratings simple and to become familiar with a few questionnaires. It is best to choose a questionnaire of known reliability and validity wherever possible. It is also important to ensure that the measure used will actually assess what you want to check. This may sound obvious, but it is common for someone to use a measure of personality trait, for example, when trying to assess a change in the patient's state.

Examples of useful measures

Problems and targets

This questionnaire is printed in Marks (1986) and is an extremely useful measure to apply to any patient who is to receive CBT. It should be completed by the therapist in collaboration with the patient.

The first section asks for up to two main problems which the patient wants treated. This is often a useful measure to use before planning treatment with the patient as it gives an idea of how the treatment should be structured. The idea of defining problems can be introduced thus: 'What I want to do now is to try to describe the main problems which you want treated. I have only a small amount of space on this form so we will have to be brief and reduce this to a sentence or two for each problem.' The problem is then written down in a form as close to the patient's words as possible, although the therapist may have to help the patient by summarising their words or prompting them to speak. The patient and the therapist are then asked to rate how much each of the problems upsets them or interferes with normal activities on a 9-point scale, where 0 means 'does not' and 8 'very severely/continuously' (these ratings are done with the therapist masked to the patient's ratings and *vice versa*; the therapist rates each problem as it relates to the patient.)

After defining the problems, the patient is asked to devise up to four targets. Targets are clearly defined tasks or items of behaviour which demonstrate improvement and which are considered desirable by the patient. They can be explained to the patient in this way: 'What I want us to do now is to define up to four targets for treatment. Targets are specific kinds of behaviour which would be useful for you to achieve and which would demonstrate to both of us that you are improving or treated when you achieve them. We will define them quite carefully in terms of frequency, duration and situation, so that there is no confusion.'

'I want to feel better' is not a good target at all as it is not precisely defined and is open to confusion as to when it is achieved. The patient with moderate depression who gave this answer when asked to define a target of treatment was then told: 'I am sure that is your main aim but as a target it is difficult to know when it is achieved. What I would prefer is if you could describe to me some of the things you would be able to do regularly if you did feel better and which you cannot do regularly now.' The patient then described how he would return to his work full time, go out with his wife twice weekly for dinner and attend his squash club for a game of squash with a friend at least once a week. The following targets were therefore agreed:

- to go to work and remain there for 8 hours a day, 5 days a week
- to go out to a restaurant in the town centre with my wife twice a week and eat a two- or three-course meal
- to play a full hour-long squash game with a friend once a week.

Once obtained, these targets are also rated by the patient and by the therapist (masked to the patient's answer) on a 9-point scale which assesses discomfort and behaviour from 0 meaning 'no discomfort or complete success', to 8 meaning 'very severe discomfort or no success'.

Visual analogue scales or verbal numeric scales

Although a visual analogue scale could just consist of a straight line on a piece of paper with no subdivisions, it is often more useful to give a scale on the line. Once a patient is familiar with rating in this way, it is no longer necessary for them always to have a written scale but verbal ratings can be used to give useful information. A popular scale is the 9-point scale as favoured by Marks (1986). This can be used to measure anxiety as shown in Fig. 2.6. Similarly, using the same gradations, the 9-point scale may be applied to measure other factors, including sexual arousal, discomfort, pleasure or indeed almost any emotion that is required. It will already be noticed from the description of the problem and target questionnaire that this scale can be used to measure percentage of success in performing a particular task.

There is, however, no particular magic in using a 9-point scale and some therapists prefer to use an 11-point scale. The important point is that the therapist is consistent with the scale, and that both patient and therapist are clear about the meaning of the gradations. Indeed, in the cognitive therapy described by Beck, therapists most usually use a scale from 0 to 100 to ask a patient to rate their strength of belief in a NAT. This scale with a large number of gradations gives more flexibility for ratings but may, at times, be more confusing to the patient.

Some patients have difficulty in understanding numbers. In these cases a straight line of defined length can be used to ask them to rate anxiety or stress. This system has been used in my unit to aid communication of distress in a young man with acalculia and with people with intellectual disabilities.

Measuring socioeconomic functioning

- *Sheehan Disability Scale* (Sheehan *et al*, 1996; Leon *et al*, 1997) is a self-rated instrument measuring impairment in work, family and social functioning during the past month. Using an 11-point scale the patient is asked to rate their work/school, social and home life/family responsibilities. On each of the three scales, 10 represents severe impairment, 7–9 marked impairment, 4–6 moderate, 1–3 mild and 0 no impairment.
- *Areas of Social Impairment Questionnaire* (Marks, 1986) is similar to the Sheehan Disability Scale but has four domains: work, home management, social leisure and private leisure. Each is rated on a 9-point scale.

Anxiety and phobias

- *Fear Questionnaire* (Marks & Matthews, 1979): this questionnaire of known reliability and validity is useful in assessing patients with phobia and gives separate scores for agoraphobia, social phobia, blood/injury phobia, generalised anxiety/depression as well as global phobic scores.
- *Hamilton Anxiety Scale* (Hamilton, 1959): this scale has been widely used for more than 50 years and is well researched in terms of reliability and validity. It was originally developed in the 1950s and is a useful measure for patients with an anxiety disorder, as it is known to detect mostly state rather than trait anxiety, and to be sensitive to change. One difficulty is that it is scored by a clinician, and its reliability is greater in those who are experienced in its use.

Depression and dysphoria

- *Beck Depression Inventory* (BDI): this comes in two main forms used in clinical practice and is useful as either a screening instrument for depression or as a way of assessing depth of depression or response to treatment. Both forms have been subjected to rigorous tests of reliability and validity.
  - *BDI short-form* (Beck *et al*, 1974) consists of 13 items which are rated by the patient. It has the advantage that being short it can be used as a screening tool for depression in all patients, but it is also useful in individuals with severe depression and intellectual impairment who may find a longer questionnaire too much to complete. I have also found this a useful questionnaire to give

to patients with OCD, as often a longer questionnaire can take them too long if they have the urge to repeatedly check their answers.

- *BDI 21-item* (Beck, 1978) is an alternative scale which has the advantage of being recommended in self-help manuals for depression (Blackburn, 1987).

OCD, hoarding disorder and body dysmorphic disorder

- *YBOCS* (Goodman *et al*, 1989): this is the most reported measure of obsessions and compulsions in the research literature. In order to apply this measure, clinicians need to undergo a brief training to ensure inter-rater reliability. The scale is divided into five factors concerning obsessions and five for compulsions. Each factor is scored up to a maximum of 4. Thus the maximum total score is 40, with scores over 32 representing profound OCD and a score over 24 representing severe OCD.
  - *YBOCS-BDD* measures the effect of body dysmorphic disorder (BDD). It is similar to the YBOCS but has a maximum score of 48 as it has 12 factors (Phillips *et al*, 1997).
- *Padua Inventory* (Sanavio, 1988): this is a patient-completed questionnaire (which may be difficult for patients with the most severe OCD to complete due to problems with obsessive indecision and doubt). The original version of the questionnaire consists of items with a maximum score of 240. A normal Italian population scored an average of 41 on this questionnaire (Sanavio, 1988). A problem was identified in the original version, however, as it measured worry as well as pure obsessions; a revised version was therefore produced (Burns *et al*, 1996). The revision was constructed to measure five content dimensions relevant to OCD: obsessional thoughts about harm to oneself or others; obsessional impulses to harm oneself or others; contamination obsessions and washing compulsions; checking compulsions; and dressing/grooming compulsions. This questionnaire is especially useful in identifying particular areas of impairment and problems in OCD.
- *The Hoarding Rating Scale-Interview* (Tolin *et al*, 2010): this is a brief self-completion questionnaire which gives an indication of whether hoarding is a major problem for an individual. It consists of 5 questions marked on a 9-point scale with 0 representing 'none' and 8 representing 'extreme'.

This chapter has described some of the measures and rating scales which can be used. Others will be discovered for specific problems and for many problems it may be useful to tailor-make a rating scale for the patient and to use this in addition to the standard scales. Each of the chapters in this book will also identify possible rating scales for use in a variety of different situations.

Key learning points

- CBT assessment involves taking a full behavioural and cognitive history, devising a CBT formulation, education of the patient into the nature of their condition and its treatment, and establishing baseline and subsequent measures of the problem.
- A good CBT history is similar to a good thorough medical or psychiatric history.
- Mnemonics can be helpful to ensure all aspects of the history are covered. Examples include: antecedents, behaviour and beliefs, and consequences (ABC); affect, behaviour and cognition (ABC); predisposing, precipitating and perpetuating factors (the three Ps); behaviour, affect, sensations, imagery, cognition, interpersonal relationships and drugs (BASIC ID).
- A CBT formulation is a hypothesis about a disorder, behaviour or symptom which attempts to identify any possible predisposing, precipitating and perpetuating factors. The formulation may alter as treatment progresses.
- Patient education about their condition and its treatment is a cornerstone of CBT.
- The patient is always involved in helping the therapist plan the treatment.
- Measurement of the problem has the advantage of helping the therapist understand what the patient wishes from treatment and avoids time-wasting; it also allows both therapist and patient to monitor progress and to call a halt to ineffective types of therapy. It ensures that objectivity about progress can be maintained by both patient and therapist.
- Although direct observation of target behaviour by an independent observer is the 'gold standard' for measuring change, in practice rating scales are often the most useful and independent measures available.
- Whereas rating scales of known reliability and validity are generally preferable in assessing change, *ad hoc* tailor-made ratings can also be useful.

References

Beck AT (1978) *Depression Inventory*. Philadelphia Center for Cognitive Therapy.

Beck AT, Rial WY, Rickels K (1974) Short form of depression inventory: cross-validation. *Psychology Reports*, **34**: 1184–6.

Beck AT, Rush AJ, Shaw BF, *et al* (1979) *Cognitive Therapy of Depression*. Guilford Press.

Blackburn I (1987) *Coping with Depression*. Chambers.

Burns GL, Keortge SG, Formea GM, *et al* (1996) Revision of the Padua Inventory of obsessive compulsive disorder symptoms: distinctions between worry, obsessions, and compulsions. *Behaviour Research and Therapy*, **34**: 163–73.

Goodman WK, Price LH, Rasmussen SA, *et al* (1989) The Yale-Brown Obsessive Compulsive Scale: development, use and reliability. *Archives of General Psychiatry*, **46**: 1006–11.

Hamilton M (1959) The assessment of anxiety states by rating. *British Journal of Medical Psychology*, **32**: 50–5.

Lazarus AA (1973) Multimodal behaviour therapy: treating the 'Basic ID'. *Journal of Nervous and Mental Disorders*, **156**: 404–11.

Leon AC, Olfson M, Portera L, *et al* (1997) Assessing psychiatric impairment in primary care with the Sheehan Disability Scale. *International Journal of Psychiatry in Medicine*, **27**: 93–105.

Marks IM (1986) *Behavioural Psychotherapy: Maudsley Pocket Book of Clinical Management.* John Wright.

Marks IM, Mathews AM (1979) Brief standard self-rating for phobic patients. *Behavior Research and Therapy*, **17**: 263–7.

O'Leary KD, Wilson GT (1975) *Behavior Therapy: Application and Outcome.* Prentice-Hall.

Phillips KA, Hollander E, Rasmussen SA (1997) A severity rating scale for body dysmorphic disorder: development, reliability, and validity of a modified version of the Yale-Brown Obsessive Compulsive Scale. *Psychopharmacology Bulletin*, **33**: 17–22.

Sanavio E (1988) Obsessions and compulsions: the Padua Inventory. *Behaviour Research and Therapy*, **26**: 169–77.

Sheehan DV, Harnett-Sheehan K, Raj BA (1996) The measurement of disability. *International Clinical Psychopharmacology*, **11** (suppl 3): 89–95.

Tolin DF, Frost RO, Steketee G (2010) A brief interview for assessing compulsive hoarding: the Hoarding Rating Scale-Interview. *Psychiatry Research*, **178**: 147–52.

Further reading

Grant A, Townend M, Mills J, *et al* (2008) *Assessment and Case Formulation in Cognitive–Behavioural Therapy.* Sage Publications.

Rules of reinforcement and practical examples

Overview

This chapter starts with the very first principles of behaviour therapy by examining the factors which help develop and modify behaviour. The types of reinforcement are described. How different reinforcers may shape human behaviour and result in mental health or behavioural problems will then be examined, followed by the use of altering reinforcers to improve functioning. Case examples will include the use of covert sensitisation and orgasmic reconditioning for illegal alternative sexual practices as well as more standard reinforcement techniques for unwanted or challenging behaviours.

In the introduction to this book, the history of behaviour therapy is discussed. In the following three chapters we examine the roles of reinforcement strategies and how they may be used in clinical settings. This understanding of reinforcement and its shaping of human behaviour is an important component when we examine the treatment of anxiety disorders and depression later in the book.

Reinforcement and operant conditioning

Much of this and the subsequent chapter is about techniques based on operant conditioning, a 'sticks and carrots' term. These principles are not always as obvious to apply as may seem on first sight. First there needs to be an understanding of reinforcement, the process of strengthening a directly measurable dimension of behaviour (the most obvious example will be covered in Chapter 6 examining exposure treatments). Anxiety is unpleasant and so when in the presence of an object or situation which provokes fear, most people will try to escape the anxiety by either running away or, in the case of OCD, by performing an anxiety-relieving compulsion. Both running away and performing an anxiolytic ritual cause the anxiety to reduce. This reduction in anxiety acts as a positive reinforcement, strengthening the likelihood of the individual escaping or ritualising in the future. By far the most common type of reinforcer to be used in clinical practice is positive reinforcement or rewarding a certain type of behaviour. The most common form of reward is social reinforcement or praise and encouragement. However, some individuals, such as people with some forms of autism, may not respond to praise and then alternative rewards need to be found. Premack's principle (1959) can be used to address this. This states that high-frequency preferred activity can be used to reinforce lower-frequency, non-preferred activity. In other words, if a child spends most of their time playing with its toy racing cars, this high-frequency preferred activity could be used to reinforce the lower frequency non-preferred activity of tidying their bedroom. Other types of reinforcement are shown in Table 3.1.

One key maladaptive response can be seen in phobic anxiety when a person reacts with fear to objects or situations that would generally be considered non-threatening, such as crowded places or domestic animals. In these cases treatment would involve the individual facing up to their fear without escaping and remaining there long enough for the anxiety to subside. This principle of habituation of anxiety with prolonged exposure is key to therapeutic strategies with most anxiety disorders (see Chapters 6, 7, 9 and 10). However, as well as anxiety, other maladaptive habits or behaviours may develop in response to stimuli unrelated to fear and in these cases alternative strategies may be needed. Then the therapist has the option of:

- eliminating the behaviour using aversive stimuli (only indicated if the behaviour is life-threatening or a severe public nuisance), e.g. covert sensitisation
- modifying the stimulus resulting in the response, e.g. orgasmic reconditioning

Table 3.1 Types of positive and negative reinforcements

++ Positive reinforcement	+− Punishment
• Social reinforcement (approval, praise) • Tangible rewards (monetary, food, gifts) • High frequency preferred activity	• Overcorrection (e.g. someone smashes a cup on the floor and is asked not only to clear up the mess but also to wash the entire floor) • Aversive techniques have no clinical relevance these days
−− Negative reinforcement	−+ Response cost
• (e.g. a man with illegal sexual practices is treated with covert sensitisation, i.e. he is trained to produce an aversive image following being instructed to have deviant images; relief is also gained from these aversive images by switching to neutral thoughts)	• Penalty involving some time and effort in response to certain behaviours • Positive reinforcer is removed if certain behaviours are indulged in, e.g. time out from positive reinforcement (3 min) • Behaviours designed to seek attention are ignored

- modifying the response to the stimulus, e.g. stimulus control techniques
- replacing the problem behaviour with alternative adaptive responses, e.g. habit reversal
- reducing the desirability of the problem behaviour, e.g. mass practice, response cost.

These five categories are not mutually exclusive and any therapist who tries to eliminate a particular behaviour without helping the patient to develop alternative strategies is doomed to failure.

Treatment of obesity

Obesity is a common problem in the Western world and produces a huge burden on health and health services. Diets are generally unsuccessful as the person loses weight while dieting only to gain more after the diet. Surgical procedures are increasingly used for those with morbid obesity. However, some simple stimulus control techniques combined with a healthy living approach to diet and exercise can help those with modest amounts of weight to lose (see Case example 11.1, pp. 173–175). These stimulus control techniques were developed in the 1960s and have stood the test of time (e.g. Stuart, 1967). The packages consisted of four key elements:

1 Description of behaviour to be controlled (individuals are asked to keep daily diaries of amount of food, time and circumstances of eating).
2 Modification and control of the discriminatory stimuli governing eating (individuals are asked to limit their eating to one room, use distinctive table settings and make eating a 'pure' experience unaccompanied by other activities such as reading, watching television, etc.).
3 Development of techniques to control the act of eating (e.g. counting each mouthful of food and replacing utensils after each mouthful, always leaving some food on the plate at the end of a meal).
4 Prompt reinforcement of behaviours that delay or control eating.

Treatment of incontinence using positive reinforcement

The case history of Flora (Case example 2.1, p. 11 and continued below) demonstrates the importance of having a positive attitude to the patient if any form of behaviour change is to be achieved. This 82-year-old woman had a cerebrovascular accident 2 years earlier, resulting in intellectual impairment. She had spent the past 2 years living in a care home where incontinence was a problem to the staff, who had to change her pad 8 or 9 times daily.

Case example 2.1: Incontinence treated with CBT (continued)

The therapist arranged to spend some time with the care home staff to observe Flora and obtain baseline measures for the problem. It rapidly became clear how tired the staff were with Flora's problem and how they had little or no interaction with her except when she was incontinent. The staff were very busy but were inadvertently reinforcing Flora's incontinence

The therapist asked if Flora could be taken to the toilet every hour between breakfast and evening. Smiles, praise and social reinforcement would be used whenever she managed to pass water. If she did not urinate, she would be taken back to the day room after 5 min on the toilet without any further communication.

Initially, Flora did not appear to listen to praise when given. This unfamiliarity with social reinforcement was overcome by the therapist looking Flora in the face while smiling and praising at the same time as gently stroking her hand. After 4 hours of this programme, Flora seemed to understand what she was required to do. She began passing water on almost every visit to the toilet. If wet at other times, this was ignored until her pad was changed at her next toilet visit.

All too often, busy and demoralised ward staff ask for a behavioural programme for a patient who they do not like. Inevitably, this would lead to failure as there would be a temptation to 'punish' the patient for their misdemeanours and to a likely lack of consistency between different staff. It can often be witnessed that the arrival of a new staff member on such a ward can make a world of difference to a patient without any behavioural programme, purely by the person demonstrating their interest in the patient. In other words, non-contingent positive regard for the patient is an important prerequisite to any behavioural programme. Clear examples of this truism can be seen in everyday life. If a child is brought up in a loving, caring environment, then reasonable punishment can be remarkably effective in reducing undesirable behaviours. If a child is neglected, however, punishment may have little effect on bad behaviour as the child receives attention, albeit negative, which they crave in response to being naughty.

Covert sensitisation, sexual and social skills training used to treat illegal alternative sexual practices

This will be presented in the story of Giles (Case example 3.1).

Case example 3.1: Treating illegal sexual practices

Giles (25) was referred to the clinic by the probation service. He had recently finished a prison sentence for his repeated offences of indecent exposure to young women in the local park. Despite his custodial sentence, his probation officer had reason to believe that Giles had reoffended since his release.

The full psychiatric history was difficult to obtain from Giles, who appeared a shy and diffident man, avoided eye contact and answered questions in brief, non-discursive replies. He was the only child of elderly parents and had led an isolated life. His school years had been unhappy as, although an average pupil, he had been bullied by the other children and had eventually refused to go to school, developing symptoms of school phobia and refusal. Referral to the child psychiatric services had not resolved this problem and he had been taught in a tutorial group with other 'delicate' children. Thereafter, having finished his education without gaining any formal qualifications, he had obtained a job in a warehouse, preferring his solitary life. He had never made any friends at school or in his employment and had never had a girlfriend or any sexual relationship.

The history of his sexual development was that he had reached puberty at 13–14 years. No formal sex education had ever been given to him and most of his knowledge he had picked up from the television, tabloid press and 'girlie' magazines. He masturbated once a week to heterosexual fantasies.

The history of his public genital exposure began at the age of 19 years. A sexually explicit magazine had included a story about a man who exposed himself to women and had implied that this was very erotic to many of them who had been overtaken by passion and made love to the man in the park. Giles had been enthralled by this story and began to emulate the man.

He would wait until he was alone at home and would then play some erotic music and look at a girlie magazine. Subsequently he left the house and went to the park. At this time he would be extremely sexually aroused, and would be fantasising about making love to his favourite 'porn' star. When at the park, he would wait in a secluded clump of trees near to a footpath. His ideal victim was a woman of 16–30 years with blonde hair and alone, although he would sometimes expose himself to a group of women. Once he had seen his target, he would come out from the trees and stand on the footpath exposing his genitals. If the woman appeared shocked and ran away, Giles would find this arousing as he believed that she may think about the episode and find it erotic. On occasions, however, women had laughed at him or shouted abuse, which he found deeply distressing, and which resulted in his not returning to the park for several months. If he had received a preferable response, he would return to the trees and masturbate. His masturbatory fantasies for the next few weeks would then focus on this episode until he would return to the park again 4–6 weeks later.

During the first session the assessment suggested that Giles would need four components in his treatment: sex education, reduction in illegal sexual urges, increase in socially acceptable sexual activity, and improvement in general social skills.

The illegal sexual behaviour was the urgent item which needed tackling.

A full description of the arousing situation was obtained. This included full descriptions of the surroundings in which Giles performed his activities, as well as descriptions of his thoughts, emotions and fantasies. A similarly detailed description of three aversive scenes was also obtained from him. These were:

- 'I am exposing my genitals to a woman and she starts to laugh. Her face creases with delight and mirth. She is pointing at my genitals and laughing. As she gets her breath back she says "Look at that tiddler, call yourself a man, I have seen babies that are better equipped!" She then calls to three friends who arrive on the path. They all look at my genitals and laugh uproariously. They make comments to each other like "It must be a caterpillar" and "I would not show us that, love, you may lose it!" I turn and run but can still hear their laughter and taunts in the background.'

- 'I am exposing my genitals and I suddenly feel the arm of a man on my shoulder. I turn round to see this 6-foot man with a skinhead haircut. He has tattoos on both arms and looks very angry. "What are you doing, that's my girl!", he says. "I'm going to have to teach you a lesson!" He punches me in the face, I feel the pain but immediately I feel another punch in the stomach and then in the face again. My head aches, my nose is broken, I'm on the floor, he's kicked me in the genitals. All the time he's cursing and shouting at me. I'm lying on the ground as a helpless bundle, so weak I cannot move. He takes out a long, thin knife and picks up my penis, "Now for the best bit", he says ...'

Giles had great difficulty thinking of a third aversive scene connected with his illegal behaviour, and so the third scene was non-specifically aversive:

- 'I feel dreadfully sick. My stomach is churning and my hands and forehead feel cold and clammy. I'm having difficulties in standing up straight. My legs are weak. I collapse and fall into a large vat of liquid. I go under and realise that it has a revolting pungent smell. The liquid is semi-solid and sticky. I realise that I have fallen into a huge vat of vomit ..., etc.'

The therapist then recorded, using a 9-point scale, how arousing the illegal sexual scene was to Giles and how aversive the three unpleasant scenes were. It was easy for the therapist to observe that Giles looked animated and excited when describing the arousing scene and pale, tremulous and anxious when describing the aversive scenes. Indeed, if this had not been the case, the therapist would have had reason to try to identify alternative fantasies.

Giles was then asked to sit in a comfortable chair in a relaxed position. He was asked to imagine the arousing scene in detail and to verbally describe his fantasy. The therapist prompted Giles with details if he appeared to be flagging. Before reaching the end of the pleasurable fantasy, the therapist instructed Giles to switch to the first aversive scene and describe this in detail.

During the first session this pairing of pleasurable and aversive fantasies was done four times. Giles was then asked to do the same exercise himself at home three times a day. To aid his imagination, he was asked to write down a 'script' for all the scenes describing the fantasy in as much detail as he had done in the session.

In the application of covert sensitisation, it is important to establish at least three aversive scenes. This is because the patient will frequently be exposed to the aversive scene and habituation of the anxiety would render the aversive scene useless. Therefore the therapist needs to prescribe different aversive scenes and to frequently check that they remain highly unpleasant and distressing.

Over the next 6 weeks, the therapist saw Giles for weekly sessions during which the fantasy pairings were repeated at least six times in every session and were continued by Giles between sessions. The aversive scene was gradually introduced earlier and earlier in the 'pleasurable' scene.

At the sixth session, Giles reported that he no longer found the arousing scene pleasurable and had extreme difficulty in inducing this fantasy without experiencing symptoms of panic. It therefore appeared that the covert sensitisation had worked extremely well, particularly as Giles explained that he had tested this out by trying to walk to the park, but had felt so anxious he had to return home.

The next problem to be tackled was establishing appropriate sexual behaviour. Over the previous 6 weeks, the therapist had asked Giles to read some basic educational books about sex, because all his prior sexual knowledge had been obtained from girlie magazines and was thus inadequate and biased. These new books were discussed with Giles to ensure that he had understood the information. Appropriate sexual fantasies which were acceptable to him were then discussed. It transpired that although Giles had previously masturbated, he had always used the unusual technique of lying face down on the floor and rubbing his genitals against the carpet. This produced low levels of arousal which had been increased by his illegal fantasies. The therapist explained the technique of masturbation using manual stimulation, and Giles was asked to practise this at home while using 'appropriate' fantasies.

While Giles was being instructed in sexual education and masturbation training, he was also attending a social skills group which used the techniques of rehearsal, modelling, feedback, role-play and homework practice, as described in Chapter 4. Three months after the commencement of treatment, Giles reported that he had a girlfriend whom he had met at an evening class he had been encouraged to join by the social skills group. This later developed into a sexual relationship which was satisfactory to both of them. He had no illegal urges and fantasies any more, and reported that he was much happier and enjoying a social life.

It was clear that Giles' antisocial sexual behaviour was causing a public nuisance that required immediate action to prevent him being arrested and given a further custodial sentence. In these cases, rapid treatment to suppress illegal sexual urges based on aversion therapy is justified. Even in this case, however, a successful treatment plan incorporated other elements to increase the patient's general levels of social functioning. Not all cases of illegal sexual behaviour are so clear cut. If a patient has a sexual preference that worries them and is a cause of concern to their sexual partner, but is not in itself dangerous or causing a public nuisance, then less radical treatments may be used.

Orgasmic reconditioning was originally described by Marquis (1970). In this treatment, the patient is asked to masturbate regularly to their troublesome target fantasies but, at the point of orgasmic inevitability, to switch to the desired fantasy. As treatment progresses the desirable stimulus is introduced earlier and earlier in the arousal process, until masturbation is achieved using only the goal fantasy. Following this, further sexual or social skills training is usually needed to ensure benefits in therapy are maintained.

When dealing with troublesome sexual urges it is important to set realistic goals with the patient. Whereas a bisexual man who wishes to become exclusively heterosexual may be helped by appropriate orgasmic reconditioning and sexual skills training, it is not possible nor usually desirable to change the orientation of an exclusively homosexual individual. In this case, counselling to help such a person accept their sexual preference may be needed. Similarly, if a homosexual paedophile is referred for treatment, it would be unrealistic to set the goal of regular adult heterosexual contact, but adult homosexual orientation is more likely to be achievable. The next case history (Case example 3.2) demonstrates some pitfalls in using inappropriate positive reinforcement programmes.

Case example 3.2: Inappropriate positive reinforcement

Daryl, a deaf, blind and mute boy of 15 years with severe intellectual impairments, lived in a local authority children's home. He was a tall boy (over 6 feet), which caused the staff some difficulties when they tried to restrain him if he was doing anything dangerous. Nevertheless, they had coped well with him and demonstrated a loving and caring attitude towards him.

Over the previous 6 months, however, Daryl had developed a new behavioural problem which was causing great concern to the staff. Initially, he had discovered masturbation which had caused few problems as the staff would remove him to his own room whenever he began to masturbate in a public place. However, Daryl seemed to increase the frequency of masturbation over the next few weeks and was currently masturbating 15 to 20 times a day. The consequence of this problem was that he had been banned from his training centre as his behaviour distressed the staff, who were concerned about the reaction of other pupils' parents. He also was unable to go on outings with the home as there had been complaints from the public about him.

One of the staff members had read about contingent reinforcement programmes and decided to try one with Daryl to reduce his masturbatory behaviour. She decided that as Daryl enjoyed eating chocolate beans, these could be used as reinforcers. Every 15 min staff were to check on Daryl and if he either was not masturbating or if he was masturbating in his room, he was to be given a chocolate bean. This programme was applied for 3 months before the staff admitted defeat and requested help from a CBT therapist. By this time, Daryl was not only masturbating as frequently as before, he had also gained a considerable amount of weight, which meant that it was almost impossible to restrain him when he did start masturbating in public. It was explained to the staff that the reinforcement programme used was not ideal for two main reasons. First, it would inevitably lead to Daryl becoming obese, and second, chocolate beans were clearly not as rewarding as masturbation to him.

An alternative programme was suggested by the therapist. This involved using masturbation (a high-frequency preferred activity) to reinforce periods of appropriate social contact. In other words, Daryl was allowed to masturbate on his own for 10 minutes for every hour in which he did not indulge in this in public. Staff were to initially ensure this by holding his hands whenever he was in a public place. As Daryl would need rapid reinforcement for any behaviour, it was arranged that he could not only be taken to his own bedroom, but there would also be a quiet room available for him at his training centre, and he could retire to a corner of the minibus when on outings. This programme was much more successful, and soon staff no longer needed to hold Daryl's hands in public, as he would wait until he was alone. Any relapse required a staff member to firmly take Daryl's hands away from his genital area, and hold them firmly for 10 minutes, which was an activity Daryl disliked.

Treatment of alcohol misuse where abstinence was advisable

A full discussion of addictive behaviours will be found in Chapter 12, here I present just one vignette (Case example 3.3). This describes a very rare situation where aversive techniques may be used.

Case example 3.3: Treatment of alcohol misuse

Shug, a 55-year-old unemployed Glaswegian labourer, had a 40 years' history of excessive drinking. This problem had resulted in the loss of numerous jobs, separation from his wife and children, and his social and financial deterioration. When referred to the clinic, he had already been detoxified from alcohol, but as this had been a frequent occurrence in recent years, he had attended to see if we could improve his situation in the longer term.

His physical health had been greatly affected by his drinking behaviour. His liver function tests were grossly abnormal, and he had a history of duodenal ulceration and haematemesis. Previous treatment had included referral to self-help groups and a 6-month attendance at an out-patient clinic for supportive psychotherapy.

Full cognitive–behavioural analysis of Shug's problem demonstrated that, although he had achieved abstinence in the past for several days and weeks, if he once took a drink he felt that he had lost control and would then continue to drink until he passed out or his money ran out. He would drink at any time of the night or day and whether he was alone or in company. Previous periods of abstinence had broken down when he had received his social security benefit and had seen friends going into a pub or an off-licence.

Treatment commenced with the therapist discussing ways in which Shug could avoid some of the stimuli which precipitated a drinking bout or to control his access to alcohol once he had started drinking. Plans were made with him to move into a hostel and to attend Alcoholics Anonymous to try to increase his social contacts with people who were abstemious. He also agreed to carry a maximum of only £5 at any time.

Shug, however, felt that these actions would be insufficient to maintain his motivation to remain alcohol free. He said that he felt he would need to be 'locked up' for 6 months if he were to be able to permanently stop drinking. It was therefore decided that he should be prescribed disulphiram to help his willpower.

Disulphiram causes vomiting or, occasionally, more severe reactions if alcohol is taken following its administration. Owing to these potential reactions, it should only be prescribed in a hospital, specialised unit or by clinicians experienced in its use. A test dose of alcohol following disulphiram is a useful test and demonstration of the effects to the patient, but should be performed in the controlled setting of the clinic. For this reason it was decided to admit Shug to hospital for a day for a test dose of alcohol. This caused Shug to vomit profusely and to feel nauseous for 6 hours after its ingestion. Theoretically, this experience acted as an aversive stimulus which was paired with the previously pleasurable activity of drinking alcohol. Future temptation to drink alcohol reminded Shug of the likely consequences of drinking following disulphiram and increased his 'willpower'.

Although the pairing of the extremely aversive experience of nausea and vomiting with alcohol might be thought to be a sufficiently noxious experience to produce abhorrence of alcohol forever, this is unfortunately rarely the case. Whereas many people have long-lasting aversions to certain foods if they have symptoms of gastroenteritis following their ingestion, the previously pleasurable associations of alcohol seem to impair such 'one-trial learning'.

Shug did not react by permanent avoidance of alcohol. Generally, he was able to reduce his drinking, but at times of stress would stop the disulphiram for a few days and he would go on a drinking binge. These binges occurred at a frequency of approximately 3-month intervals.

Four years after starting therapy, Shug has considerably reduced his drinking, but has not achieved the goal of abstinence. His drinking is sporadic but of a 'binge' and out-of-control pattern. Attempts to introduce controlled drinking have failed. On the positive side, however, he is now working as a night watchman and has held this job for 2 years. His employers have been tolerant of his occasional absenteeism due to alcohol. The general physician is less worried about his physical health but would still wish him to be alcohol-free.

Habit reversal

Problem behaviours may also take the form of bad habits which have been learnt in response to a whole range of stimuli. Azrin & Nunn (1973) pioneered the treatment of habit reversal, which has been used to treat a range of conditions and habits, including multiple and facial tics, skin picking and neurodermatitis (lichen simplex chronicus) and excessive scratching related to skin pathology. This treatment has four components:

1 awareness training
2 competing response training
3 habit control motivation
4 generalisation training.

There is currently renewed interest in the use of habit reversal for the treatment of conditions including trichotillomania (hair-pulling) (Huynh *et al*, 2013) and skin-picking (Grant *et al*, 2012), since these conditions are newly defined and included in DSM-5 under the heading of obsessive–compulsive and related disorders (American Psychiatric Association, 2013). The four elements are illustrated in the case history of Sarah (Case example 3.4).

Case example 3.4: Treatment of facial tics using habit reversal

Sarah, an attractive and lively 24-year-old games mistress, was referred to the clinic with a 14-year history of unsightly and embarrassing facial tics. The onset had occurred at puberty, but was not related by Sarah to any particular life event. Over the years she had received treatment with a variety of medication, including haloperidol and benzodiazepine drugs, with no effect. She had also received individual psychodynamic psychotherapy which had not helped.

The tic could occur at any time but was more frequent if she was anxious or bored. Close observation of the movements revealed that it commenced with Sarah screwing up both eyes, followed by crinkling her nose, and then making a sharp downward movement of her chin, opening her mouth.

The first thing that Sarah was asked to do was to record the frequency of her tics over a few days. This awareness training is useful, as many people with habit disorders are oblivious of some of the times when they perform the undesirable behaviour. Obviously, Sarah had a busy life and so the records were made as simple as possible for her to keep. She was asked to obtain a small notebook and to divide each page into columns each representing a 1 h period. Every time she performed the tic, she was asked to place a mark in the appropriate column. She was also to record her activity at each hourly interval e.g. 'lunch with colleagues', 'lacrosse lesson with lower-sixth form'.

This diary was also useful as a baseline measure of Sarah's problem, and was maintained throughout treatment to monitor her progress. In addition, the therapist decided to use another assessment measure by recording a 20 min interview with Sarah on camera. During this interview, the therapist asked a series of 'neutral' questions about her job and hobbies and some more emotive questions about the effect of the tic on her life. The mean number of tics per minute during the 'neutral' and 'emotive' discussion was then calculated and this procedure was repeated at the end of treatment with the therapist asking identical questions. The baseline measures showed that Sarah performed the tic an average of 300 times a day or approximately 0.5 tics per minute.

At the second session the principle of competing response practice was explained to Sarah. The therapist said: 'One of the problems with a long-standing habit is that you have built up and strengthened the muscles of your face which are involved in the tic at the expense of the opposing muscles. What I will be asking you to do is to perform some exercises to strengthen these opposing muscles.

The start of every tic begins with you screwing up both your eyes. As soon as you feel that you are going to tic, I want you to raise your eyebrows, wrinkling your forehead. You may find this easier to do if you place your thumb and index finger of one hand under each of your eyebrows. I then want you to hold this position to the count of 20 or until the urge to tic passes, whichever is the longer time. At the same time as doing this I would like you to clench you teeth together very tightly and likewise to maintain this position.'

Following this description, the therapist asked Sarah to practise the competing response in the session. The therapist then asked Sarah to list all the deleterious effects of having a tic and the advantages of being tic-free. She was asked to write this list down and to read it through whenever she felt bored or disheartened by the treatment (habit-control motivation).

Finally, ways in which Sarah could incorporate the competing response movements into her everyday life without looking conspicuous were discussed. Sarah suggested that if she were outside, she could place her hand under her eyebrows as if shielding her eyes from the sun. If she was inside and sitting at a desk or table, she could use her hand under her eyebrows to 'support' her head (generalisation training).

When Sarah was seen a week later for her third session, the frequency of tics had already reduced to less than 10% of the baseline level. Difficulties were discussed with her at this session and over the following two sessions. Six weeks after her initial appointment, Sarah was discharged from active treatment. The frequency of tics was less than 1%, which was acceptable to Sarah. This improvement was maintained at 1 year post-treatment follow-up.

Tics may also be part of other conditions, most notably Tourette syndrome as well as other neurological conditions. Tourette syndrome can also be paired with obsessive–compulsive symptoms. In such cases, as well as the evidence-based treatment of dopamine-blocking medication, it may be helpful to use some habit reversal as well as graded exposure and self-imposed response prevention (ERP) for the obsessive–compulsive symptoms.

Mass practice

Mass practice involves the individual repeatedly performing the undesirable habit or behaviour to 'satiate' or encourage them to become aware of the habit and reduce its frequency (Case example 3.5).

Case example 3.5 Repetitive throat-clearing treated by mass practice

George, a 56-year-old road sweeper, had been treated for mycoplasma pneumonia. Since that time he had developed the habit of repeatedly clearing his throat despite having no phlegm to move. This habit occurred 60–80 times an hour and was causing some marital problems as it greatly irritated his wife.

Treatment with habit reversal had been unsuccessful as it was difficult to find an effective competing response for George to use.

The therapist then decided to use mass practice. George was first asked to find three half-hour periods in the day when he could retire to his room alone and would not be heard by his family. He was then told that during these times he was to repeatedly clear his throat for the entire 30 min period. At other times of the day, he was to try not to clear his throat but to 'save it up' to his next throat-clearing session.

The week after this instruction was given to George, he returned with his wife to the clinic. He reported that he had complied with the instructions for the first 3 days but that since that time the thought of clearing his throat was so averse to him that he had not been able to do it at all. His wife confirmed his improvement, and was delighted with it.

George was asked to continue monitoring his throat clearing, and to reintroduce mass practice if the frequency increased to more than five times a day.

Key learning points

- Operant conditioning involves altering behaviour by influencing the response to that behaviour.
- Reinforcement may be positive, negative, punishment or response cost; positive reinforcement is the most useful approach clinically.
- Eliminating a behaviour using aversive stimuli (e.g. covert sensitisation) is only indicated if the behaviour is life-threatening or a severe public nuisance.
- The stimulus that produces an unwanted response can itself be modified (e.g. orgasmic reconditioning).
- The response to the stimulus can be modified (e.g. stimulus control techniques).
- The problem behaviour can be replaced with alternative adaptive responses (e.g. habit reversal).
- The desirability of the problem behaviour can be reduced (e.g. mass practice, response cost).

Suggested measures to use with conditions covered in this chapter

- General measures of functioning: Sheehan Disability Scale (measuring impact on life), see Chapter 2.
- Specific behavioural problems: the measures used will need to be tailored to the individual problem in most cases. For example, in the case of treatment of obesity, the measurement of weight is a reliable indicator of success. Similarly, frequency of undesired behaviour can be measured for conditions as widespread as illegal sexual practices, incontinence and throat clearing. For skin-picking, it is possible to photograph lesions before and after interventions as well as estimating size and extent of the lesions. For substance misuse, a measure of abstinence is one option but it can also be useful to measure craving for the drug (e.g. Singleton *et al*, 1995).

References

American Psychiatric Association (2013) *Diagnostic and Statistical Manual for Psychiatric Disorders* (DSM-5). APA.

Azrin NH, Nunn RG (1973) Habit reversal: a method of eliminating nervous habits and tics. *Behaviour Research and Therapy*, **11**: 619–28.

Grant JE, Odlaug BL, Chamberlain SR, *et al* (2012) Skin picking disorder. *American Journal of Psychiatry*, **169**: 1143–9.

Huynh M, Gavino AC, Magid M (2013) Trichotillomania. *Seminars in Cutaneous Medicine and Surgery*, **32**: 88–94.

Marquis JN (1970) Orgasmic reconditioning: changing sexual object choice through controlling masturbation fantasies. *Journal of Behavior Therapy and Experimental Psychiatry*, **1**: 263–70.

Premack D (1959) Toward empirical behavior laws: I. Positive reinforcement. *Psychological Review*, **66**: 219–33.

Singleton EG, Tiffany ST, Henningfield JE (1995) Development and validation of a new questionnaire to assess craving for alcohol. In *Problems of Drug Dependence, 1994: Proceedings of the 56th Annual Scientific Meeting, The College on Problems of Drug Dependence, Inc* (ed. LS Harris): p. 289. National Institute on Drug Abuse Research Monograph Series Vol. 153. NIDA.

Stuart RB (1967) Behavioral control of overeating. *Behaviour Research and Therapy*, **1**: 357–65.

Further reading

Chance P (2003) *Learning and Behaviour* (5th edn). Thomson-Wadsworth.

Domjan MP (2004) *The Essentials of Conditioning and Learning* (3rd edn). Wadsworth Publishing.

Social skills training

Overview

The principles of coaching and reinforcement will be discussed along with case examples of the application of reinforcement, coaching skills and graded exposure for social skills and assertiveness deficits. Clinical examples demonstrating the distinction and overlap between social anxiety disorder and poor social skills will be described. Anger and poor impulse control will be examined, as will comorbidity and overlap with other treatments.

A lack of social skills may be present from childhood or only become apparent later in life. Social skills deficit may arise in response to a mental health problem such as schizophrenia or may lead to psychiatric problems in their own right. Indeed, many people may have poor social skills, which interferes with their ability to sustain relationships, succeed in the workplace and live fulfilling lives. Failure in these domains can result in psychological distress and mental health problems. Situations and conditions that can result in impaired social skills include:

- lack of general social skills
  - social anxiety disorder (social phobia)
  - social skills not developed (e.g. owing to being brought up in a different culture and lack of understanding of the social norms in the new culture)
  - secondary to a developmental disorder (e.g. Asperger syndrome or autism spectrum disorder)
  - secondary to severe, enduring mental illness and subsequent withdrawal and negative symptoms (e.g. secondary to schizophrenia)
- lack of assertiveness
  - this can lead to a build up of resentment and eventually may result in psychiatric difficulties such as depression

- lack of impulse control
  - can be comorbid with other psychiatric disorders (e.g. alcohol or drug misuse, personality disorder)
  - can be a standalone condition and part of a generally impulsive personality.

Michel Hersen was one of the most powerful figures in the development of social skills and assertiveness training in the 1970s and 1980s. Although much of this work is now forgotten, many of the skills developed from this time are used in a variety of clinical and non-clinical settings (Miller, 2012; Thase, 2012). Social skills training techniques are part of packages used to treat patients with psychotic illnesses and depression (Bellack, 2004). They are also now widely used in the fields of autism and Asperger syndrome (Patrick, 2008; Weiss *et al*, 2013; Chang *et al*, 2014).

As well as applying social skills training to improve the outcomes with people using mental health services, various components have also been used to increase the efficacy of healthcare workers, for example assertiveness skills have been widely applied to improve effectiveness of nursing staff on general wards (e.g. Hodgetts, 2011). Coaching involves similar principles to social skills training and may be useful in developing skills in healthcare practitioners (Mortlock, 2012). Recently, there has been increasing interest in using these type of skills to try to develop leadership skills in doctors in the National Health Service (NHS) and other healthcare systems (Drummond & Hattersley, 2008).

Bellack & Hersen (1979) defined social skill as 'the ability to express both positive and negative feelings in the interpersonal context without suffering consequent loss of social reinforcement'. This definition, however, may overlook some of the complexity of human social interaction and particularly the complexities of team, society and family work and activities. In such situations people need to be influenced by others and react to the needs of other members of the group.

In 1983, Shepherd suggested that competent social skills involve:

- the observed behaviour during a social interaction
- the cognitive responses a person makes in a social interaction, i.e. their subjective thoughts and feelings, and how competent they feel themselves to be
- the ability to sustain social roles and relationships, e.g. as a parent, employee, employer, colleague or friend.

The first stage in this process, however, is skill acquisition.

Development of skills and coaching

To develop a new skill, the therapist or coach needs to first observe the current level of skill. The learning sequence is thus:

1 Observe the person's current level of performance.
2 Demonstrate the new skill to be learnt
   • divide complex tasks into a series of smaller actions.
3 Ask the person to practise the skill
   • as well as within the therapy/coaching session, they should practise between sessions.
4 Feedback on performance
   • feedback should start with positive comments followed by positive suggestions of how to improve the performance.
5 Repetition of all of the above.

An easy example to demonstrate this is teaching a child to tie shoelaces. First, the parent gains the child's attention. They then divide the steps involved in tying a bow into several easy steps and demonstrate this several times. They ask the child to copy this using prompts, positive feedback and encouragement. After several trials the child may be able to perform the task and may then practise alone in their own time. See Case example 4.1.

Case example 4.1: Individual social skills training

Jeffrey was hiding behind a newspaper in the waiting room, and when called for his appointment did not look up but kept his eyes firmly fixed on the floor. During the interview he did not look at the therapist and his voice was barely audible. In muted tones he described how he had always been shy, even at school, and that at university shyness had prevented his joining in with social activities. Then he had trained as a librarian and enjoyed his job, except when this brought him into contact with the public. His shyness in this situation had been noticed and was threatening to hold up his promotion. He always ate lunch alone to avoid dining with colleagues, and his social life was very poor as he feared going out into social situations and so had become a complete recluse. His main spare time activities were watching television alone or playing chess with a computer. The most fearful situation for Jeffrey was talking to a young woman when he would become lost for words and feared blushing.

During the assessment it became clear that Jeffrey had very low self-esteem. He believed he would fail situations before he tried. This expectation of failure had become a self-fulfilling prophecy, and that was why he never met young women. He now totally avoided the feared situation. This made him think even more badly of himself and so the vicious spiral continued. The therapist wondered whether cognitive therapy for this low self-esteem would be necessary but felt the best course of action was to start by building up his skill and to see whether with new skills and some success, his idea of self-worth would increase.

Treatment followed the four steps for all new skill acquisition:
• description of new behaviour
• guidance and demonstration
• practice of the new behaviour with feedback
• transfer of the new behaviour to the natural environment.

Description of new behaviour

This was achieved by asking Jeffrey in what ways he thought his behaviour ought to be changed.

Therapist: 'Tell me Jeffrey, what would you like to do that you find too difficult or painful at the moment?'

Jeffrey: 'I suppose I ought to be able to look you in the face. Then I'd like to be able to talk to people without blushing. I would like to be able to eat in front of other people, especially at work.' Finally, in a whisper, he admitted: 'It would be great if I could chat to women like other blokes do.'

These four statements were taken as goals to be aimed for in the next phase of treatment.

Guidance and demonstration

The problem of gaze aversion was dealt with by guidance and demonstration. First, the therapist demonstrated with a co-therapist how they looked at each other during a conversation and Jeffrey was asked to watch this.

It was discussed with him how, if a person is talking, they will tend to look away for much of the time but will periodically check the face of the listener to see how they are responding. This looking at the listener compared with looking away is approximately 1:3. If someone is listening to another person, they will look at the speaker's face more intently. In this case the ratio of looking at the speaker's face to looking away is approximately 2:3.

The therapist and Jeffrey then tried to hold a conversation and practise these various ratios for looking and looking away. Jeffrey found this very difficult and it was noted that if he looked the therapist straight in the eye, he would immediately drop his gaze. To assist with this the therapist asked him to look the therapist in the eye and to try and 'outstare' each other. This is similar to a game often played by children and Jeffrey soon grasped this and found he could perform it very well.

After this, Jeffrey found he could gain eye contact in a conversation without immediately dropping his gaze. He was asked to try this during the week and to report back on how this went.

Practice of the new behaviour with feedback

It was agreed that Jeffrey would look at a recording of himself engaged in conversation. This was a very frightening prospect for him initially but he agreed to do it. The video was made with the unit occupational therapist. The occupational therapist was a socially skilled, attractive young woman who asked Jeffrey all about his work in the library. When the recording was played back to Jeffrey, he was seen to make good eye contact and was praised for this. However, it was noted that he had poor conversational skills and that he spoke so quietly that he was barely audible. This was fed back to him by suggesting that he try and speak louder and by discussing with him other possible topics of conversation that he felt he could use.

It was then suggested to Jeffrey that for the next recorded session he should prepare some questions to ask the occupational therapist, for example, how she chose to be an occupational therapist and what she liked and disliked about the job.

When he attempted this last task he became completely inaudible on the recording, and attention was now focused on his problem with voice production. Before this he was given positive feedback for the things he was doing well, for example his posture was better. It was then suggested that he try and speak a little faster and also the use of a more varied tone with the pitch of the voice getting higher at the end of a question was demonstrated. After the therapist's demonstration, Jeffrey was asked to try to repeat that.

Whenever he used a good expressive tone, spoke fluently, spoke faster or more powerfully, the achievement was pointed out and he was praised.

Three more recorded sessions were necessary using a variety of female students and staff to role-play with Jeffrey before all the skills had been mastered.

Transfer of the new behaviour to the natural environment

Jeffrey had done well so far and had exceeded his own expectations, but he still worried about his performance in a real-life situation. However, he now agreed to meet his colleagues in the work cafeteria and coped with eating in front of them with little difficulty, possibly because they all happened to be men at the time: his greatest difficulty remained talking to young women.

There were very few situations where he came into contact with young women, and his social skills deficit was partially responsible for this self-perpetuating situation. One possibility, however, was on his weekly visit to the launderette.

Jeffrey: 'I dread having to speak to someone, so I usually take a book along. I know I would not be able to say anything to a young woman.'

Therapist: 'Leave the book behind and initiate a planned conversation with a young woman which we will have previously rehearsed.'

This was along the lines of 'Could you show me how to work this machine?' This turned out to be very successful, as the young woman then talked to Jeffrey in a non-threatening way about the neighbourhood and he was able to practise his new-found voice production and conversational skills.

Later on some sessions were spent with the aim of improving Jeffrey's lifestyle, and he realised that playing chess with computers was not helpful. He joined a social club for university graduates and in this way was able to meet young women in a non-threatening environment where his new skills soon generalised, his social roles expanded, and he continued to improve at follow-up at 1 year.

Variations on the basic training

In some cases therapy is not as straightforward as just described and if difficulties are encountered, more complicated techniques can be used.

Role play and role reversal

This is where the patient plays the role of someone they fear encountering, for instance in the case of Jeffrey he could have pretended to be a young woman and the therapist could have taken his role. In this way the therapist would have acted as a competent model so that the patient could be exposed to a useful learning situation. In the next stage the patient plays himself again and the therapist plays the young woman.

Use of an ear microphone

This is a device for the patient to receive prompting from the therapist, who watches the session through a one-way screen. It could have been used in Case example 4.1 if Jeffrey had been totally lost for words, as is the case with some patients.

Use of a script

Once again, for the patient who becomes speechless in certain situations a script can be useful. The patient can be encouraged to write the script as a homework exercise and it can be discussed and edited with the aid of the therapist. Reading from the script in practice sessions is gradually faded out, so that it is eventually not necessary in practice sessions before carrying out real-life practice.

Use of a self-help book or online resources

Many people with social anxiety and a lack of social skills will have already tried the self-help route before seeking professional advice. However, targeted information on specific problems can be useful. The therapist must always check the content of whatever is 'prescribed' and must ensure that this is likely to be useful.

The next two examples describe some of the techniques discussed (Case examples 4.2 and 4.3).

Case example 4.2: Assertiveness training using role play, role reversal and homework practice

Jo was a 35-year-old woman who described herself as lacking in self-confidence since birth. She had been 'shy' as a child and remembered being teased at school. The presenting complaint was that she felt she could never stand up for herself. When asked for a current example she described how people took advantage of her at the office where she worked as a supervisor in a computer factory. Both her boss and also some of her junior staff would always ask her to take on extra work. Consequently, she worked late most evenings and felt that she was unable to engage in her hobbies during the week.

Plan of treatment

During the assessment, it became clear that Jo had always been 'easy-going', even as a child. Her siblings also tended to rely on her and would expect her frequently to babysit for them at the expense of her own social life. Jo was unmarried but enjoyed long-distance walking, which she rarely found time to do and had hardly managed to go out with her rambling club over the previous year. The thought of standing up for herself made her anxiety increase, so she took the least line of resistance in a situation of conflict and became compliant. However, her compliance then made her angry and frustrated with herself, and she often became depressed as a result.

The aim of therapy was to establish some realistic targets for Jo to learn to increase her self-confidence.

Treatment

During the first session, Jo was asked to imagine that the therapist was her boss who wanted her to work late. Jo was asked to politely refuse this. Initially she was unable to think of a way to do this. The therapist therefore asked Jo to pretend to be her boss while the therapist pretended to be Jo.

The therapist said: 'I'm sorry but I really can't do this extra work tonight as I am going out.'

The 'boss' tried to argue but the therapist looked the 'boss' in the eye and said, 'I am really sorry but I really do not have time to take on this extra work.'

Following on from this, Jo was asked to decide if the therapist had been rude or disrespectful to the 'boss'. She was also asked to describe how she had felt as the 'boss' on hearing the therapist decline. Jo admitted that she had not felt angry but had felt that the response was reasonable.

Over the next week, Jo was asked to practise this in the office. Prior to this, she was asked to practise certain scenarios by herself in front of the mirror at home. She was asked to speak the words out loud so that she could practise a range of refusals. She also was to practise refusals to her siblings.

Jo progressed very well but then became worried that she had refused to help her sister at a time when she would have liked to have looked after the children. The therapist and Jo discussed how it was fine for her to say 'yes' but only if this was something she wanted to do. The aim of assertiveness training was to ensure she was able to say 'no' appropriately and when she wanted to but she could still help out at work and in her social life if this was in her own interest.

It is worth noting that in the past it was often suggested that people should 'release their aggression' by punching a pillow or engage in a similar 'safe' aggressive activity. This is now strongly discouraged as it can be demonstrated that these activities tend to overall raise the urge to act aggressively rather than reduce it (Bushman *et al*, 1999).

Case example 4.3: Anger management using role play

Bill was 20 years old and unemployed, and had recently been cautioned by the police following a fight in the local job centre. A full history was taken and it was found that, in general, Bill lacked assertiveness and tended to let his frustration build up until he occasionally 'lashed out'. These episodes when he did 'lash out' were often usually completely out of proportion to the situation which appeared to provoke them.

One of the complicating factors was Bill's alcohol consumption. He did not drink on a daily basis but would sometimes binge drink, consuming 5–6 pints of lager at one time. Several of his violent outbursts had been after he had been drinking. At the end of the assessment, it was decided that treatment should consist of:

- working on Bill's assertion skills to prevent the build-up of anger and resentment in the first place
- stopping all binge drinking and restricting alcohol intake to 1–2 pints of beer as a maximum at any one time
- developing alternative strategies if Bill felt his temper was increasing.

Bill reluctantly agreed to reduce his binge drinking but did not feel he wished to do this long term. He was advised to stick to this for the duration of therapy and to see what difference this made to the way he felt. He then embarked on a course of role play, examining certain situations where he felt resentful and angry but where he was unable to assert himself.

The therapy progressed well but Bill was convinced it would be impossible for him to be assertive in the job centre. He said he regularly would be standing in a queue and one or two people who he had heard were 'hard cases' would push in. The therapist suggested strategies but these were rejected by Bill. The therapist then decided to accompany him to the job centre. When this occurred, it became clear that normal assertive social skills were unlikely to be useful in this situation as the men who pushed in were indeed extremely intimidating. It was therefore decided that assertion was unlikely to help in this situation and that other ways of diffusing Bill's anger were more likely to be helpful.

This anecdote emphasises the need for the therapist to totally understand the patient's social situation and the environment in which they live. It is not helpful to superimpose generic values in inappropriate situations!

Some of Bill's recent temper outbursts were examined. Bill was very ashamed and embarrassed by some of these as they often involved his family members. He was asked to describe in detail the 'worst-case' scenario for each of these episodes. He was then asked to write these down on some cards to use as 'cue cards' if he felt his anger increasing. In addition, Bill was asked to think of alternative strategies to reduce his anger. He was a keen runner and always found he felt better after going for a run. For this reason, Bill readily agreed to go for a run whenever he felt his anger starting to increase. Going for a run was not always possible and so a number of other strategies were also devised, such as making an excuse and leaving the room for 10 min when he would read his cue cards or speak to someone else if a person was upsetting him.

More recently, it has been demonstrated that third generation CBT treatment of mindfulness can be useful in reducing aggressive behaviour (Hepner et al, 2008). Mindfulness is described fully in Chapter 8 (p. 126 onwards). It consists of teaching the patient to relax and then to fully focus on their surroundings and things in the 'here and now' rather than ruminating about the past or future. People with aggression often ruminate on the past and let their anger escalate. If they learn to be mindful, they are taught to experience and accept their emotions without escalating them.

The range of applications of social skills training

Social interaction is at the centre of much human activity, and the range of applications of social skills training is wide. Social skills problems may be comorbid with a range of psychiatric disorders. These may include social anxiety, developmental disorders, including autism and Asperger syndrome, schizophrenia and depression. In mild autism or Asperger syndrome, social skills training can be used. For those with more difficulty in interpreting other people's emotions, a more specialist intervention may be required.

In chronic schizophrenia the lack of social skills may be a function of the disorder, the effect of strong medication, preoccupation with delusional beliefs and hallucinatory experiences, or the result of frequent hospitalisation. The emphasis for social skills training is on the deficit aspect of the disorder, though many techniques are similar, for example practice, rehearsal and praise are used in both conditions. In addition, there is some suggestion that some people with schizophrenia may have impaired awareness of the social implications of their own and other people's behaviour. This may be amenable to social cognitive therapies that are beyond the scope of this book.

The person with depression may be unable to show behaviour that is positively reinforced by others, will generally lack assertiveness and will show a low level of activity. The management of these problems in general is described in Chapter 8, but may also include a social skills training component, as described here.

Individual *v.* group treatment

Many of the techniques used in treating individuals can be applied cost-effectively in a group setting. There is a potential saving in therapist time if patients are treated in groups, but the treatment goals must reflect the needs of the whole group, and in practice it may take some time to put such a group together. A specific advantage of the group is that individual members may role-play for each other and can provide feedback and reinforcement for each other. However, the progress of the group can only go as fast as its slowest member.

Key learning points

- Social skills training applies to social phobia and lack of social skills acquisition.
- The principles of skills acquisition include: analysis of problem, demonstration of new behaviours, practice and constructive feedback.
- These principles can be applied in all learning situations, including coaching, clinical and also professional development of new skills.
- Lack of assertiveness requires specific techniques such as role play and homework practice, directed at the low level of assertiveness.
- Lack of impulse control can be dealt with by anger management: a package of techniques directed at training recognition of early cues triggering the impulse.
- Aggression can be exacerbated by activities designed to 'let off steam' – distraction and mindfulness can be more useful.

Suggested measures to use with conditions covered in this chapter

- For all conditions: Problems and targets, Sheehan Disability Scale (measuring impact on life) (both in Chapter 2).
- Social skills: Specific Level of Functioning Assessment (SLOF) (Schneider & Struening, 1983).
- Assertiveness: Adult Self-Expression Scale (Gay *et al*, 1975).
- Anger: Spielberger State-Trait Anger Inventory (Spielberger *et al*, 1983).

References

Bellack AS (2004) Skills training for people with severe mental illness. *Psychiatric Rehabilitation Journal*, **27**: 375–91.

Bellack AS, Hersen M (eds) (1979) *Research and Practice in Social Skills Training*. Plenum.

Bushman BJ, Baumeister RF, Stack AD (1999) Catharsis, aggression, and persuasive influence: self-fulfilling or self-defeating prophecies? *Journal of Personality and Social Psychology*, **76**: 367–76.

Chang YC, Laugeson EA, Gantman A, *et al* (2014) Predicting treatment success in social skills training for adolescents with autism spectrum disorders: The UCLA Program for the Education and Enrichment of Relational Skills. *Autism*, **18**: 467–70.

Drummond LM, Hattersley N (2008) Leadership training: what is it for? *BMJ Careers*, **337**: 83–4.

Gay ML, Hollandsworth JG, Galassi JP (1975) An Assertiveness Inventory for Adults. *Journal of Counseling Psychology*, **22**: 340–4.

Heppner WL, Kernis MH, Lakey CE, *et al* (2008) Mindfulness as a means of reducing aggressive behavior: dispositional and situational evidence. *Aggressive Behaviour*, **34**: 486–96.

Hodgetts S (2011) Being assertive benefits everyone. *Nursing Times*, **107**: 41.

Miller PM (2012) Michel Hersen and the development of social skills training: historical perspective of an academic scholar and pioneer. *Behavioral Modification*, **36**: 444–53.

Mortlock S (2012) Coaching skills: take the driving seat. *Health Service Journal*, **122**: 28–9.

*Patrick NJ (2008) *Social Skills for Teenagers and Adults with Asperger's Syndrome: A Practical Guide to Day-to-Day Life*. Jessica Kingsley Publishers.

Schneider LC, Struening EL (1983) SLOF: A behavioral rating scale for assessing the mentally ill. *Social Work Research and Abstracts*, **19**: 9–21.

Shepherd G (1983) Chapter 1: Introduction. In *Developments in Social Skills Training* (eds S Spence, G Shepherd). Academic Press.

Spielberger CD, Jacobs GA, Russell S, *et al* (1983) Assessment of anger: the state-trait anger scale. In *Advances in Personality Assessment, Vol 2* (eds JN Butcher, CD Spielberger). Lawrence Erlbaum Associates.

Thase ME (2012) Social skills training for depression and comparative efficacy research: a 30-year retrospective. *Behavioral Modification*, **36**: 545–57.

Weiss JA, Viecili MA, Sloman L, *et al* (2013) Direct and indirect psychosocial outcomes for children with autism spectrum disorder and their parents following a parent-involved social skills group intervention. *Journal of the Academy of Child and Adolescent Psychiatry*, **22**: 303–9.

*Suitable to recommend to patients.

Recommended treatment manuals and other reading

Agresta J, Bellack AS, Gingerich S, *et al* (2004) *Social Skills Training for Schizophrenia: A Step-by-Step Guide*. Guilford Press.

Bellack AS, Hersen M (eds) (1979) *Research and Practice in Social Skills Training*. Plenum.

Relationship, communication and sexual skills training

Overview

This chapter will look at human interaction and how skills can be developed to improve it. Although often described as 'marital', many of these techniques can be used in any relationship and between people of any gender and age. The chapter will start by examining behavioural exchange methods and then move on to examining communication skills and how these may be improved. Mention will be made of the newer integrative couple therapy and how this can be used in treatment. Finally, there will be a description of sexual skills acquisition using graded exposure and sexual skills training. Although the case histories cited involve heterosexual couples, identical techniques can be used with homosexual couples.

People are sociable beings and thus tend to live together. In general, most people are happiest when living in close proximity to other people with whom they have a close bond. However, these relationships can frequently be marred by simple misunderstandings or basic lack of skills. In this chapter, we will be examining three different aspects and approaches to improving poor relationships. Much of the research in these mainly behavioural techniques was performed in the 1970s and 1980s and with married couples. There is no reason why the techniques should be restricted to such a group, however, and many can be extended beyond the marital relationship as well, of course, as being useful in same-sex couples. These three approaches are:

- behavioural exchange therapy (reciprocity negotiation training)
- communication skills training
- sexual skills training.

In recent years these simple behavioural interventions have tended to be overlooked in favour of more complex paradigms, such as those used in systemic therapy. A review of the literature in 1996 (Wesley & Waring) performed a meta-analysis examining the outcome of behavioural marital therapy, cognitively oriented marital therapy, emotionally focused marital therapy and insight-oriented marital therapy. The authors found good evidence for the efficacy of each of these four methods but were unable to demonstrate any clear advantage of one rather than any other and also found no evidence for particular problems responding preferentially to any one type of therapy. Behavioural interventions are simple to learn and effective and thus can be widely applied, often in combination with other treatments.

Behavioural exchange therapy

This technique was developed from the pioneering observations of Stuart (1969, 1973, 1980), who applied social learning theory to marital therapy. He recognised the power of the patterns of mutual reinforcement that married couples set up. From these observations he proposed that in any partnership the existing status quo was the most rewarding and least costly in terms of effort. All relationships involve rewards as well as 'costs' for the individuals. Most people expect an approximately equal sharing of these. In problematic or unhappy relationships these rewards or costs are either at a very low level or are clearly unequal. He also suggested that the way to enable one partner to change behaviour is for each to change their behaviour first, and the way to initiate change was to reward the partner for carrying out whatever behaviour they liked in their partner.

Following the work of Stuart, Azrin *et al* (1973) described a similar technique they labelled 'reciprocity counselling'. There is clearly a plethora of terms with similar meaning; so for the sake of simplicity we shall call all such interventions behavioural exchange therapy. See Case example 5.1.

Case example 5.1: Behavioural exchange marital therapy

Mary and Ron were a couple in their 30s with a 3-year-old daughter, Rosie. Ron worked in a firm of accountants and was successful at his high-powered job. Mary had given up her equally successful career to look after their child, and was happy to do this for a few years. The couple described their problem as 'constant rows', and they gave the following account when seen together and asked to say what they considered to be the main difficulty.

Mary: 'He is becoming impossible to live with. I never know what time he will be home at night, and in what condition. I mean how much he will have been drinking.'

Ron: 'I know I have behaved badly but when I come home all I get is complaints. I don't seem to ever do anything right in her eyes. Most of the people I work with go out for a few drinks, one thing leads to another, and before long I just forget all about coming home and frankly it is a relief to come in late and not be faced with a barrage of criticism.'

Therapist (to Mary): 'You have said Ron is impossible to live with, and then you specified his coming home late and then his drinking too much. Is that the main thing that you would like to change about Ron?'

Mary: 'Not just that. I could cope with that. When I found out about the womanising, that was the last straw.'

Therapist (to Ron): 'Do you know what she means by this?'

Ron: 'It was one of those things all the lads did at the office. After a few drinks we would go on to a club, and one thing led to another. Mary would not have found out except that I had to tell her when I got a sexually transmitted disease. I don't blame her at all for being angry about that. We have talked about it all but I do feel that if she didn't get at me all the time this wouldn't have happened. She isn't the same person I married who was interesting and carefree.'

Assessment

It was clear from the assessment that the relationship was at a low ebb of negative feelings. Mary felt that Ron did not take his fair share of household responsibilities but went out as he had done as a single man before he was a father. Ron felt that every time he came home, there were a list of demands from Mary who 'kept nagging' him.

Treatment

After each of the couple had been given sufficient time to vent their feelings and anger, the therapist asked them to think of two behaviours which they would like from the other. Mary started by saying that she wanted Ron: 'Not to go out drinking' and 'To do more around the house'. Ron asked that Mary: 'Stop nagging' and said that there was no other task that he could think of.

None of these tasks are suitable as behavioural goals for therapy. To be effective goals should be:

- specific rather than general
- repeatable
- positive rather than asking people to stop doing something
- acceptable
- realistic.

The therapist explained these rules to the couple and tried to help them reformulate their wishes so that they complied with these rules. First, the therapist asked Mary to think of some tasks that met the criteria above. After some discussion she agreed that: Ron will do the washing up after the evening meal every day whether or not he is eating at home, and Ron will come home early one day a week (prearranged between them) and care for Rosie, allowing Mary to go out with her friends.

When the therapist turned his attention to Ron's wishes, he found that all he would say was 'stop nagging'. It was explained to the couple that it is very difficult for people to stop a behaviour and much easier to replace it with something else. The problem also with this as a task was that it was vague rather than specific. Eventually, it was agreed that the following were suitable asks: 'When I come in from work (assuming this is not late at night but is at the normal 7.00 pm), Mary will sit down with me and have a cup of tea. I will tell her about my day at work and she can tell me about her day. This conversation will last for half an hour, after which I will bathe Rosie.'

Although this meant that Ron had two tasks to Mary's one, both agreed that this represented an equal share for the week. These tasks were written down for each of them and a further appointment made.

As the weeks progressed the couple added another few small items on a reciprocal basis. One week both arrived very angry with each other and it transpired that Ron had again been out late and had not telephoned and so Mary was unaware of his whereabouts. She had retaliated by not speaking to him the next day. Ron felt indignant by this as he was entertaining an important client who had just arrived from abroad. When this was discussed it was agreed that Ron would always telephone Mary prior to any impromptu meetings of this sort and would inform her of his likely arrival time home.

Overall, these small tasks improved the relationship between the couple. The therapy was effective in this case as both were keen to continue the marriage and to work together for the sake of their daughter. Such an approach is likely to be less successful if one of the couple is less committed to continuing the relationship.

It is worthwhile thinking again about the nature of the therapeutic tasks allocated to each of the couple:

- positive rather than negative behaviour is emphasised, e.g. 'Stop criticising my appearance' could be translated into 'Say if you approve of my hair or clothes'
- repeatable rather than once-only behaviour is used, e.g. 'Go to my sister's wedding' is an unsuitable target, but 'Go out socially with me once a week' is acceptable
- specific rather than general behaviour is preferred, e.g. 'Help me more with the housework' is too general a target, whereas 'Wash the dishes after the evening meal five nights a week' is suitable
- the tasks should be acceptable to both parties
- they should be realistic rather than overambitious
- complaints should be translated into positive wishes.

Communication skills training

Although behavioural exchange training can be usefully employed with many couples with relationship problems, there are some couples whose recurrent communication skills problems lead to resentment and misunderstandings. Most of the work on communication skills training has focused on teaching couples communication problem-solving skills as this appears to be the area where conflicts most frequently arise.

In their description of marital therapy, Jacobson & Gurman (1986) emphasised that three behavioural techniques be used in communication skills training:

- therapist issues instructions of what is required (this may be verbal instruction or via modelling)
- behavioural rehearsal, i.e. practice makes perfect
- feedback (verbal, audiotaped, videotaped); positive reinforcement should always be given before any suggestions for change.

The first thing the therapist must do in communication skills training is to ask the couple to discuss something themselves and not to talk to the therapist. The therapist then looks for any 'destructive' communications, such as listed below, and makes interventions designed to reduce these:

- destructive criticism (e.g. 'You are fat and ugly')
- generalisation (e.g. 'You always behave so immaturely')
- mind reading (e.g. 'I know what you are thinking, so you don't need to say anything')
- bringing up the past (e.g. 'Just look at the way you behaved to me at Bob and Sally's wedding last year')
- putting oneself in the right and one's partner in the wrong (e.g. 'You make me so angry by what you say that I have no option but to go and smash up the kitchen')
- using logical argument as a weapon (e.g. 'I understand you are upset just now and it is likely to be due to the fact you are premenstrual')
- raising the voice or using other threatening body language
- using 'the sting in the tail' (e.g. 'That's really brilliant that you got the work promotion, you should be really pleased with yourself. I guess you will neglect us even more now').

Observing this list of destructive communications, it becomes immediately obvious that these are not just relevant to couples but have wider relevance in all human interactions, in both work and social life.

The new, more positive communication patterns which should be encouraged to replace these problem communications should aim to:

- express one's own feelings instead of imputing feelings in the other partner or using 'logical argument'
- use specific examples and stick to the point – do not bring up the past or generalise about matters
- avoid mindreading – allow the other person to express themselves; however well you may believe you know someone, you may find you are surprised if you just stop and listen
- take responsibility for own actions; other people cannot force you to behave badly, it is down to you
- avoid monologues; say what you need to say and then stop and listen to others
- examine non-verbal communication.

These rules may sound difficult to remember but are usually easy to spot in practice. Of course, all of us use poor communication skills at some time, but with some couples it is a persistent habit. The next case history (Case example 5.2) illustrates how faulty communication can ruin a marriage.

Case example 5.2: Communication skills training

The following argument was witnessed between Dawn and Monty, a married couple who were debating what colour to paint the kitchen:

Dawn: 'I would like it painted white, although you would think that was clinical and boring.' (*Mind reading*)

Monty: 'White wouldn't look too bad in the kitchen but I'm not happy painting it white after that accident you had when we were first married – you remember how you poured the strawberry jam down the wall! (*Bringing up the past*) You always are a messy person.' (*Generalisation*)

Dawn: 'Me, messy? What about you; you are always spilling things!' (*Not sticking to point; generalisation*)

Monty: 'Stop being so touchy, you always are at these times of the month.' (*Using 'logical' argument*)

Dawn: 'Oh, shut up, you self-opinionated idiot!' (*Abuse; raising of voice*)

In a case like this, any therapy would involve pointing out the errors, modelling appropriate responses with the couple, getting them to practise such responses and feedback on the progress.

Caring days

Most couples entering marital therapy do not care greatly for each other. However, Stuart (1980) has suggested that if they act 'as if' they do care the relationship can improve. The therapist uses the word 'care' rather than 'love' because the former does not have the same mythical and impenetrable qualities as the latter. It is also difficult to encourage people to love each other but perfectly possible to ask them to construct a list of ways each could care for the other. These behaviours must be:

- positive
- specific
- small behaviours occurring at least once daily
- not the subject of recent conflict.

The couple should try to select at least 18 care items, and then each partner makes a commitment to carry out at least five of the behaviours on the list each day. In this task, each person is asked to carry out the behaviour regardless of whether their partner has kept their side of the arrangement. The idea behind the caring days technique is that the couple can begin to reverse the often long-standing negative patterns of their relationship, without any apportionment of blame for what might have gone on in the past. Small changes brought about in this way can often be used as an introduction to more fundamental changes in behaviour that were addressed earlier in this chapter.

Integrative couple therapy

Early behavioural couple therapy concentrated on the therapist teaching new skills and then encouraging the couple to practise them. During the 1990s, integrative couple therapy (Christensen *et al*, 1995; Jacobson & Christensen, 1998) was devised, whereby the couple were encouraged to examine the personality characteristics of their partners.

This therapy combines all the previously discussed interventions but also looks at the basic dialectical dilemma of relationships. This is that the very traits in our partners which draw us to them and make us love them are the same traits that we can also hate. The first theory on which this is based is that most couples enter therapy in a state of confrontation with each other and thus the therapist needs to alter this to a state of empathy. As well as general marital therapy techniques, each of the couple are encouraged through discussion to understand and accept their partner's personality traits.

First, this is done by working with the therapist on a guiding formulation. This states that in a relationship the problem is not one person's fault. The couple need to identify a central theme and the characteristic interaction pattern. Once these have been identified, the therapist needs to point out how this may have become a 'trap'. The goal is to put things in a less adversarial context. A formulation can be created which emphasises emotions and attempts to make the person's behaviour understandable to the other partner.

As therapy progresses, this empathy can be developed using:

- *empathic joining* (this refers to the therapist encouraging each of the partners to express the emotions that they feel with each of their problems and to explain them to their partner; the therapist must ensure that this is done equally and that both partners are given equal attention)
- *unified detachment* (the therapist describes the problem in a detached way by referring to the problem as 'it' rather than 'what you do'; humour and even exaggeration can be used so that the couple understand the problem)
- *tolerance building* (this involves demonstrating the negative behaviour to the couple, even using role play and employing alternative strategies; the idea is to promote independence, self-reliance and alternative ways in which their needs could be met).

In our first case example, Ron was a powerful and ambitious man, whereas Mary was a caring and concerned woman. When they arrived for therapy, however, it was Ron's assertive and inconsiderate behaviour which Mary found difficult to cope with, even though she admitted to always being attracted to 'powerful men who know what they want'. Ron, on the other hand, admired Mary for her compassion and concern but was irate when this translated into her wishing to know where he was and what he was doing. The couple needed not only to adapt their behaviour but also to accept the limitations of each other and return to loving the very characteristics which were causing conflict.

More recently emphasis has also moved to the individuals in the relationship looking at their own self-regulation. This kind of approach allows work where one of the partners has a particular problem with regulating their behaviour, such as borderline personality disorder or substance misuse. In this approach there is encouragement for the individual to work on controlling their own reactions and emotions as well as looking at increasing the rewards in the marriage.

Treatment of sexual dysfunction

The treatment of sexual dysfunction developed from different origins than most other behavioural or cognitive treatment. In the time of Freud, sexual problems of any type were considered to be deep-seated neuroses which would take many years of individual psychoanalysis to rectify. Although there had been attempts to challenge this idea by several clinicians, it was the work of the American duo, W. H. Masters and V. E. Johnson which finally demonstrated that sexual problems could generally be treated quickly and effectively with sexual skills learning packages. In 1966, they published the first extensive scientific examination of the physiology of human sexuality (Masters & Johnston, 1966). This work was ground-breaking as it described a four-stage model of human sexual response and demonstrated the similarities in this response between men and women. This four-stage model of response is demonstrated in Table 5.1. and Figs 5.1 and 5.2.

Following on from their work on describing human sexuality, Masters & Johnson then published the work of a trial in which they successfully treated couples with sexual dysfunction using a time-limited behavioural approach (Masters & Johnson, 1970).

There were many criticisms of their work but the fact remains that it still forms a firm basis of treatment of sexual dysfunction to this day. The limitations of their work include that they advertised for couples

Table 5.1   Four stages of human sexual arousal

Stage	Female	Male	Comments
Arousal	• Increased blood flow to genital organs • Vaginal lubrication • Increased muscle tension	• Increased blood flow to genital organs • Erection of penis	• Failure can cause dyspareunia and lack of lubrication in women, erectile failure in men
Plateau	• High sexual tension • Retraction of shaft of clitoris behind the symphysis pubis	• High sexual tension	• Prolonged in female anorgasmia • Short in premature ejaculation and prolonged in delayed ejaculation
Orgasm	• Preceded by orgasmic inevitability • 5–15 pubococcygeus and general muscle spasms	• Preceded by ejaculatory inevitability	
Resolution	• Slower with age and parity • Slower if no orgasm	• Refractory period when no further sexual arousal can occur; with age increases in length dramatically	

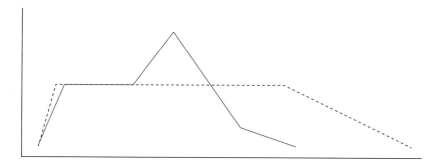

Fig. 5.1   Female sexual response.

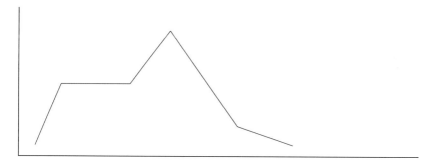

Fig. 5.2   Male sexual response.

with sexual problems in a magazine with a predominantly middle-class readership, thereby skewing their sample to the highly motivated and educated section of society. Second, the trial was conducted in a hotel in Florida, which undoubtedly produced a 'second honeymoon' atmosphere as well as further excluding those clients who were not extremely motivated as well as well-heeled. Finally, each of the couples worked on their problems for several hours each day, both with their therapists (two therapists worked with each couple) and on their own, a situation which would be impossible for most patients who attend a publicly funded health clinic.

Despite the criticism of the scientific merit of their treatment trial, Masters & Johnson produced dramatically successful results which were impossible to ignore. Thereafter, many workers were swept along with a wave of enthusiasm for this new treatment, which was then applied by many who knew little about the subject and many who believed it was a panacea. Inevitable disappointments followed, but now we know that these techniques can be modified to apply in less-controlled settings and can be used to help the majority of patients with sexual difficulties. It has also been shown that there is little advantage in using a co-therapist rather than a single therapist (Crowe *et al*, 1981). The basic treatment package consists of the following steps:

1   ban on sexual intercourse throughout treatment
2   education about sex, basic anatomy and physiology of sexuality, and exploring the couple's sexual vocabulary plus providing a vocabulary for future sessions
3   teach relaxation
4   non-genital sensate focus
5   genital sensate focus
6   penetration (initially without pelvic thrusting; this is generally performed in the female superior or lateral positions for most problems except for male retarded ejaculation)
7   use of different sexual positions and resumption or commencement of full sexual life.

These steps in treatment are demonstrated in the case history of Michael and Lorraine (Case example 5.3).

Case example 5.3: Treatment of low sexual drive

Michael and Lorraine were a 23-year-old couple who had been living together for 2 years when referred to the psychiatric clinic with a complaint that Lorraine had never enjoyed sex and would only tolerate Michael's advances to her approximately once every 2 months. This situation was intolerable to Michael, who felt rejected and unloved. Frequent arguments had ensued as Lorraine would refuse any physical contact with Michael, fearing it might lead to a sexual advance.

Initially, a full history was taken from each of them. Lorraine, who worked as a primary school teacher, had never had any previous sexual experience prior to living with Michael. She was the youngest of six children and had been raised in a happy and loving Roman Catholic family. From the age of 5 years, she had been sent to a convent girls' school. She had progressed well at this school and had ultimately gained good examination passes, enabling her to go on to teacher training college to take up her chosen career. She received no sexual education at home, and felt that her parents would have been far too embarrassed to discuss such matters with her. At school the only formal education was from a nun who explained in vague terms that women had to endure 'humiliation' in marriage to experience the joy of having children. Information from school friends had also hardly been enthusiastic and encouraging about sex. There had been a general belief that sex was a painful and frightening event for the woman, who would tolerate it purely for the sake of her partner. Elicit copies of D. H. Lawrence's *Lady Chatterley's Lover* and some 'soft porn' which had been smuggled into the school did little to dispel this myth and sex was still generally held to be something which men inflicted on women for their own pleasure.

Lorraine's menarche had commenced at age 12 years and had distressed her greatly as she had not been expecting it and she found it a frightening and embarrassing event. She had never masturbated as she believed this was 'sinful'. At teacher training college, Lorraine had met Michael and had started dating him. Their relationship had never been physically passionate, although after a year she had allowed him to touch her breasts, but they had not engaged in 'heavy petting' until they had started to live together. She had agreed to live with Michael when she left college but felt guilty about this decision, which her parents disapproved of, despite the fact that she no longer felt she was religious. When Michael made any sexual advance to her, she felt 'numb with fear' and wished to end it as soon as possible. She had never been orgasmic.

Michael was a teacher at a comprehensive school. He had been the only child of elderly parents, had had a happy childhood and had attended local state schools. Sex had been freely discussed in his household but he still believed that for successful sex the man was responsible for his own and his partner's pleasure. His first sexual experience had been at age 15 years with a girl of similar age that he met at school. This episode had not been enjoyable but he thereafter had several casual relationships which he had found satisfying. At age 20 years a girlfriend had commented that his penis was small and he had started to worry about this and whether he could thus satisfy any woman. He masturbated twice a week to heterosexual fantasies and had done so since the age of 14 years. He described his relationship with Lorraine as being good and close despite the sexual problems.

After the histories of Lorraine and Michael were taken, it was possible to make a formulation.

'Lorraine has always been brought up to believe that sex is an unpleasant experience for a woman. Therefore, whenever sexual advances are made to her, she expects it to be non-enjoyable and nasty. These thoughts lead her to feel anxious and tense, and so instead of being able to relax and enjoy sex, she is constantly preoccupied with her own catastrophic thoughts. This means that sex is never enjoyable to her, which strengthens her negative beliefs, and so the vicious circle becomes complete.

Michael has previously enjoyed sex, but recently has become overly concerned about his sexual performance and ability to satisfy a partner. This means that whenever he starts to make a sexual advance, he is constantly thinking and worrying about his own performance instead of relaxing and enjoying sex. As with Lorraine, these anxieties mean that sex is never fully satisfying and a vicious circle is again formed. Also, Lorraine's present inability to enjoy sex reinforces Michael's feelings of inadequacy.'

Both Lorraine and Michael agreed with this formulation. The therapist then explained to them that therapy would be structured to enable both of them to gradually learn to enjoy sex, and would be conducted at their own speed. The ban on intercourse was also explained and imposed. An arrangement to see them in a week was made.

Whereas in most couples presenting with sexual disorders full physical examination of both partners is necessary to exclude an organic cause for the problems (for further details of possible organic causes of sexual dysfunctions see Hawton, 1985 or Bancroft, 1983), in this case the factors seemed clearly psychological and they had both recently undergone full physical examinations.

In the second session, sexual education was commenced. This was started by using pictures of male and female genitalia and asking the couple to give their words for the different structures and functions with the therapist providing words for them when they could not think of any. These words were written down by the therapist so that words with which the couple were happy and familiar could be used throughout therapy. The therapist then discussed the function and physiology of the sexual organs and the mechanics of sexual intercourse. Care was taken to correct any faulty information believed by the

63

couple. For example, it was explained to Michael that the size of a man's penis had little to do with his ability to give sexual pleasure to his partner and that in any case, a relatively small penis tends to enlarge more during erection than a larger one. Michael's faulty belief that a man was solely responsible for his own and his partner's pleasure was also addressed, as was his idea that a man should always initiate sex. Lorraine's view of sex as something which women were 'subjected to' without personal enjoyment was also challenged.

Relaxation instructions were then given to them and a practice run of relaxation was performed by the therapist together with the couple.

For homework, they were asked to set aside 1 hour a day and to lie on the bed wearing comfortable clothing such as night clothes in a warm room with soft lighting and gentle background music and to practise relaxation. This was to encourage a hedonistic and relaxed view of their sexual activity. When they were both fully relaxed they were to read an educational book about sex. For this couple the classic book *The Joy of Sex* (Comfort & Quilliam, 2008) was suggested, as it provides no-nonsense sexual information in a sensitive manner with excellent illustrations. In addition, Lorraine was asked to read a book about women's sexuality on her own (Friday, 2002). Michael was reminded of the ban on sexual intercourse and told that if he felt very sexually aroused during the homework he was to masturbate. Lorraine expressed interest in this, and said that she would be happy for Michael to do this while lying next to her. The question of birth control was also raised with them and Lorraine admitted that this had always frightened her as she did not like to ask the family doctor, who had known her as a child. It was therefore recommended that they attend a local family planning clinic together to obtain information. It was agreed that as they had a large amount of homework, they should not meet the therapist again until 3 weeks later.

At the third session, Lorraine and Michael appeared much more at ease. First, their homework was reviewed with them. Whereas initially Lorraine had been tense and unable to relax, once she realised that she could trust Michael not to attempt sexual intercourse, she had relaxed and found the exercises pleasant and soothing. They had both found the books interesting and useful and Michael had started reading Lorraine's book. Lorraine had been interested in Michael's obvious pleasure during masturbation and asked if it were possible for her to do likewise. She, however, explained that she did not know how to masturbate. The therapist showed her a picture of female external genitalia which she could take home with her. It was suggested that she might then examine her own genitals using a hand mirror. Then, she could start to touch her genitals and to try to gently rub her clitoris and to insert her finger into her vagina. At all times she should monitor the sensation and continue whatever felt pleasant to her. As she felt unable to do this in front of Michael, it was suggested that she could do this after a warm bath, at a time when Michael would agree not to come into the bedroom, lying on the bed after she had performed the relaxation exercises.

The next stage in therapy was to introduce non-genital sensate focus. Michael and Lorraine were asked again to set aside some time every evening when they would not be interrupted by anyone or anything. They were asked to again lie on the bed wearing either no clothes or underwear only. Again the room should be warm, softly lit and with some pleasant background music. After their relaxation exercises, they were to each take turns in touching their partner's body and could do this anywhere except they were NOT to touch Lorraine's breasts or either of their genitals. This touching should be gentle, and could take the form of rubbing, stroking in circular movements or caressing, and could also be performed with the lips and tongue as well as the fingers and palms. The therapist then asked them to try out these movements with their hands on the back of their partner's hand. Once this was done satisfactorily, the therapist explained that a vital part of the exercise was that the partner who was being fondled should give verbal feedback as to what was pleasant, less pleasant and how they might prefer this to be done. Each of them was to take turns in being the active participant and the recipient. In other words, it was to be performed on a 'give to get' basis with open communication and feedback to practise discussing sensual and sexual matters freely. It was also suggested that, whereas these exercises could be performed with dry hands, they might also like to try using lotion. Baby oil, body creams and lotions or even lubricant jelly were all suitable for this purpose and the couple were encouraged to try these out and to find which was best for them.

As this is an extremely important step in treatment which should be performed correctly before moving on to the next stage, an appointment was then made to see them again in a week.

At the fourth session, the couple reported that they had progressed well. Both were enjoying the non-genital sensate focus and were learning more about what was exciting and pleasurable to their partners and themselves. Lorraine had been shy in giving feedback but this was gradually improving. The therapist praised them for their progress and urged them to continue with this exercise, which was agreeable to both.

Lorraine then asked if she could see the therapist on her own. Michael was happy with this and left the room. She then reported that she had successfully performed self-exploration of her genitals and found this enjoyable. However, she had stopped doing this when she felt that her excitement was increasing as she was not sure what might happen if she 'lost control'. The therapist asked her to think of the last time that this happened and to report what went through her mind at this time. Lorraine reported that she had thought: 'I may lose control and go out of my mind'. This thought had immediately caused her to stop the masturbation exercises.

Thus it appeared that Lorraine's negative automatic thought about losing control was severely interfering with her sexual pleasure. The therapist decided to use a cognitive approach (see Beck's cognitive model of depression in Chapter 8, pp. 119–125) to challenge these thoughts and said: 'Can you think of any evidence to support or refute this belief?'

After much consideration and discussion, Lorraine came up with the following evidence (the figure after each statement is a measure of her belief in each statement rated from 0%, untrue to 100%, absolutely certain).

Initial belief: 'I may lose control during sexual arousal and go out of my mind' (80%)

Evidence for:
- 'I feel strange, as if I may go mad' (20%)
- 'People in novels do sometimes go mad' (10%)
- 'My cousin had schizophrenia, therefore madness runs in the family' (15%).

Evidence against:
- 'Thousands of women have frequent orgasms and I have never heard of anyone going mad' (75%)
- 'My friend Elizabeth has a brother who has schizophrenia and is always talking about her sexual experiences' (65%)

- 'I have seen Michael have orgasms many times without any ill effect' (85%)
- 'I have got excited about many things and never gone mad' (20%).

At the end of this exercise, Lorraine rated her belief that she might lose control and go mad as less than 5%. She was, therefore willing to continue with the self-exploration programme. The therapist then raised with her whether or not she would be able to discuss her worries in front of Michael, but she felt this would be too embarrassing, and so Michael was brought back into the room and another appointment made for 1 week later.

When the couple arrived for the fifth session, they both looked cheerful. Lorraine immediately reported that she had masturbated on her own to orgasm. The non-genital sensate focus had progressed well and they had both enjoyed using body lotion in this. The next stage of genital sensate focus was therefore explained to them. It is useful for the therapist to be very explicit when explaining this stage as it is important to ensure that the couple understand the exercise and it can also serve as a model of talking about sexual experience without undue coyness. The therapist therefore said: 'The next stage of genital sensate focus is exactly the same as the previous exercise except that I now want you to include the genital and breast regions. Once again you should start with the relaxation exercises and then start to take turns in caressing your partner's body. You can then also include the breasts and genitals. The partner who is being touched should tell the other what is enjoyable or how they would prefer this to be done. You can also demonstrate this by guiding your partner's hands and demonstrating what gives you the most pleasure.

Michael, Lorraine will then guide you as to what feels best for her. You may like to start by caressing her breasts and nipples gently and may also use your lips and tongue. Then you could move to the outer and inner labia and try gently rubbing her clitoris and eventually try to insert your finger into her vagina if it is sufficiently slippery and lubricated. You may find that it is even more enjoyable for Lorraine if you gently use your lips and tongue. Lorraine can guide you in this and also the rhythm and amount of pressure which feels best to her.

Lorraine, you too should try caressing gently Michael's scrotum and penis. The top of the penis is particularly sensitive, so be careful to check that you do not press too hard there. You have watched Michael masturbate and so have a good idea of what pleases him but you may like to experiment with other movements and sensations. Again, Michael may find this even more exciting if you also use your lips and tongue.'

Michael and Lorraine felt happy with these instructions, although Lorraine was unsure as to whether she liked the idea of oral sex. It was explained that this was not mandatory, but that many couples found this extremely pleasant and that they may like to try it even if they decided against it later. A further appointment was made for 1 week later.

When the couple returned they said that they had been successful using the exercises. Michael had been orgasmic on each occasion but Lorraine had not been so yet. The therapist urged them to continue and explained that women were frequently slower to get aroused than men. For this reason it was particularly important that they made sure that the room was comfortable and relaxing, and that the relaxation and non-genital sensate focus exercises were performed first to ensure Lorraine had time to become aroused.

By the seventh session both reported that they had enjoyed several sessions of genital sensate focus, both reaching orgasm, and were keen to move on to the next stage. The idea of penetration was then introduced. The therapist said that it should be performed after all the previous steps in the exercises. This was to be carried out with Lorraine in the female superior position, so that Lorraine felt she had greater control. Once both of them felt happy with this, Michael could try some gentle pelvic thrusts, but should stop if Lorraine felt uncomfortable, and then try again when she felt content to continue.

After Lorraine and Michael successfully achieved enjoyable intercourse with Lorraine in the female superior position, a repertoire of sexual positions was suggested to introduce variety into their sex lives. Generally, they progressed extremely well. Lorraine was concerned as she found that she was not orgasmic during penetration, although she was during genital sensate focus. It was explained to her that a high percentage of women cannot reach orgasm without additional direct clitoral stimulation during penetration. Despite this fact, she could try by initially commencing penetration immediately prior to orgasmic inevitability and then gradually introducing penetration earlier in the arousal chain. This technique is known as the bridge manoeuvre (Kaplan, 1976).

The case history of Lorraine and Michael demonstrates how even fairly deep-seated sexual problems can be dealt with in as little as 10 sessions of therapist's time spread over 4 months. Although the basic package of treatment illustrated here can be used to treat many couples, some specific sexual problems require additional techniques (Table 5.2 and Case example 5.4).

Table 5.2 Additional techniques for specific sexual problems

Problem	Technique	Comments
Vaginismus	Individual treatment of woman may be necessary Possible use of 'vaginal dilators'	
Premature ejaculation	Either use (a) the stop–start technique (Semans, 1956) or (b) the squeeze technique	(a) before ejaculatory inevitability the man should signal and *all* stimulation must stop until excitement levels reduce
		(b) man squeezes the base of the corona of the penis before ejaculatory inevitability to reduce excitement
Erectile dysfunction	Waxing and waning (Friedman, 1968)	Stimulation occurs and then stops so that the couple learn that erections can be gained and lost and to reduce the pressure to use the erection immediately for fear of erectile failure

Case example 5.4: Vaginismus

Faith, a 22-year-old married woman, was referred to the clinic accompanied by her husband with a 2-year history of unconsummated marriage. She had been raised as an only child and had had little or no sexual education. She described herself as totally naive when she married Calvin, her 24-year-old husband. Further details of the history revealed that when Calvin attempted penetration, he felt a marked 'barrier' to his penis entering the vagina. These attempts also seemed to cause Faith distress and pain and so he had stopped, not wishing to hurt her. Faith also described a tense feeling in her inner thighs at these times. She had never used tampons for menstruation as, when she had tried, she had discovered the same hard ridge which prevented insertion.

The initial step in treatment was to ensure Faith had an appropriate physical examination from her GP, the local family planning clinic doctor or a gynaecologist. This examination must include the attempt at a vaginal examination.

Physical examination of Faith was normal but attempts at vaginal examination proved impossible. Having firmly established the diagnosis of vaginismus, the therapist then started by giving relaxation instructions and sex education as in the previous case of Lorraine and Michael. An appointment was then made to see Faith alone for the next session.

Traditionally, treatment of vaginismus using the partner from the outset has been described. Although this can be a very valid approach with some couples, better results can often be achieved with very anxious women if they are taught to control their own bodies first before introducing the partner. Of course, some women with vaginismus do present without a partner, having noticed the problem themselves or in previous relationships, and consequently need to be treated alone.

The first session with Faith alone was used to check that she had understood the sex education. Then she was asked to perform self-examination and self-exploration exercises at home using a hand mirror after she had had a warm bath and was relaxed and comfortable without fear of interruption. She was also given instructions in performing Kegel's exercises. These are contractions and relaxation of the pubococcygeus muscles. The easiest way to explain these to a patient is to ask them to stop mid-stream while passing urine. Once they can do this, they can try making the same movement when not passing water. If they make this movement slowly, they should be aware that they can contract these muscles to varying degrees. When the muscles are fully contracted, the muscles surrounding the anus are involved and these can be relaxed so that just the anterior muscles are contracting, which in turn can be fully relaxed. The purpose of these exercises in vaginismus is to increase the woman's awareness of the muscles involved in the problem and to establish some control over them.

At the second individual session, Faith reported some success with the Kegel exercises and self-examination, but had not done any self-exploration. She was asked to start self-exploration and to try to monitor pleasurable sensations, including trying to gently rub her clitoral region, and to continue anything which was pleasurable. When she was feeling completely relaxed and was enjoying the sensations of touching herself, she was asked to try to gently insert the tip of her finger into her vagina, using a lubricant jelly. While doing this she should try to perform some Kegel exercises a few times and monitor the effect on her vagina. Once she could do this, she was asked to gradually insert more and more of her finger and if she felt able before her next visit, to try with her ring finger and later, her middle finger.

When Faith arrived for her next appointment a week later, she reported that although she had managed to insert each of her fingers in turn, she was concerned that this was a 'filthy' thing to do. Further questioning revealed that she still believed that the top of her vagina was 'full of dirty slimy stuff like pus'. The therapist then explained again all about vaginal lubrication and normal female anatomy. As Faith seemed reassured by this explanation, the therapist asked her to continue with the exercises as previously but to try inserting two and then three fingers into her vagina. She was also asked to practise inserting the smallest size of tampon into her vagina and keeping it there for up to 2 hours (the smallest tampons are those labelled for light menstrual flow).

Three more sessions were needed with Faith alone, by which time she could happily insert three fingers into her vagina and also insert a medium tampon. Before this stage was reached, a joint session had been held with Calvin and Faith and they had been started on non-genital sensate focus.

Once Faith was happy with her ability to insert three fingers into her vagina, the couple were seen and given instructions for genital sensate focus. Faith was to demonstrate to Calvin how she was best aroused and how to gradually work up to the insertion of his smallest finger. At her own speed, they could move on to larger fingers and eventually more than one finger.

An encouraging sign happened after four weeks of genital sensate focus, when Faith reported that she had been orgasmic and that Calvin could insert three fingers without causing her pain or distress. The next stage was to move on to penile penetration without movement with Faith in the superior position. Once this was achieved, the therapist gave instructions for penetration plus gentle pelvic thrusts and thereafter, alternative sexual positions. The couple continued to progress well with therapy and to maintain their gains at follow-up.

In Case example 5.4, the therapist used gradual increasing size of fingers to build up Faith's self-confidence. Masters & Johnson (1970) recommended the use of 'vaginal dilators'. Clearly, this is a misnomer as they do not 'dilate' anything and so many people prefer to call them 'trainers'. These are glass or, more commonly, plastic rods of graduated diameter which can be inserted into the vagina, starting with the smallest. They do have some advantages including their smooth texture, which eases insertion, their clear, even graduation from one size to the next (unlike fingers), and their ability to remain in situ for long enough for the woman to get used to them. There are, however, disadvantages, including their 'clinical' nature reminding some patients of the doctor's surgery rather than an erotic experience, in addition to their expense. They mainly have a place, therefore, when the use of fingers fails.

The next example discussed is a story of a man with sexual problems following long-term drug misuse (Case example 5.5).

Case example 5.5: Treatment of retarded ejaculation

Raymond, a 30-year-old ex-drug addict, came to the psychiatric clinic owing to his concern that he could take up to one hour during sexual intercourse to reach orgasm. He had no regular girlfriend at the time of presentation but had found this problem extremely embarrassing in the past. He had not masturbated for 10 years, initially due to his reduced sexual interest while he had been using heroin and more recently because he feared that it would 'use up his sexual energy and make me even slower next time I have sex'.

His history was typical of many heroin users. He had enjoyed sex in his teens and had had no problems then. The first involvement with heroin had been at age 20 years at a party, but he had found that he soon began to use it regularly, losing his girlfriend, previous social life and job in the process. During the period of his addiction, he had lived rough and turned to petty crime and drug dealing to support his drug habit. At this time he had a girlfriend who was also a drug user. Sex had occurred infrequently due to the reduction of libido produced by heroin and when it had occurred, he had frequently taken up to an hour to reach orgasm.

Five years ago he had been treated for his drug addiction, and after a difficult 2 years, he had obtained a good steady job, non-drug using friends and a flat-share. He had a live-in girlfriend at this time who left him after 1 year. It was then that he noticed that he still had retarded ejaculation. Initially he thought this would improve with time, but he became increasingly worried when this failed to occur. For the past 2 years, he had avoided any sexual relationships for fear of embarrassment owing to his problem. He did not masturbate but frequently had spontaneous nocturnal emissions.

First, the therapist explained to Raymond how during his period of heroin misuse he had learned that it took him a long time to reach orgasm. Although delayed ejaculation is part of the pharmacological action of heroin, because this lesson was learnt, expectation and anticipatory failure led this to persist even after he had stopped using the drug. In the same way as he had learned retarded ejaculation, he could relearn normal ejaculation.

Next, the therapist discussed male sexual anatomy and physiology with him and generally talked about areas of sexual education.

During the second session, instructions in masturbation were given to Raymond. He was asked first to perform relaxation exercises and then to start gently stimulating himself. It was explained that a 'waxing and waning' approach, whereby periods of stimulation were interspersed with a period of stopping stimulation, was usually more arousing. Raymond was also asked to use erotic fantasies to aid his arousal and advised that, if he found them exciting, 'girlie' magazines might increase his arousal at this time.

In fact, Raymond proceeded very well with these instructions. To his surprise, he found that once he had relaxed and was in the mood for sexual excitement, he had an orgasm fairly rapidly. He realised that anxiety and anticipation of failure had caused his problem in the past. As there was little else that could be done at this time, Raymond was discharged, although asked to return for therapy if he needed to.

One year after Raymond had been last seen in the clinic, the therapist received a letter from him which stated that he was soon getting married, and that he had had no other problems since he had realised the role that anxiety played in his difficulties.

Finally, it must not be forgotten that although all the examples cited in this chapter have been of couples or individuals with heterosexual orientation, these techniques could be adapted to homosexual couples of either gender.

Suggested measures to use with conditions covered in this chapter

- Relationship satisfaction: The Golombok–Rust Inventory of Marital Satisfaction (Rust *et al*, 1990).
- Sexual satisfaction: The Golombok–Rust Inventory of Sexual Satisfaction (Rust & Golombok, 1985).

Key learning points

- There are many models of marital therapy but no one model has been shown to be superior to any other.
- There are three main types of behavioural intervention which can be used to help marital or family problems: behavioural exchange therapy, communication skills training and sexual skills training.
  - The principles underlying behavioural exchange therapy are rebalancing of the rewards and costs in the relationship.
  - Behavioural exchange therapy is based on definable tasks which are allocated to each of the partners and are performed on a reciprocal or 'give to get' basis.
  - In communication skills training, the therapist asks the partners to talk to each other to identify any faulty communication patterns.
  - The therapist issues instructions of required behaviour which may be a verbal instruction or via modelling. This is followed by behavioural rehearsal and feedback.
- New treatments such as integrative couple therapy have been developed in which the partners are encouraged to examine the personality characteristics of their partners. The therapy examines how the very traits in a partner which may have initially attracted them can sometimes be the traits which cause friction. Methods of coping with this are then developed.
- Treatment of sexual dysfunction in a couple can be combined with behavioural marital therapy.
- Human sexual response can be divided into four stages: excitement, plateau, orgasm and resolution.
  - Dysfunction may occur in any of the four stages of sexual response.
- The standard treatment for sexual dysfunction begins with a ban on sexual intercourse throughout treatment, followed by education about sex and the basic anatomy and physiology of sexuality, and exploration of the couple's sexual vocabulary as well as providing a vocabulary for future sessions.
- The basic stages of treatment for sexual dysfunction comprise: non-genital sensate focus; genital sensate focus; penetration; and penetration with movement. Penetration is initially without pelvic thrusting and performed in the female superior position; experimentation with different sexual positions then proceeds.
- The treatments can be applied to dysfunctions arising in homosexual as well as heterosexual couples.
- Additional techniques in sexual dysfunction may be needed for specific problems.
- Sexual dysfunction techniques may be used for an individual where no partner is available.

References

Azrin NH, Naster BJ, Jones R (1973) Reciprocity counselling: a rapid learning based procedure for marital counselling. *Behaviour Research and Therapy*, **11**: 365–82.

Bancroft J (1983) *Human Sexuality and its Problems*. Churchill Livingstone.

Christensen A, Jacobson NS, Babcock JC (1995) Integrative couple therapy. In *Clinical Handbook of Couple Therapy* (2nd edn): 31–64. Guilford Press.

Comfort A, Quilliam S (2008) *The Joy of Sex*. Crown Publishing Group.

Crowe MJ, Gillan P, Golombok S (1981) Form and content in the conjoint treatment of sexual dysfunction: a controlled study. *Behaviour Research and Therapy*, **19**: 47–54.

Friday N (2002) *My Secret Garden*. Quartet Books.

Friedman D (1968) The treatment of impotence by brietal relaxation therapy. *Behaviour Research and Therapy*, **6**: 257–61.

Hawton K (1985) *Sex Therapy: A Practical Guide*. Oxford University Press.

Jacobson NS, Christensen A (1998) *Acceptance and Change in Couple Therapy: A Therapist's Guide to Transforming Relationships*. Norton.

Jacobson NS, Gurman AS (1986) *Clinical Handbook of Marital Therapy*. Guilford Press.

Kaplan HS (1976) *The Illustrated Manual of Sex Therapy*. Souvenir Press.

Masters WH, Johnson VE (1966) *Human Sexual Response*. Churchill.

Masters WH, Johnson VE (1970) *Human Sexual Inadequacy*. Churchill.

Rust J, Golombok S (1985) The Golombok–Rust Inventory of Sexual Satisfaction (GRISS). *British Journal of Clinical Psychology*, **24**: 63–4.

Rust J, Bennun I, Golombok S (1990) The GRIMS: a psychometric instrument for the assessment of marital discord. *Journal of Family Therapy*, **12**: 45–57.

Semans JM (1956) Premature ejaculation: a new approach. *Southern Medical Journal*, **49**: 353–7.

Stuart RB (1969) Operant-interpersonal treatment for marital discord. *Journal of Consulting and Clinical Psychology*, **33**: 675–82.

Stuart RB (1973) *Premarital Counselling Inventory*. Research Press.

Stuart RB (1980) *Helping Couples Change*. Guilford Press.

Wesley S, Waring EM (1996) A critical review of marital therapy outcome research. *Canadian Journal of Psychiatry*, **41**: 421–8.

Further reading

Gurman AS (2008) *Clinical Handbook of Couple Therapy* (4th edn). Guilford Press.

Jacobsen N, Christensen A (2000) *Reconcilable Differences*. Guilford Press.

Leiblum SR (2007) *Principles and Practice of Sex Therapy* (4th edn). Guilford Press.

Phobic and social anxiety

Overview

This chapter will give a full description of the exposure principle and habituation. Case histories of treatment using graded exposure (both therapist-assisted and self-exposure) will be presented. Comparison will be made between phobic anxiety and social anxiety disorder. There will be an examination of the role of safety signals in the maintenance and treatment of agoraphobia and social anxiety. The role of cognitive therapies in social anxiety disorder will be discussed. Finally, there will be a brief look at third generation CBT treatments of mindfulness and acceptance and commitment therapy for social anxiety disorder.

In DSM-5 (American Psychiatric Association, 2013) anxiety disorders are included under the heading of mood disorders. This is because of the noted interlinkages of anxiety and depression (Clark & Watson, 2006). Whereas in DSM-IV-TR (American Psychiatric Association, 2000) panic disorder was linked with agoraphobia, it is now recognised that some patients have symptoms of agoraphobia without panic. The two disorders are now separated in DSM-5 and both agoraphobia and panic disorder can be separately recorded.

Fear is a universal and essential emotion. Without it the human race would have fallen over cliffs and failed to run from sabre-tooth tigers until we became extinct. However, not all fear is rational and based on a threat to survival. People differ in the background level of fear (trait anxiety) and the situations which provoke fear (state anxiety). All of us have some morbid fears which we know to be irrational but which we cannot stop. These fears may be embarrassing but they do not lead us to change our lifestyle in any major way. They can be seen as on a continuum with phobic disorder.

Phobias have been defined as morbid fears which are involuntary, cannot be reasoned away and lead to avoidance of the feared object or situation (Marks, 1969). Clearly, they do overlap with morbid fears. Most patients with phobic disorder, however, have made multiple adjustments to their

Table 6.1 Types and characteristics of phobic disorder and social anxiety

Disorder	Prevalence	Onset	Gender incidence	Description	Comments
Agoraphobia	One of the most common and most handicapping phobias in psychiatric practice	Early adult life	Females more frequently affected than males	Fear of crowded places, travelling by public transport, supermarkets, enclosed spaces	Can present with or without panic disorder
Specific animal phobia	Rarely seen in psychiatric practice and more likely by GPs (or person will try self-help)	Early childhood, usually before age 7	More common in adult women but equal gender incidence in childhood	Dogs, cats, spiders, insects, etc.	Specific to the animal
Miscellaneous specific phobia	May present in variety of ways	Varies	Overall equal	Heights, enclosed places, flying, thunder, etc.	
Blood and injury phobia	Possibly more common than ever recorded as these patients tend to avoid all clinical situations	Often starts in adolescence and may improve with onset of middle age	Equal	Medical or dental procedures, blood	Parasympathetically mediated fainting response rather than sympathetically mediated fight, flight or freeze reaction
Social anxiety disorder	Previously categorised as social phobia, this condition is second only to agoraphobia in its prevalence in mental health clinics	Adolescence	Equal	Can be generally fearful of all social situations or specific, e.g. eating, drinking, blushing, vomiting	Psychological therapy will vary depending on whether the disorder is general or specific Extensively studied from the psychopharmacological standpoint

GP, general practitioner.

lifestyle to avoid the phobic stimulus. For example, a patient with spider phobia was so fearful of even hearing the word 'spider' that they had left a well-paid job and avoided all parties.

A useful working definition of the most commonly seen types of phobic disorder is given in Table 6.1.

Social anxiety disorder (social phobia) has often been separated from the other types of phobic disorder as it is the one which has been most extensively studied in terms of its psychopharmacology and also in terms of cognitive therapy in recent years. It is a chronic, disabling disorder characterised by the fear of negative evaluation by other people in social or performance situations. Unlike other phobic anxiety disorders, there is good evidence that CBT produces better results in the treatment of social anxiety (Ougrin, 2011).

Avoidance model of phobic anxiety, exposure principle and habituation model

If an individual is fearful of dogs, then the sight of a dog in the distance will cause them anxiety. High anxiety is unpleasant and the person will normally try to escape the dog and run away. Once the dog is out of sight, anxiety will reduce. This reduction in anxiety is like a reward and thus reinforces the escape behaviour and, in turn, any behaviour which is rewarded tends to be repeated. Thus the escape and avoidance worsen the phobic anxiety. In reality people do not tend to repeatedly escape and be rewarded but tend to focus on avoidance of cues which cause anxiety. This is demonstrated in Fig. 6.1.

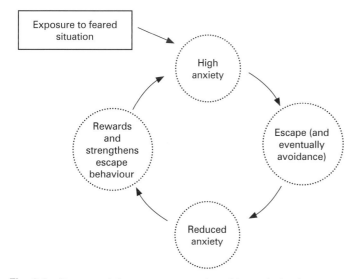

Fig. 6.1 Escape reinforces escape and avoidance behaviour.

Treatment therefore involves asking the person to remain in feared situations until the anxiety reduces. This reduction in anxiety takes approximately 1 hour in the first instance and is called habituation. This is shown in Fig 6.2.

It can be seen that anxiety reduces within an exposure session, and if the session is repeated regularly, the anxiety will tend to be less severe and last for a shorter period over time (habituation between sessions).

This observation that reliable methods of reducing fear involved exposure to the feared situation led to the development of the exposure principle as the rationale for the success of behavioural treatments for phobic and also obsessive–compulsive disorders (Marks, 1973). This development concentrated research and clinical treatment on the important variables of the exposure and elimination of redundant components, such as relaxation.

The most effective exposure has been shown to be:

- prolonged rather than of short duration (Stern & Marks, 1973)
- real-life rather than fantasy exposure (Emmelkamp & Wessels, 1975)
- regularly practised with self-exposure homework tasks (McDonald *et al*, 1978).

Although the flooding *v.* desensitisation debate has now sunk into oblivion, there is still concern and confusion in clinical practice about the optimal pace of exposure programmes. Taking a highly anxious patient who has not been out of the house for the past 20 years on a train may be effective in dealing with their agoraphobia, but any therapist who adopts such tactics is likely to have a high dropout and low adherence rate. Also, painstakingly working through a very structured hierarchy with a patient experiencing little or no anxiety at each step is likely to lead to boredom and despondency in the therapist and frustration in the patient, who sees little improvement after many hours of treatment. It makes sense to tailor the speed of treatment to the needs of individual patients. Some patients

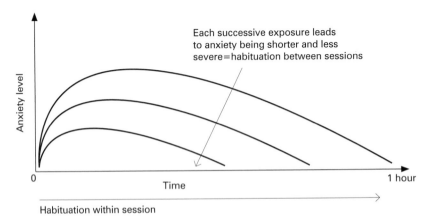

Fig. 6.2 Habituation.

are highly anxious and need hours of exposure before they arrive at their treatment goals, whereas others may need little more than having the rationale of exposure explained to enable them to tackle their most feared situations. Let us now turn to a story of a young woman with agoraphobia and anxiety (Case example 6.1).

Case example 6.1: Treatment of agoraphobia with graduated exposure

June, a 22-year-old married lady, was brought to the clinic by her husband. They had married 1 year previously and since that time June had been unable to go to work owing to her fear of travelling alone. Her husband, a security man, needed to work shifts and was often out all night. On these occasions June would ask her elder, unmarried sister to sleep in the house with her. Once, when her husband had been called out unexpectedly at night, June had a panic attack and had called her GP as she believed she was going to die. Following this episode, the couple had been referred to the local psychiatric services, where they had received marital counselling which they felt to have been unhelpful.

First, a full history of the problem was obtained. It was found that June, the youngest of a family of two girls and three boys, had always been an anxious and shy person. At the age of 14 years and when recovering from influenza, she had fainted during morning assembly at school. Following this, she had been unwilling to return to school. After a week at home, she had eventually been persuaded to return, on condition that her elder sister accompanied her to the gates and met up with her at break and lunch times. Thereafter she was always accompanied on the journey to and from school until she left at the age of 16.

After leaving school she had started work as a typist in an insurance office. This office was close to where her sister worked and so she always walked to work with her. She avoided travelling on buses or trains for fear that she might faint. Immediately prior to her marriage, she had passed her driving test, but was unable to drive unaccompanied as she feared fainting at the wheel.

She married her childhood sweetheart at the age of 21. Her husband, Barry, was understanding but believed her anxiety problems would improve once she was settled in her own home. They had moved into their flat following the wedding. The flat was 5 miles away from June's family home and to get to work she would have to catch either a bus or a train. She had attempted to get to work on the first day after moving, but had panicked at the bus stop and returned home. Since that time she had remained off work.

After the history was obtained, a working hypothesis for the origin and maintenance of June's symptoms was established. The therapist explained:

'Although you have always been a shy and nervous person, it seems that your problems really began after you had fainted at school. This was an unpleasant experience, which you learned to associate with being away from your family. Following this episode, you avoided going anywhere alone, and this strengthened the belief. You never allowed yourself to discover whether or not you could be alone without fainting.

Currently, whenever you are in danger of being alone, you take precautions to prevent this. When you went to the bus stop to go to work, you were tense because of your expectation that something dreadful might happen. Owing to your tense state, you began to notice the physical symptoms of your anxiety, for example your heart pounding, and believed that this was evidence that something terrible was about to happen and you might die.'

It was next necessary to educate June and Barry about anxiety. First, the possible physical and emotional symptoms of anxiety were explained to them. Then it was described how avoidance of feared situations led to further avoidance, and this was illustrated with a diagram (Fig. 6.3).

Second, it was explained that during exposure to fear-provoking situations, anxiety does eventually reduce, even though this may take up to an hour. This was illustrated to June by using a diagram similar to Fig. 6.2. Third, they were reassured that if this exposure exercise is practised regularly, the anxiety experienced gradually reduces in both intensity and duration. To help them remember all this information it was summarised as 'three golden rules' for exposure treatment:

- *anxiety is unpleasant but it does no harm* i.e. I will not die, go mad or lose control
- *anxiety does eventually reduce,* i.e. it cannot continue indefinitely if I continue to face up to the situation
- *practice makes perfect* i.e. the more I repeat a particular exposure exercise, the easier it becomes.

Following this explanation of the rationale of exposure treatment, it was necessary to identify the targets of treatment with the patient herself. June chose five specific tasks which she would like to be able to perform by the end of treatment and which would demonstrate to both herself and her therapist that she had improved:

- to drive alone on the motorway to visit an old school friend in a nearby town
- to travel to work alone on the bus during the rush hour
- to travel to work alone on the train during the rush hour
- to travel alone by bus and underground train into the city centre and to visit the main shopping areas
- to remain in the flat alone overnight while Barry is on a night shift.

June decided that it would be easiest for her to start by tackling her problem of walking alone. Barry agreed to be involved in the treatment and to act as her co-therapist. As there was insufficient time at this first meeting for any therapist-aided exposure, June and Barry agreed to start the programme during the week. Every evening, when Barry returned from work, they were to go out for a walk. June was to leave first and to travel along a predetermined

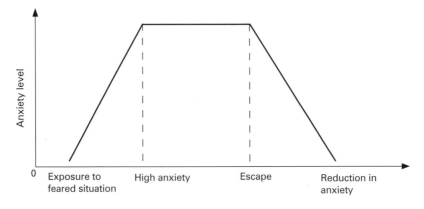

Fig. 6.3 Reduction in anxiety rewards escape behaviour.

route, while Barry was to wait for 5 min and then follow in her footsteps. They were to take care that the exposure time was long enough for June's anxiety to reduce (habituation), which usually takes approximately an hour. June was to record the details of the exposure exercises in a diary, and to also note down her anxiety levels at the beginning, middle and towards the end of the exposure task. To introduce some consistency into the anxiety ratings, she was asked to record the level of anxiety using a 0–8 scale where 0 meant no anxiety and 8 extreme anxiety or panic (see Fig. 2.6, p. 18). If June found her anxiety levels reducing during the week, she was to go out for a long walk alone, while Barry remained in the house.

At the second session the following week, June and Barry were delighted with the progress. June had managed not only to walk alone, but had even visited the local shops and carried out some shopping while Barry remained at home. The therapist praised her for this excellent progress. It was suggested to June that, with her consent, the session could be used to start tackling bus travel. At first, June asked if Barry could sit next to her, but she eventually agreed to sit at the front of the bus, while Barry and the therapist sat at the back. After a few minutes, June became very anxious and came to the therapist complaining of symptoms of panic. She was gently reminded that this feeling, although unpleasant, would eventually pass, whereas if she gave up now, her anxiety might be even worse next time. She returned to her seat and after a further 45 min looked much more relaxed and cheerful. At the prearranged stop all three left the bus. June was praised by the therapist who said: 'You have done extremely well. Despite feeling panicky you have managed to face up to your fear, and have learned that these frightening and nasty symptoms do eventually reduce.'

Following the praise from both the therapist and her husband, June expressed her feeling of delight with her achievement and requested that she might go alone into a nearby supermarket and buy some shopping while Barry and the therapist remained outside. She was again praised for this decision, and succeeded in buying a basket of groceries despite the crowds in the store.

On the return journey, June sat alone upstairs on the bus while her husband and the therapist sat downstairs. Again, she coped excellently and readily agreed to continue this practice with Barry during the following week. She was to try to tackle bus travel alone while Barry remained at home. It was explained to her that this may be easier if they initially went out in the car together and then Barry left her to come home. This is because it is usually easier for people with agoraphobia to approach home or another 'safe' place than it is to travel away from 'safety'. Once this is overcome, it is usually possible to move on to travelling away from home as well as towards it.

For the third session, it was arranged that the therapist would meet June alone outside an underground station. Barry was at work and unable to attend that week. June travelled to the station alone on a bus. During this session exposure to underground travel was performed in a similar way to the session with bus travel. The fourth and fifth sessions were given at the out-patient clinic. June and Barry gradually increased the homework exposure, so that June practised travelling alone to her place of work by bus and train, and was able to return to work before the end of the fifth week. She also travelled up to the city alone when Barry was at work. During this time, June began working on her fear of remaining alone in the house overnight. Initially, she stayed alone in the house during the day and evening, and then progressed to remaining alone overnight when she knew that her sister was at home. She was pleased and surprised with herself when she did not feel the need to telephone her sister, and felt able to try being alone without taking these precautions. Throughout this time the therapist monitored her progress, praised her for her success and suggested tasks which she should attempt.

By session six, most of the treatment targets had been achieved, however driving alone had proved more difficult. Barry was concerned that she might become very anxious when driving and 'do something silly', and so had been unwilling to encourage her to practise driving. As June found it easier to drive on quiet roads, the therapist and Barry sat in the car while June drove from the clinic into the country. Again, she found this easier than she had anticipated and agreed that after 45 minutes of driving, she would stop at a station and leave the therapist and Barry to catch a train while she drove herself back to the clinic. This demonstration proved to both June and Barry that she was able to drive sensibly and safely. Following this session, June continued to practise driving over the next 3 weeks. Initially, she continued on quiet roads, and then on increasingly busy roads in town. Driving in lines of traffic when she was in the right-hand lane and felt unable to 'escape' was particularly difficult for her, and so she devised some routes which involved doing this. Her confidence increased as she practised, and she began travelling on motorways. Once again, she began by driving on motorways at relatively quiet 'off-peak' times and then progressed to busier times.

Session seven was used to reiterate the principles of treatment, which June had successfully learned and applied. She had achieved all her targets of treatment. The therapist warned her that she would still need to continue practising over the following months. Everyone has good and bad days, weeks or months and the important thing would be for June to continue to face up to difficult situations even during the 'bad' times when she felt more anxious. Any periods of illness which restricted her activities might well lead to a slight increase in fear when she returned to normal. Finally, she was congratulated for all her success and hard work. Arrangements were made for her to be reviewed at 1, 3, 6 and 12 months to ensure that her gains were maintained.

June's case demonstrates how a young woman with a moderately severe phobia was treated with the help of her husband and 14 hours of therapist's time over a 7-week period. Some patients, however, may require more or less time and not every patient has a helpful and willing spouse, relative or friend who will act as co-therapist. Indeed, most patients with mild to moderate phobic anxiety can be treated using self-exposure. Such self-exposure methods will be discussed later in the chapter and may include self-help books, therapist instruction or computer programs. However, no therapist should attempt to give self-exposure instructions until they have witnessed first-hand exposure in real life. Helping and witnessing a patient in extreme anxiety is a powerful learning tool and will help a therapist to problem-solve treatment with the patient (Case example 6.2).

Case example 6.2: Flight phobia

Adrian was a 27-year-old unmarried civil engineer. He worked for a large successful firm. Recently he had been promoted at work and was asked to take responsibility for a job the firm was to undertake abroad. This required him to make frequent trips abroad for meetings with the clients. Adrian had a 4-year history of fear of travelling by plane. He had so far managed to keep his fear secret by arranging meetings for Monday mornings and then travelling to the city by boat and train on Sunday. However, he realised that he would not be able to maintain his pretence for long without being discovered. His concern was that if his problem were known at work, his future career might be jeopardised as his bosses would think him 'a nervous wreck'.

The onset of Adrian's problem had occurred 4 years ago, when he was returning to England from a holiday in India. The flight had been particularly turbulent, and he had suddenly remembered some details of a similar aircraft being involved in a crash a few months previously. He had felt anxious and nauseous throughout the remainder of the flight. Since that time, he had felt unable to travel anywhere by plane unless he took diazepam (prescribed by his GP) and alcohol until he had almost total amnesia for the journey. Whereas he had managed to travel in this state in the company of relatives or friends to go on holiday, he realised that he could not do this if travelling to attend a business meeting.

After the history was obtained and he was given the rationale of exposure treatment, Adrian agreed to start a programme of self-exposure by visiting the airport every evening and remaining there to watch aircraft take off and land and the passengers checking in their luggage. He was asked to imagine that he was actually about to travel while at the airport and to remain there until his anxiety subsided. It was explained that taking alcohol or tranquillising tablets were forms of avoidance, and so although initially reducing anxiety, in the longer term they strengthened and increased his fear.

Ten days after this initial assessment, the therapist received a call from Adrian who was at the airport. He reported that he had initially felt extremely anxious and nauseous when visiting the airport, but that this had improved as he continued to practise. While there he had noticed that he could obtain a cheap flight abroad and return the same day and wondered if the therapist would be willing to accompany him on such a flight. The therapist agreed, and a mutually acceptable date was arranged so that Adrian could book the seats.

On the day the flight was arranged, the therapist met Adrian at the airport. He appeared anxious and rated his anxiety as 6 on a 9-point scale. Previously, he said that he would have gone immediately to the bar 'to settle his nerves' when he felt anxious, but managed to remain in the queue to check in on the flight, and then accompanied the therapist to the departure lounge. The trip involved just over 1 hour's flying time, which when considered with the delays and return journey, would allow sufficient time for Adrian's anxiety to reduce.

When the flight was called, Adrian developed symptoms of panic. He appeared flushed, sweaty and tremulous. He said that he felt he had made a mistake and that he wished to leave the airport, return home and continue practising the visits to the airport before attempting to fly. The therapist responded by pointing out: 'I can see that you are extremely anxious and realise how unpleasant that must be. However, if you go home now, it will be much more difficult for you the next time you try. Although you feel very anxious now, you will remember that the first time you came to the airport you were also quite panicky. No matter how dreadful you feel now, that feeling will pass as long as you continue.'

Following this, Adrian stood still and did not appear to be about to run from the lounge. The therapist noticed that he was breathing very rapidly and felt that this hyperventilation was likely to be contributing to Adrian's discomfort. Instructions for taking slow deep breaths were given to him in this way: 'I see that you are breathing very rapidly and shallowly. This kind of breathing often makes people feel much worse and adds to their symptoms.

What I would like you to do with me now is to place your hand on your abdomen. You should be able to feel it moving in and out if you are breathing correctly using your diaphragm. Now, drop your shoulders down and try to relax them and keep them still – you do not need to use your shoulders if you are breathing correctly. Good, you have done that well. I am now going to count slowly to 5 several times. I want you to breathe in slowly and feel your stomach push out for the first count to 5. Then, I would like you to hold your breath for the next count to 5 and last to breathe out slowly and regularly for the final count to 5. We will then repeat this a few times until you can do it on your own.'

After a few trials, Adrian had slowed his breathing and reported that he was feeling a little better. By this time there was an announcement for the remaining passengers to board the aircraft immediately. Adrian agreed to continue and boarded the plane. The flight was moderately turbulent throughout. Adrian reported that he was tempted to have a drink when the air hostess arrived with the bar, but realised that this would worsen his problem. Despite this, he appeared much less anxious by the time they landed.

On the return flight, Adrian was much more confident. He asked if he could change seats with the therapist to sit next to the window and look at the clouds and the view. At the time of landing in London, he reported that he was enjoying the flight. Following this therapist-aided session, Adrian arranged to fly for a business meeting. At 6-month post-treatment follow-up, he was flying regularly to Europe and had recently booked a holiday in California. He reported that he still found it helpful to avoid alcohol prior to or during a flight as he felt that any feeling of 'light-headedness' increased his anxiety.

Adrian's success illustrates how even one session of therapist-aided exposure can effect a significant and lasting change in phobic anxiety. Not all phobias are dealt with so easily and quickly, however. A more severely disabling phobia which took several months to treat is illustrated in the next vignette (Case example 6.3).

Case example 6.3: Severe blood and injury phobia

Gwen, a 35-year-old married woman, was referred to the clinic owing to her extreme fear of any medical or dental procedures. For years she had avoided any contact with the medical profession, but recently had forced herself to attend her GP because of marked and sudden abdominal swelling. She had been referred to the local hospital and had only been able to attend there after taking 40 mg of diazepam to lower her anxiety. A large ovarian cyst was diagnosed and her gynaecologist advised that a laparotomy operation was needed. Gwen felt unable to consent to this, and had refused to attend the hospital or her GP again. Indeed, she was reluctant to come to a psychiatric clinic and would only attend when reassured that the building was separate from the general hospital and that there would be no medical equipment in the room.

The onset of her fear was at the age of 14 when she had been required to give a blood sample following a routine medical examination in school. She felt anxious, nauseous and light-headed. The medical officer had not been sympathetic and had gruffly told her to 'pull herself together'. The nurse had then held tightly on to her arm to prevent her from moving. The blood sample

Table 6.2 Example of therapist-aided exposure in the clinic

Session	Details of clinic exposure	Length of exposure (hours)	Homework for next session (tasks repeated 3 times per day)
1	• In hospital environment until anxiety reduces • Looked at pictures of medical procedures	2	• Visit hospital waiting rooms, GP surgery waiting room, hospital ward, A&E department, look at medical pictures
2	• Applied tourniquet and sphygmomanometer to therapist's, husband's and own arm • Used alcohol swab on arm	1.5	• Apply tourniquet and alcohol swabs to own arm 3 times/day
3	• Examine and handle a variety of needles and syringes	1.5	• Handle needles • Inject an orange
4	• Watched therapist and husband have subcutaneous injections • Had injection herself	2.5	• Visit GP and receive inoculations as required • Commence course of dental treatment
5, 6	• Watched husband and therapist have phlebotomy performed	1	• Watch video of therapist undergoing phlebotomy (3 times/day)
7, 8	• Had blood sample taken	1.5	• Visit GP and have blood sample taken
9	• Watched therapist and husband donate blood and then donated blood herself	2	• Continue watching video and applying tourniquet to arm
10	• Visited gynaecology ward; met nursing and medical staff and discussed planned surgical procedure	3	• Admission to hospital for laparoscopy

A&E, accident and emergency; GP, general practitioner.

had been taken, but Gwen had fainted immediately after the procedure. From that time, she had felt faint whenever visiting her GP or a hospital. This had deteriorated over the years until she avoided these situations. She had painful dental carries as she had avoided attending the dentist for the past 10 years.

The assessment interview was complicated by Gwen's extreme fear. She frequently retched and complained of feeling faint. Much of the interview was performed with Gwen clutching a sick bowl lying flat on the examination couch. Luckily, her husband was able to supply many of the details for her.

As with the previous cases, Gwen and her husband were educated about anxiety and exposure. In addition, it was necessary to explain to them that phobias of blood, injury and medical interventions were often different to other phobias because as well as the anxiety reaction (predominantly mediated by the sympathetic component of the autonomic nervous system), there was additionally a fainting reaction (mediated by the parasympathetic component of the autonomic nervous system), which meant that exposure therapy would be performed with Gwen lying flat at first. Another useful technique for such patients is to teach them applied muscle tension, which involves the patient contracting their calf muscles and their biceps when feeling faint to raise the blood pressure.

As Gwen progressed with exposure and her physiological responses reduced, she would be gradually raised into an upright position. Because Gwen was extremely anxious, it was important to emphasise that nothing would be done without her prior consent, and that the therapist and her husband would not try to trick her in any way. Her husband agreed to act as co-therapist.

Gwen's main target was to undergo the necessary laparotomy operation, but her intermediate targets were:

- to have my blood pressure taken
- to visit a hospital ward and remain there for several hours without fainting
- to have an injection
- to have a blood sample taken
- to give a pint of blood at the blood transfusion centre.

The details of Gwen's exposure programme and her homework practice are shown in Table 6.2.

This case shows how exposure can sometimes be a slow process with a highly anxious person, but that ultimately success can be achieved. In these cases, it is important to obtain objective measures of anxiety and goals of treatment. Otherwise, the slow but sure progress may have been overlooked by both patient and therapist, who might have abandoned treatment in the belief it was unsuccessful.

The use of therapist modelling

Modelling is a procedure often used to facilitate exposure therapy. The therapist models an activity that the patient is afraid to perform and asks the patient then to follow suit (Bandura, 1969). This procedure was combined with exposure in the treatment of the patients presented in this chapter, but is illustrated in a more obvious way in the treatment of dog phobia (Case example 6.4).

Case example 6.4: Dog phobia

Lauren, an 18-year-old student teacher, since childhood had avoided situations where she might come into contact with dogs. The family protected her in this way and someone always had to check the garden at her home to ensure that no dogs had strayed in before she went there. She had to cross the road to avoid dogs and never went into public parks for the same reason. Her mother told her that, at the age of 2, she had been frightened by a large dog jumping onto her pushchair. Although family members had told her about this, Lauren had no recollection of it.

The first session was spent gaining a full history from Lauren and creating a formulation. It was explained to her that by avoiding and escaping from situations where she might come into contact with dogs, she was exacerbating her anxiety. Lauren realised she could not go through life with her family checking for her all the time. She had tried to help herself and after researching what treatments might be helpful to her had read about graded exposure. Therefore, she had recently been looking at a book of dog breeds and trying to find out more about the characteristics of different breeds. Initially she had found just looking at pictures was very anxiety-provoking but had persisted. After this, she had managed to watch TV programmes which featured dogs and had ended up being fascinated by sheepdogs.

After a full discussion and agreeing a hierarchy of feared situations with the therapist, Lauren decided that the first treatment session should be being in the room with a small dog but that the dog would always be on the other side of the room and would remain on a leash. When she entered the room, Lauren was visibly shaking and tearful, but she persisted and remained in the room. After speaking with the owner, the therapist sat close to the dog and petted and stroked it. Lauren was encouraged to watch this and not to avoid looking at the dog. The therapist talked to Lauren as well as the dog and the owner throughout the session. After 20 min Lauren agreed that she might be able to approach the dog. She was given instructions as to what the dog liked and was able to imitate the therapist's stroking action along the dog's back. In the first session, she could not be persuaded to touch the head of the dog and was insistent that it remained on a leash.

At the end of the session, Lauren was delighted with her progress. She was given the homework task of learning more about dog behaviour. This is because people who are very anxious with dogs are often at risk of being bitten as the anxiety is sensed by the dog and this in turn makes the dog anxious and less predictable in its behaviour. She also agreed to visit a local animal shelter and talk to the staff there.

At the next session, Lauren was very pleased with her progress. She had talked to the volunteers and staff at the animal shelter and had walked near to dogs that were being walked on leads. Although she had not had any direct contact with any of the dogs, she was delighted that she had been able to remain in the vicinity with little anxiety.

There then followed four more therapist-aided exposure sessions. The therapist modelled and demonstrated to Lauren the best way to approach and handle a dog. This was confirmed by Lauren's experience at the animal shelter. The therapist showed how the dog may 'play bite' where it would pick up the therapist's hand in its mouth without causing any harm or pain to the therapist. Eventually, Lauren was able to touch the dog even when it was off the lead. She also continued to visit the animal sanctuary and was working with the cats there. Although working with cats, this still meant she was in the proximity of dogs. Lauren expressed that she would not wish to own a dog but that she did not wish to see one harmed in any way and that, although cautious, she could admire some of their characteristics.

Social anxiety disorder or social phobia

Social anxiety disorder (social phobia) is often confused with agoraphobia or generalised anxiety disorder. Panic attacks can occur in all of these syndromes. Identifying the reason behind the fear (i.e. fear of social interaction rather than fear of anxiety symptoms) will help the clinician differentiate. In the case of social anxiety disorder, the person experiences intense, excessive or unreasonable and distressing social anxiety, leading to avoidance of social situations. To distinguish social anxiety disorder from agoraphobia, it can be helpful to obtain very thorough descriptions of the fear. For example, if someone is fearful of visiting shops, this could be part of an agoraphobic syndrome, a generalised anxiety or a social phobia. In social anxiety the person will tend to be more fearful of small shops, where social interaction is more likely to occur, than the large impersonal supermarkets often feared by the patient with agoraphobia. A patient with social anxiety disorder may also experience anxiety in the supermarket queue, owing to fear of talking to the checkout clerk, whereas a patient with agoraphobia may fear feeling trapped in the queue.

Social anxiety disorder is the preferred name (rather than social phobia) and the disorder is listed in DSM-5 (American Psychiatric Association, 2013) under the category of anxiety disorders. This change in nomenclature was made after a group of US psychiatrists campaigned, believing that the name social phobia trivialised the condition. This appears to be due to a lack of understanding of how handicapping a true phobia can be! There has been some criticism of DSM-5, mostly in the UK media, for expanding the definition of social anxiety disorder too far and incorporating a range of normal 'shyness'. What the critics seem to fail to understand is that, like most conditions, these traits exist on a continuum. Only when the symptoms are distressing or intolerable to a person should treatment be offered. The worry remains, however, that overdiagnosis could lead to drug companies pushing the usage of increasing numbers of drugs to treat these conditions.

Behavioural treatment of social anxiety disorder

In cases of discrete social anxiety, where individuals are only fearful of a small component of social activity (e.g. public speaking or eating in public; Case example 6.5) and have otherwise developed appropriate social skills, exposure therapy should be effective.

Case example 6.5: Fear of eating and drinking in public

George was a 40-year-old company executive with a lifelong fear of eating or drinking in public. This fear had led him to avoid all social situations since leaving university. He had successfully worked for the past 19 years but had never attended any social events at the company. At a recent appraisal his boss had remarked about this and had urged him to attend the company dinner. George had gained the impression that his lack of socialisation was holding his career prospects back. He also felt that this fear had made it difficult for him to have a social live and he had not had a girlfriend since leaving university. His fear was that he might shake with anxiety while eating or drinking and that this shaking would be noticeable because it could either cause him to spill his food or drink or make a rattling noise with crockery. He believed others would think he was an alcoholic owing to his shaking. Thus the easiest situation for him to handle would be to drink out of a paper cup and eat with his hands rather than more formal occasions requiring the use of utensils and crockery.

Although he had always been anxious, the onset of his fear was during his time at university. He had a professor who was noted to shake in the morning and was known to be a problem drinker. The students would make jokes and pour scorn on this man. George became fearful that if his hands shook, he would be subjected to the same ridicule. At university he had coped by avoiding any formal situations and felt that spilling beer in the students' union was a normal practice unlikely to raise suspicion. It was when he started his job that his problems really started to restrict him. Over the years his fears had grown until he did not eat or drink anything in public.

After a full assessment and education session, George was asked to construct a hierarchy of fears. These ranged from eating in a local fast-food restaurant to the top of his hierarchy, which was to attend the company formal dinner. It was agreed that the first step was for George to eat in the fast-food restaurant near his work daily. Visiting with a therapist would have been unhelpful for George as he felt that the therapist represented 'safety' to him. For this reason he was asked to perform the exposure tasks on his own. Although apprehensive at first, George found that his anxiety habituated rapidly and he was able to move from fast-food restaurants to chain restaurants and increasingly formal settings.

After 10 weeks, George was able to attend a formal dinner and managed to invite a female colleague to accompany him. This was a big change for George, who would have previously feared she would ridicule him. In reality, during the course of the evening, she confessed she was very anxious accompanying him as she saw him as a very successful and powerful person.

In cases of generalised fear of all social situations, however, the patient may have avoided social contact for many years, to the extent that normal adult social skills have not been developed. In these socially maladroit individuals, if exposure therapy is used alone, the feedback from other people may be so discouraging that it reinforces the patient's fear and promotes further avoidance. In these cases it is helpful to include social skills training before attempting real-life exposure to social situations. Social skills training is described fully in Chapter 4.

An excellent self-help module for the treatment of mild to moderate social phobia can be found on the website of the Clinical Research Unit for Anxiety and Depression at Sydney University, New South Wales, Australia (https://crufad.org/index.php/learn-about/social-phobia).

Safety behaviours

Exposure therapy is the treatment of choice for most patients with phobic anxiety disorders. Cognitive therapy can be useful for treating those patients who have failed exposure therapy or who have extreme fears and are unable to undertake exposure immediately. Cognitive therapy requires a greater level of therapist training and supervision. These techniques are discussed in more detail in Chapter 7 and subsequent chapters.

Patients with the generalised phobic disorders such as social anxiety and agoraphobia often learn a number of safety behaviours designed to guard against the feared situation. For example, a young woman who is concerned that she may faint in a public place may have developed a pattern of continually flexing her calf muscles in social situations. Normal exposure to social situations will not result in habituation because this safety behaviour is a form of avoidance. Thus she needs to be encouraged to face social situations without performing the safety behaviour. Safety behaviours are also found in some patients with agoraphobia. A typical example would be a woman with agoraphobia who would only travel on a bus when carrying her handbag. This bag always contained smelling salts in case she felt faint, mint sweets in case she felt sick, sunglasses in case she found it too bright and a bottle of unopened diazepam tablets which had been prescribed 2 years earlier in case she panicked. Again explanation of the maintaining role of such safety behaviour may be sufficient for the patient to instigate effective exposure, or they may need some initial cognitive work.

On the other hand, it is possible to use safety signals to aid an exposure programme. For example, for many people with agoraphobia, home is a strong safety signal. Therefore it would be easier for the patient to be accompanied by the therapist travelling away from home and it may be then easier to encourage them to travel alone back home, towards their safety signal. Once this has been mastered it is often easier for the patient to make the similar journey away from their safety signal (see Case example 6.1, pp. 77–80).

Cognitive therapy

There is evidence that patients with social phobia may benefit more from cognitive therapy than those with other phobic disorders. With some patients it is necessary to use cognitive techniques to encourage an individual to abandon their safety behaviours (Wells *et al*, 1995).

Studies have demonstrated that individuals with social anxiety are more likely to interpret social signals as evidence that a socially negative event will occur, for example that they will make a social gaffe or will be the subject of ridicule or opprobrium (Clark & Wells, 1995; Rapee & Heimberg 1997; Hirsch & Clark, 2004). Examples of this type of thinking error are in a situation where someone laughs when someone else has spoken. A socially anxious person is more likely to interpret this as embarrassing and assume that something inappropriate or stupid has been said. A non-anxious individual may have a much wider repertoire of possibilities including:

- what was said was witty or amusing
- the person who laughed may themselves be anxious and have an anxious laugh
- the person may be trying to be pleasant and encouraging,

as well as thoughts that something inappropriate or stupid has been said. People with social anxiety make these negative evaluations of events not only related to their own social behaviour and performance but also with respect to others. In addition, it has been shown that such people have a very negative evaluation of their own social performance. Once they are in a social situation, they will tend to try to avoid and turn their attention away from social interactions which they see (rightly or wrongly) as negative. They focus instead on their own performance to the exclusion of others. This can then lead to the difficult social interactions which they fear in the first place (Roth & Heimberg, 2001) (Case example 6.6).

Case example 6.6: Cognitive techniques for social phobia

George was a 25-year-old man who worked as a caretaker at a warehouse. He had always been isolated as a child and had had few friends. Subsequently he was bullied at school owing to his lack of friends and general awkwardness. George reacted to this bullying by spending increasing amounts of time alone. Although he claimed that his real desire would be to marry and have children, George had never had a girlfriend. Recently he had tried online dating, which had worked well until George had met up with the women. At this time he had become very anxious and described how 'women never want to see me again'. He described how anxious he would get when going out and how at the beginning he felt the whole evening would be 'a disaster, as always'.

When asked about his social skills, George felt that he was 'terrible', saying 'no one would want to go out with me as I am boring and have nothing interesting to say'.

First, George was asked to role-play a general going out for a coffee with a friend. At first he was almost silent. The therapist then asked him about one of his hobbies, which was birdwatching. George became immediately animated and started talking about a recent trip he had taken to Dungeness to observe birds. Initially, George demonstrated appropriate social skills but when the therapist asked a question about a particular bird, he became very flustered and stammered for a while before starting to raise his voice and talk in a monologue loudly. This appeared quite threatening and so the therapist asked George to stop and to say how he felt things had gone. It became apparent that from the outset he had had thoughts such as 'This will be a disaster. I am being really boring. No one wants to know about my bird watching trips'. These thoughts meant that George was getting increasingly anxious. When the therapist interjected to ask him a question, George's immediate thoughts were 'Why is she interrupting me, I must be even more boring than I thought. I am a total failure'. This was quickly followed by thoughts such as 'It is rude to interrupt me, how dare she?'. This then led to George becoming annoyed and starting to shout to ensure that he finished everything he wanted to say without any interruptions. A vicious circle was thus set up (Fig. 6.4).

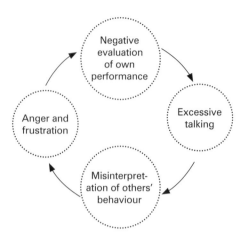

Fig. 6.4 Vicious circle regarding George's anxiety.

Treatment of George involved, first, encouraging him to really observe other people's reactions. This can be difficult as it has been shown that some people with social anxiety misinterpret various emotions and expressions in others, including smiling and laughing, as threatening. In George's case he mainly switched off from other people and did not observe them in any way as he was convinced they would be hostile. He was also encouraged to examine some of his beliefs about his performance and to examine the evidence for his belief that he was a total social failure (the theory and techniques of challenging beliefs and negative automatic thoughts are fully discussed and demonstrated in Chapters 7 and 8 of this book). Much of the work was done with George using video feedback. It can be very difficult to persuade a person with social anxiety to allow themselves to be filmed and this should not be attempted as a first step. Everyone tends to be very critical and embarrassed when first seeing themselves on film. This can be even more difficult for someone with social anxiety and so must be introduced gradually and when the individual has sufficient social skills to perform reasonably well.

A recent study has demonstrated that a simple computer program can be useful in developing more realistic social evaluation in people with social anxiety disorders (Amir *et al*, 2010). Volunteers who were anxious about public speaking were asked to give their interpretations of various social interactions. The program gave positive feedback for responses which were not catastrophic and disastrous but were positive interpretations. After only one session on the computer, participants were more quickly able to ignore perceived threat. Although this was a preliminary study and with volunteers rather than patients with social anxiety, it does suggest that teaching people to attend less to threat cues and more to positive cues may be helpful for treating social anxiety.

Third generation CBT

The whole concept of third generation CBT (sometimes known as third wave CBT) will be fully explored in Chapter 8. These therapies, which were developed in the 1990s, represent a move back to more behavioural methods of treatment. Two key treatments of possible relevance to social anxiety disorder are mindfulness and acceptance and commitment therapy. These involve teaching the patient to accept their emotions and concentrate on what is really happening around them in their environment at the present time. With faulty attentional bias and misinterpretation being thought to be integral to the genesis of social anxiety, it would seem logical to try methods which divert the thoughts away from emotions and misinterpretations and concentrate on what is actually occurring in the 'here and now'. Although this is intellectually attractive, there is currently a lack of strong evidence to support these approaches in social anxiety. However, some recent controlled trials have been positive, with mindfulness and acceptance and commitment therapy producing superior results to standard CBT (Kocovski *et al*, 2013).

Key learning points

- Graduated exposure *in vivo* is effective in the management of phobic anxiety.
- Exposure should be tailored for the individual patient and performed at the maximum speed that they can tolerate.
- Realistic treatment targets must be decided with the patient at the commencement of treatment.
- A helpful spouse, relative or friend can often be usefully incorporated in the exposure treatment.
- 'Homework' practice between treatment sessions is vital.
- Modelling can be used to facilitate exposure.
- Education about the rationale of exposure is important, so that the patient can learn to become their own therapist and deal with any recurrence of fear before deterioration occurs.
- Social anxiety disorder has some differences from other phobic disorders but graded exposure can still be useful for those with specific social fears.
- Safety behaviours may act as a form of avoidance and need to be examined.
- Cognitive therapy has a role to play in many patients with social anxiety disorder.
- People with social anxiety often misinterpret social signals and fail to attend to positive and negative social cues, which leads to further social difficulties.
- Third generation CBT approaches such as mindfulness and acceptance and commitment therapy may have a role in social anxiety disorders.

Suggested measures to use with conditions covered in this chapter

- Problems and targets, Fear Questionnaire and Hamilton Anxiety Scale, all discussed in Chapter 2.

References

American Psychiatric Association (2013) *Diagnostic and Statistical Manual for Psychiatric Disorders* (DSM-5). APA.

Amir N, Bomyea J, Beard C (2010) The effect of single-session interpretation modification on attention bias in socially anxious individuals. *Journal of Anxiety Disorders*, 24: 176.

American Psychiatric Association (2000) *Diagnostic and Statistical Manual for Psychiatric Disorders* (DSM-IV-TR). APA.

Bandura A (1969) *The Principles of Behavior Modification*. Holt, Rinehart & Winston.

Clark DM, Wells A (1995) A cognitive model of social phobia. In *Social Phobia: Diagnosis, Assessment, and Treatment* (eds GG Heimberg, MR Liebowitz, DA Hope, *et al*): 69–93. Guilford Press.

Clark LA, Watson D (2006) Distress and fear disorders: an alternative empirically based taxonomy of the 'mood' and 'anxiety' disorders. *British Journal of Psychiatry*, 189: 481–3.

Emmelkamp PMG, Wessels H (1975) Flooding in imagination v. flooding in vivo in agoraphobics. *Behaviour Research and Therapy*, 13: 7.

Hirsch CR, Clark DM (2004) Information-processing bias in social phobia. *Clinical Psychology Review*, 24: 799–825.

Kocovski NL, Fleming JE, Hawley LL, *et al* (2013) Mindfulness and acceptance-based group therapy versus traditional cognitive behavioral group therapy for social anxiety disorder: a randomized controlled trial. *Behaviour Research and Therapy*, 51: 889–98.

Marks IM (1969) *Fears and Phobias*. Heinemann.

Marks IM (1973) The reduction of fear: towards a unifying theory. *Journal of the Canadian Psychiatric Association*, 18: 9–12.

McDonald R, Sartory G, Grey SJ, *et al* (1978) Effects of self-exposure instructions on agoraphobic outpatients. *Behaviour Research and Therapy*, 17: 83–5.

Ougrin D (2011) Efficacy of exposure versus cognitive therapy in anxiety disorders: systematic review and meta-analysis. *BMC Psychiatry*, 11: 200.

Rapee RM, Heimberg RG (1997) A cognitive-behavioral model of anxiety in social phobia. *Behaviour Research and Therapy*, 35: 741–56.

Roth DA, Heimberg RG (2001) Cognitive-behavioral models of social anxiety disorder. *Psychiatric Clinics of North America*, 24: 753–71.

Stern RS, Marks IM (1973) Brief and prolonged flooding: a comparison in agoraphobic patients. *Archives of General Psychiatry*, 28: 270–6.

Wells A, Clark DM, Salkovskis P, *et al* (1995) Social phobia: the role of in-situation safety behaviors in maintaining anxiety and negative beliefs. *Behavior Therapy*, 26: 153–61.

Recommended treatment manuals and other reading

Beck AT, Emery G, Greenburg RL (2005) *Anxiety Disorders and Phobias: A Cognitive Perspective*. Basic Books.

*Butler G (2008) *Overcoming Social Anxiety and Shyness: A Self-Help Guide Using Cognitive-Behavioural Techniques*. Basic Books.

Marks IM (1981) *Cure and Care of Neurosis*. Wiley.

Marks IM (1987) *Fears, Phobias and Rituals*. Oxford University Press.

*Marks IM (2001) *Living with Fear: Understanding and Coping with Anxiety*. McGraw-Hill.

*Suitable to recommend to patients.

Treatment of obsessive–compulsive disorders

Overview

This chapter will include discussion of obsessions and compulsions as well as a description of graded exposure combined with self-imposed response-prevention (ERP). Case histories of treatment using ERP (both therapist-assisted and self-exposure) and examples of treatment of obsessive ruminations using ERP will be presented. There will then be a discussion and case histories focusing on hoarding, both as a symptom of OCD and as a stand-alone disorder, as well as a brief discussion about animal hoarding. Finally, there will be a short discussion about the various theories, treatments and possible roles of cognitive therapy in OCD and the pitfalls to be avoided.

The key features of OCD are the existence of both obsessions and compulsions. Most of us do experience obsessions and compulsions from time to time. We all know people who set themselves extremely high standards. These people often have the obsessive traits of high achievement, meticulousness, punctuality, extreme neatness or cleanliness. Indeed, traits such as striving for perfection and meticulous hygiene can be seen to have a survival advantage. This advantage may help to keep these traits in the gene pool. In OCD, however, these tendencies have become an end in themselves, with the person feeling compelled to perform compulsions even to the detriment of everything else in their life. For example, whereas general hygiene in the kitchen can be seen to be an excellent thing, in the case of a person with OCD this may have got so out of hand that every waking hour is spent cleaning the kitchen. A woman with OCD and contamination fears had financial difficulties owing to her inability to do any paid work and also her excessive spending on cleaning materials. Both she and her young son were undernourished as too much time was spent cleaning to the detriment of cooking any food.

In DSM-5 (American Psychiatric Association, 2013), OCD has been removed from the category of anxiety disorders and instead is in a separate category of obsessive–compulsive and related disorders. As well as OCD, this category includes body dysmorphic disorders (previously categorised as a somatoform disorder), hoarding disorder (new diagnosis), trichotillomania (new diagnosis), skin-picking (new diagnosis) as well as OCD symptoms arising from substance misuse and medication and other organic disorders.

Obsessions

Obsessions are thoughts, images or impulses that come into the person's mind and are distressing and anxiety-provoking. Everyone has worrying or anxiety-provoking thoughts from time to time but with obsessions they are so all pervasive or so worrying that the person feels the need to try not to have this thought ever again. Of course, this effort at trying not to have a thought means that the thought becomes more frequent.

For example, a religious person may have blasphemous thoughts. These are abhorrent and so extreme efforts are used to try to prevent them coming back. However, trying to suppress these is part of a vicious circle of constantly monitoring these thoughts and consequently increasing them. Much of the person's time and effort is devoted to trying to resist the obsessions. Later in the illness, less time may be spent resisting as the individual learns this is not successful (World Health Organization, 1992; American Psychiatric Association, 2000).

Common obsessions include (Drummond & Fineberg, 2007):

- *Fear of contamination* (particularly dirt and germs) owing to the worry that harm may occur to self or others.
- *Fear of harm occurring to self or others due to an act of omission*, for instance fear that the family may be attacked if the door or windows are left open, leading to excessive checking of them.
- *Fear of harm occurring to self or others due to an act of commission*, for instance worry that one may 'run amok' and harm someone in the presence of knives (this often causes some fear in the professionals dealing with the individual). In OCD, this is not a true urge or desire but the person really would not want to perform the act at all and is frightened by the thought.
- *Blasphemous or religious obsessions* which are repugnant to the individual.
- *Fear of loss of objects or inadvertent disclosure of information*. For example, inability to throw household rubbish away for fear that secret information may get into the wrong hands to the detriment of the person. This can result in a house virtually uninhabitable and filled with empty packets and papers.
- *Hoarding.* This is described as a new separate category of disorders in DSM-5 and it is likely that ICD-11 will also include a separate category for this condition. Although this can occur without OCD, some individuals hoard objects for a variety of reasons related to their

obsessional fears. For example, a man wanted to keep up to date on all book reviews so he bought four newspapers a day and would repeatedly read over these reviews. He was unable to cut out the reviews for fear he may have missed some of the information. His house and garage were completely full of newspapers and he had consequently rented a flat, resulting in financial hardship. The new flat was rapidly becoming uninhabitable owing to continued hoarding of newspapers.

- *Perfectionism* is a common theme for people with OCD. Because nobody is perfect, these individuals are bound to fail. This failure leads to anxiety. Instead, the opposite to perfection often occurs, as the person cannot even start to perform an action for fear of failure. For example, a woman felt the need to have a perfectly tidy house. She managed to achieve a pristine environment for a brief time. However, as the exacting standards become impossible to maintain, she was found existing in squalor in an extremely anxious state.

Obsessions are usually recognised by the person with OCD as being a product of their own mind. Importantly, however, obsessions are anxiety-provoking and abhorrent. For example, a person with OCD who has obsessive concerns that they may sexually abuse young children will not do so. A true paedophile enjoys the thoughts of abuse and finds them sexually rewarding rather than repugnant.

People with OCD also recognise that their obsessions are irrational, at least early in the illness. However, DSM-5 does recognise that some individuals have little or no insight but are still classified as having OCD. If a person has recently been in a situation that has provoked the obsessions, they will be more likely to claim to believe in their rationality. However, in any periods of calm reflection, most people will admit the irrationality of the obsessions.

The key factor is that obsessions are anxiogenic and raise anxiety levels or at least a sense of discomfort and being ill at ease.

Compulsions

Compulsions are thoughts, words or deeds that are designed to reduce or prevent the harm of the obsessive thought. However, they are either not realistically connected to the obsessive concern or else are clearly excessive (World Health Organization, 1992; American Psychiatric Association, 2013).

For example, an individual with blasphemous thoughts may feel the need to repeat prayers following a blasphemous thought. These prayers may be performed in set numbers such as three that may be perceived as a 'good' number. Thus stopping at a number that is not divisible by three would cause further anxiety.

Sometimes, though, the compulsions are not connected with the obsessions in any logical way but are an example of 'magical thinking'.

Most of us do have some examples of irrational magical thinking in superstitious behaviour to prevent bad things occurring. In OCD, however, these behaviours are more extreme. For example, a man had the thought that catastrophe may befall his close family members. This was extremely anxiety-provoking to him and he developed a compulsion which involved his standing on his right leg and hopping up and down in multiples of twelve until he felt that he had 'undone' the bad thought.

As well as compulsions, some people with OCD repeatedly seek reassurance from others as a way of abating anxiety. This works in an identical way to compulsions. For example, a young woman had a fear that she might inadvertently push a child on the road whenever she went out. She would, therefore, avoid going out unaccompanied but would insist a family member accompany her. While out and on returning she would constantly seek reassurance that she had not performed these acts by asking the observer to account for every movement and every minute of her time.

Although compulsions reduce anxiety, they do so inefficiently. They tend to reduce the anxiety a little but their effect is short-lived. For example, a man who has fear of contracting diarrhoea from dirt and germs may wash his hands in a stereotyped way every time he touches a door handle used by others. This activity will reduce his anxiety a little but it will not be long before he feels he may not have washed his hands sufficiently well and he feels the urge to repeat this. The end result is that people with OCD spend most of the time being highly anxious and distressed.

Treatment of OCD using ERP

Obsessive–compulsive symptoms often resemble phobias but there are also some important differences, as shown in Table 7.1.

At first this may seem a complicated distinction, but some examples will demonstrate the differences. In Chapter 6, we related the case history of the student teacher Lauren who had a fear of dogs (Case example 6.4). This fear is an example of a specific animal phobia as the fear was purely related to the presence of dogs in her vicinity. Contrast this with the story of Eleanor (Case example 7.1). It demonstrates that the keystone of treatment for OCD is exposure to the anxiety-producing obsessions or the stimuli which

Table 7.1 OCD and phobias

Similarities	Differences
Anxiety and discomfort usually accompany the obsessional thought	In OCD the fear is not of the object itself but of its consequences
Avoidance of certain situations or stimuli	Elaborate belief systems develop around OCD compulsions and rituals but not around phobias

OCD, obsessive–compulsive disorder.

produce these thoughts. Self-imposed response prevention is additionally used as a way of prolonging exposure and removing the compulsions. The important thing to remember is that the patient needs to reliably and regularly face up to the feared situation in a graded fashion, while at the same time stopping the anxiolytic compulsions.

Case example 7.1: Extreme fear of contamination, I

Eleanor had a 10-year history of fear of contamination by dirt from dog faeces, as she was concerned that she might catch a variety of diseases, which could then be passed on to others and which would result in her feeling responsible for this plague. This problem caused her to avoid any situations where she had seen dogs in the past. Even if she saw a dog through her window she would feel anxious and resort to cleaning rituals. Her anxiety-reducing rituals consisted of stripping off all her clothes, which were then considered contaminated, and washing them. She would bathe in a set pattern and would repeat this ritual washing in multiples of four, which she considered a 'good' number.

In a case discussed earlier (Case example 6.4), Lauren had a classic dog phobia which lead to avoidance of dogs or any situations which reminded her of dogs. Eleanor's problem was different in that her fear was not of dogs themselves, but of the consequences which she thought might result from contact with dogs. Unlike Lauren, whose anxiety was relieved by escaping from the dog, Eleanor would still remain anxious after the dog had left, until she had performed her washing rituals to her satisfaction. The development of elaborate belief systems in people with OCD is demonstrated here, as Eleanor performed her stereotyped washing rituals in multiples of four. However, these belief systems are only part of the phenomena, as people with OCD generally realise that their fears are irrational, and that their ritualistic patterns are unrealistic.

Treatment for both Lauren and Eleanor was similar, as they received graduated prolonged exposure to their feared situation. There was an additional component in Eleanor's treatment because of the rituals, self-imposed response prevention or, in other words, explaining to the patient the effect of rituals on anxiety and then asking them not to ritualise. After the therapist had taken Eleanor's history and talked to her about anxiety, the following explanation was given:

'When you are in contact with anything which makes you feel "contaminated", you experience extreme anxiety. A high level of anxiety is uncomfortable, and so being human, you will try to escape or avoid that experience. However, escaping from the situation is not possible if you already feel contaminated. To reduce your anxiety you have therefore developed the anxiety-reducing ritual of washing in a set pattern in multiples of four. When you perform this ritual, your anxiety reduces.

As high anxiety is uncomfortable, this reduction in anxiety is like a reward. You are therefore rewarding your ritualistic behaviour. If we reward any behaviour, we increase the chance of it recurring in that situation again. For example, if a dog sits up and begs and is rewarded with a chocolate drop, then you increase the chance of it sitting up and begging again.

In the case of obsessional rituals, however, although they reduce anxiety, there are two problems: they only reduce anxiety a small amount; and the anxiety reduction is short lived and you then have to repeat the ritual.

In practice this means that you are constantly experiencing very high levels of tension and anxiety. I am going to ask you to stop performing any rituals at all. Although this sounds difficult, I think you will soon find that your anxiety eventually reduces much further than when you ritualise. Old habits die hard and you may, on occasion, find yourself ritualising. That is fine as long as you stop once you realise and then "recontaminate" yourself.'

The therapist drew a graph (Fig. 7.1) for Eleanor during this explanation.

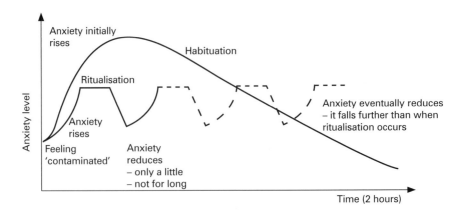

Fig. 7.1 Eleanor's diagram.

Therapists often make the mistake of asking the patient to produce a hierarchy of compulsions. This will not work and it is often easier for a person with OCD to stop a behaviour completely or replace the pathological behaviour with a new, more adaptive behaviour. Another difference between exposure for phobic disorder and exposure for OCD is that whereas the anxiety generated by exposure for phobic situations generally takes up to an hour to habituate, in OCD this can often take up to 2 hours. This slower habituation is thought to be due to small pieces of compulsive thoughts or behaviour creeping in and slowing down the habituation process (see Case example 7.2).

Case example 7.2: Extreme fear of contamination, II

Mike was a 30-year-old electrician who had always had minor obsessive–compulsive difficulties. Five years earlier he was visiting a large shopping centre with his wife and went to the toilet in there. While in the toilet he noticed some dried blood on the cubicle door. Following on from this, he became convinced he had contracted HIV from the blood. He visited his local genito-urinary clinic to have an HIV test. Unsurprisingly, the test was negative but this did not reassure him and he started returning there on a weekly basis 'in case they'd missed something'. In addition, he became concerned about anything that he might have touched since he went to the shopping centre or that he might have become 'contaminated' in another way.

These problems grew and Mike eventually was forced to stop seeking reassurance from the genito-urinary clinic and his GP, as the former refused to see him again and the GP threatened to discharge him from his books unless he stopped seeing him concerning HIV. Although Mike was very anxious to begin with, the anxiety did reduce eventually but he continued to perform extensive 'decontamination' compulsions. These involved asking anyone who had been outside (and thus potentially in contact with somebody who may have been to the shopping centre) to take off all their external clothes, which were placed in plastic bags. They were then asked to wash and bathe extensively. The clothes were sprayed 10–15 times with antibacterial spray before being allowed to be washed on a hot wash several times. Clothes were often thrown away if Mike did not feel they were 'clean'. He had been unable to work for the past 5 years and, owing to the stress of his compulsive rituals, had stayed in bed for the past 6 months. As getting out of bed resulted in so many urges to start his 'decontamination rituals', he was frequently incontinent of urine in the bed. In addition he restricted his fluid consumption to avoid visiting the toilet. At the time of assessment, he was drinking only 500 ml of fluid a day. Bathing took him up to 5 h and consequently he only bathed once a month. His wife was tired and distraught and was considering divorce.

The first stage of treatment was to fully assess Mike and to discover the obsessional fear at the root of his problems. This was identified as 'A fear of catching HIV primarily from the shopping centre or anyone who has been in contact with the centre'. This fear resulted in extensive avoidance of leaving the house and extensive decontamination compulsive rituals concerning items which were brought into the house. In addition there were widespread decontamination compulsions concerning the house and Mike's personal hygiene. Owing to the extreme nature of these problems, Mike was avoiding basic personal care of washing and bathing. In addition, he was restricting his fluid intake to reduce his use of the toilet.

Mike was educated about OCD and the principles of treatment were explained to him. It was described how he would be asked to face up to his fear and 'contaminate' himself without engaging in his 'decontamination' behaviours. The first thing that needed to be addressed, however, was his avoidance of drinking sufficient fluid. It was explained to Mike and his wife that such fluid restriction could lead to permanent damage to the kidneys. Although we would normally expect Mike to produce a hierarchy of fears, it was felt so important to address this that any therapy would need to start by tackling this. Mike agreed he would drink 1–1.5 litres of fluid a day, if he could use tissues to touch any item in the bathroom. The therapist and his wife agreed to this but he was told that he must also go to the toilet at least every 3 h during the day to avoid any incontinence. Before the therapist saw him again, he was asked to produce a list of situations which would cause him to feel 'contaminated' and anxious and to give these an anxiety rating, with 0 representing no anxiety and 8 representing panic. It was explained that these anxiety ratings needed to determine how he would feel if he did not engage in any compulsive rituals or any avoidance to 'put right' the fear. Although he was being allowed to use tissues to visit the toilet initially, this was to ensure his health and he would be asked to forego them ultimately.

Mike was very anxious about what he might be asked to do but did realise that his concern about the shopping centre was 'completely over the top'.

At the therapist's next visit, Mike had produced a hierarchy of fears (Table 7.2).

At the next session, it was agreed that first it was important to look at changing the compulsive behaviours and devising a reasonable self-care

Table 7.2 Mike's hierarchy of fears

Exposure item (without washing/decontamination rituals)	Predicted anxiety level (0–8 scale)
Touch walls, door knobs, taps, etc., in house without hand-washing after or 'decontaminating' before	3–4
Touching clothes that have been outside	4
Using bathroom and toilet without 'decontaminating' first and by touching flushers and bathroom taps using bare hands	5
Walking to the high street and seeing other people; returning home without changing clothes or bathing immediately	5–6
Deliberately touching red marks on paintwork or walls	7–8
Travelling on public transport	8
Travelling to shopping centre	8

regime. It was established that Mike had been drinking very well over the previous week and looked well hydrated and well fed. Next the therapist enquired about his bathing and the reason it took so long. As well as cleaning everywhere before going into the bath, Mike also had a set 'routine' of showering whereby he washed starting from the top of his body and worked down. If he felt any area had not been washed 'properly' he would repeat this. These repetitions often occurred 8–9 times, so that each part of his body was red raw. To break this pattern, the therapist asked him to take a shower twice daily but that he was to only stand under the shower for a maximum of 5 min and was not to use soap or try to 'wash' any area. He was also asked not to clean the shower before use. Mike agreed to try this and predicted his anxiety would be 6–7 for this. The therapist also showed him a new way of washing his hands (which at present could take 5–10 min): the therapist asked him to place the plug in the basin and to quarter fill it with water; 'normal' hand washing taking 30 s or less was then demonstrated. This involved only the hands and not up to the forearms as Mike had previously been doing. Mike was then asked to try this out with the therapist watching. He was asked to only wash his hands after going to the toilet and at no other times. It was agreed that at the next session the therapist would come to Mike's house and they would 'contaminate' themselves by touching items around the house which Mike believed to be contaminated.

When the therapist visited the house, Mike was delighted as he had bathed in the prescribed fashion all week, continued to maintain his fluid levels and had washed his hands as demonstrated. The therapist praised him and then demonstrated the way to expose himself to 'contamination'. This involved touching the 'contaminated' object with both hands, rubbing the hands together and then touching his hair, upper torso, lower torso, legs, lips and mouth, and then licking his hands to ensure that he felt 'contaminated'. Mike was extremely anxious about this but was reminded of the habituation curve (Fig. 6.2, p. 76) and agreed to give it a go. In fact he did extremely well and during the session agreed to go further and touch the toilet flusher and taps without washing. He was praised and asked to continue performing these exposure exercises three times a day for the next week.

Treatment continued in this way. Mike was asked to touch the toilet seat and contaminate himself in the prescribed manner. This often surprises new therapists but in OCD, as with phobic disorder, it is often useful to over-learn to prevent slipping back once therapy stops. After nine sessions, Mike agreed to accompany the therapist to the shopping centre. They travelled round the centre touching as many items as possible. They went into the toilets and touched the taps and toilet flushers as well as various marks on the door. Following this, they went to the burger shop and ate a burger without washing their hands. Mike was anxious but settled as the day progressed. This exposure session lasted a total of 4 h, including travel on public transport to get there.

Some people worry that exposure exercises such as those described above are 'risky' and that it is unethical to ask someone to risk contracting an illness by not washing. The risk of contracting HIV by such activity is almost zero but there is a small possibility of catching another less serious infection. It is important to remember however that all of us perform risky behaviours every day when we drive a car or cross a road on foot. Patients with OCD can be restricted in all aspects of their lives for decades. If I were asked to weigh up the cost–benefit analysis of taking an extremely small risk of catching a minor illness or suffering from OCD with its life-impacting consequences, I know which one I would choose. When explained this way, most patients and most potential therapists are prepared to use exposure in this way.

Obsessions with covert compulsions (ruminations)

Therapists often become confused about so-called obsessive ruminations. This is because they are used to the idea of anxiogenic obsessive thoughts followed by anxiolytic compulsive behaviours. However, compulsions can be behaviours, thoughts or images. Once this is remembered, the therapist needs to establish what the anxiety-provoking thoughts are and encourage the patient to expose themselves to those while stopping the anxiety-reducing compulsive thoughts. An example of a patient with obsessive ruminations who was successfully treated with the use of prolonged exposure is presented in Case example 7.3.

Case example 7.3: Prolonged exposure therapy for obsessive ruminations

Ethan, a 42-year-old unmarried ex-schoolteacher, had a 15-year history of distressing obsessions which occupied him 10–12 hours a day and had led to his early retirement from work. Whenever he saw anyone he would have the thought 'I would like to have sex with them'. This thought was repugnant to him as he was a devout 'born-again' Christian who did not agree with extramarital sex, and the ideas of homosexuality, paedophilia and incest which his thoughts implied were abhorrent to him.

In order to reduce his anxiety, he had developed the habit of repeating the Lord's prayer and following this by saying 'Jesus, forgive me' seven times. If he was interrupted by any sound or movement in his environment, he would have to repeat it until performed perfectly. This problem had led him to seek the life of a recluse and he had even stopped attending church. He had contemplated suicide to rid himself of the problem but felt this was an even greater sin.

Initially, treatment took the form of graduated prolonged exposure to situations he avoided. However, he only made limited progress as he could not stop himself automatically starting his 'praying ritual', which helped to maintain his anxiety. It was decided that he needed to experience prolonged exposure to his anxiety-provoking thoughts without ritualising. This was achieved by getting him to record the thoughts ('I want to have sex with her. I want to have sex with him') on a continuous feedback loop on the audio device on his smartphone in his own voice. After recording this, Ethan was asked to play this to himself via the earpiece for at least 1 hour three to four times a day while in the company of other people, e.g. on the bus.

Ethan found this so aversive initially that he had difficulty in complying. The therapist, therefore, advised him to start with the volume turned down low, and to increase the volume as he became more confident. This procedure worked extremely well and within 2 weeks of starting to use the digital tracks, Ethan reported that he had little anxiety and was able to go out at other times. Despite having the thought, he no longer carried out the ritual. After 2 months he was able to return to work as a 'supply' teacher. At 6-month post-treatment follow-up, he reported that he had a girlfriend, was planning to marry, and he laughed at the thoughts which he now considered to be 'stupid'.

Treating obsessive ruminations

Two issues appear to be of particular importance. First, the tape should be recorded in the patient's own voice, and second, it should be played through the earpiece. The effect of both of these seem to make it virtually impossible for the patient to ignore the sound of the recording or to ritualise at the same time.

Hoarding

Hoarding and OCD

Hoarding can be a symptom of several disorders, including schizophrenia (inability to structure life sufficiently to organise disposal of excessive objects), depression (somatic retardation leading to a lack of normal self-care functions), dementia (inability to work out what is necessary), and OCD (fear of loss of objects, fear of contamination, excessive checking). Hoarding can also exist as a stand-alone disorder, though this was not classified as a separate category until recently. People with hoarding disorder who were not clearly suffering from another psychiatric disorder were classified as having either obsessive–compulsive personality or OCD. This means there is very little known about people who hoard but do not have another disorder. There are suggestions that hoarders are more likely to be female (Frost *et al*, 2011*a*), older than the average person with OCD (Saxena *et al*, 2011) and live alone (Rodriguez *et al*, 2012). Hoarding disorder is a separate category in the new DSM-5 and is likely also to be included in ICD-11. See a case example of a person with OCD and hoarding symptoms (Case example 7.4).

Case example 7.4: OCD and hoarding problems

Joan was a 42-year-old lady who lived with her husband and two teenage children. She reported that she had suffered from a series of obsessive worries all her life but these had not been overly problematic until the birth of her youngest child 15 years earlier. This had been a difficult delivery and Joan had suffered from a massive haemmorrhage during labour. There had been concern about the baby following this and he had stayed on the paediatric intensive care unit overnight. Although there had been no long-lasting effect on his health, Joan had understandably found this a very difficult experience.

Following the birth, she had post-natal depression. This depression was eventually noted and treated with antidepressants 9 months after the birth, but Joan was left with residual obsessive fears. These fears were that she might inadvertently disclose information which would lead to her losing her children. She was not worried about verbally giving away information but was worried that she might write something down which was incriminating and, as a written word, would be more difficult to explain away.

Initially, this problem had meant that Joan had felt the need to meticulously check all pieces of paper in the house for fear they might contain some detrimental information. All labels, receipts, letters and papers which came into the house were repeatedly checked. Over the past 8 years this problem had exacerbated and Joan was now unable to throw away any written material, including empty food packets. The family lived in a large, detached four-bedroom house but this was fast becoming uninhabitable owing to Joan's hoarding. At first, the double garage had been filled from floor to ceiling, but now the spare bedroom was becoming full and Joan was wanting her sons to share a room so that she could continue to hoard her items. Over the past 3 years, as well as paper items which came into the house, Joan had collected pieces of paper and detritus left on the pavements in case they contained damaging revelations about her.

After the full assessment was performed and Joan was educated about her problem, it was agreed that the first issue to be tackled would be working on preventing more extra items being brought into the house. With any patient who hoards, the first thing to establish is that no more items will be brought into the house while the clearing of items is taking place. Otherwise the exercise of clearing the house is pointless as the hoard will rapidly re-accumulate. Obviously, in a situation like Joan's, some items would continue to come into the house in the form of letters and food packaging. It was thus decided that therapy would start with an exposure programme involving Joan's fear of revealing information. It was very difficult for Joan to create a hierarchy of her fears as all related to her fear of revealing detrimental information. Throwing away a food packet was as anxiety-provoking as throwing away a piece of paper with her writing on it, as she felt both might contain damaging information. Eventually it was agreed that the therapist would write on several pieces of paper 'I declare that I am a bad mother and that my children should be taken away from me'. These pieces of paper were then signed by the therapist. Joan and the therapist then walked into the town's main high street and deposited these pieces of paper in litter bins, on the table of a fast food restaurant and on the table in a local library. Joan found this very anxiety-provoking but agreed that she would not return to the high street to collect these pieces of paper later. She also agreed to go out every day and to throw away blank pieces of paper in the way the therapist and she had done during the session.

103

Over the next week, Joan was feeling very pleased and had already been able to throw away printed paper. She was praised for doing this. It was agreed that, in light of this, therapy should move on to throwing away some of the hoarded items. Initially Joan wanted to check all of the papers she threw away. A reminder of how this checking was likely to lead to more checking and more anxiety was discussed with her. Eventually, she agreed that the therapy could start with throwing away items in the garage which had been there for over 2 years. During the first session, the therapist and Joan managed to discard six large rubbish sacks full of paper. Joan agreed to let the therapist take these to the local tip so that she could not check them. She also agreed to put out at least two sacks per day for her husband to discard on his way to work.

Over the next few weeks, Joan cleared most of her house. Dealing with newer post was difficult initially but she was reminded of the principle that she should read any post, act on it immediately if necessary and then discard it.

Hoarding without OCD

In Joan's situation (Case example 7.4), her hoarding was clearly related to an OCD fear of revealing information. Some patients have hoarding problems without OCD symptoms. In these cases people are frequently living in dangerous situations with risk of fire from hoarded items or even structural collapse. Frequently, individuals are not referred to the medical or psychiatric professions and are instead dealt with via the courts. Many are made homeless because of eviction as a result of their problems. These individuals can be very difficult to treat. Unlike in OCD, drugs such as serotonin reuptake inhibitors and/or dopamine blockers may not have major beneficial effects. One of the most striking characteristics of patients with hoarding is their absolute belief that their hoards are 'valuable'. An elderly lady who lived in a house which was falling down due to structural damage secondary to hoarded newspapers and letters suggested that to start throwing any of these items away would be tantamount to 'committing grievous bodily harm'. People with pure hoarding disorder are more likely to be older than people with OCD, live alone, be male and many have a history of deprivation in childhood.

In these situations, the first thing that needs to occur is establishing trust between the therapist and patient. Second, there needs to be an agreement that no more hoarded items must enter the house. Only after these steps can any clearing take place. Once the trust has been built between patient and therapist and no further items are accumulated, it is time to start persuading the individual to discard hoarded objects. This needs to be done by agreeing the rules for objects that should be discarded, recycled or saved. When making this decision, the patient should be encouraged to only hold the object once and not to go back on the decision. It appears that prolonged handling of the object leads to greater attachment of the individual to that object. Once an object is discarded, the person is less distressed if they do not see the discarded item again (Saxena & Maidment, 2007), like in Case example 7.5.

Case example 7.5: Hoarding

Albert was a 65-year-old unmarried man who lived alone in a housing association flat. He had worked previously as a builder but retired 5 years ago. Referral was made to local psychiatric services via the housing association. Although they were keen to help Albert, his excessive hoarding was putting other residents at risk as objects had spilled out into communal areas, causing a risk that someone might fall; there was concern that the weight of his hoarded items would shortly put the building structure at risk and there was fear of fire owing to the excessive papers including in kitchen areas.

For the first meeting, Albert was insistent that he should meet the therapist at the hospital site. He gave a history of a deprived and difficult childhood when he had had to move several times with his unmarried mother, who had had a series of relationships with different men. When he became an adult he was determined to work to be able to afford 'nice' things in his home. Initially, he had managed to keep a tidy and functional home. He was married from the age of 25 to 50 years but sadly his wife died of breast cancer 15 years ago. They had not had any children. Albert was distraught after his wife died and had never wished to form another relationship. At the beginning he worked harder, but since taking retirement 5 years ago, he had found himself very lonely and isolated. His hoarding problem started shortly after his wife died. He would visit various house-clearance shops in his area and buy a variety of objects, mostly the type of objects or furniture that he remembered from his youth. In addition, he would buy multiple books in charity shops, although he rarely found the time to read them. The problem had escalated further following retirement. It was immediately apparent that Albert was very embarrassed by his problem. He described himself as 'lazy' and 'greedy' for having this problem. When it was suggested that the therapist might visit his home, Albert was adamant that this could not happen.

The first stage of therapy involved the therapist gaining Albert's trust. In addition, it was important to ensure that no more items were being brought into the house. The therapist discussed with Albert the feelings he had when he found a 'nice' item or a book. Albert described his excitement and pleasure at finding the item and said it gave him a 'buzz', but when he returned home he felt humiliated and despondent that his flat was so overcrowded. It was clear that Albert lived a very sad and restricted life and that buying items was his chief pleasure, even though this then led to deeper despair. It was important to establish a moratorium on new items coming into the house but also to try to ensure that Albert had some pleasurable activities to replace the excitement that had resulted from his shopping. First, a discussion was held about Albert's interests. He admitted that he was very interested in reading and books. It was agreed that Albert would not visit any of his usual shops during the next week; when he went out to buy groceries, he would only take sufficient money to do this (and no bank cards) and not buy anything else; in addition he would go to the local library and find out about book reading clubs as well as sign himself up as a member so that he could borrow books.

For several weeks, Albert was resistant to the therapist visiting his home as he felt deeply ashamed about the state it was in. He was encouraged to take photographs of each room but was reluctant to do this. To start therapy, he was asked to bring a bag of items so that a decision could be made about them. Albert agreed that approximately 75% of items needed to go from his flat but was extremely anxious about this. On the next appointment, he arrived with a bag of books. Together with the therapist he agreed that there were three categories of items:

- items for recycling for paper (rubbish) – books with pages missing or badly torn or mouldy
- items for disposal at charity shops/library – books in reasonably good condition but which he had read
- items to keep – books of particular significance or value, such as first editions and family books inherited from his grandfather.

To this end three large bags were made available. Albert was then asked to take out a book and decide quickly which category it belonged in. It was important that he did not handle the item for too long as this tends to increase the attachment to an object. Also it was negotiated that once a decision about disposal had been made, it was final. The session took 2 hours and Albert found it extremely distressing and very difficult to discard items. During the session, he wept at times when discarding books and said he felt as if he was losing close friends. He was reminded of his goal of having a tidy, habitable flat with sufficient good-quality items to live comfortably. Albert agreed to persevere and at the end of the session the therapist and Albert disposed of one bag in the recycling bin, another at a local charity shop and the third contained 2 books out of 30 which Albert wanted to take home. He was then given the task of continuing this process on his own until the next session.

After 4 weeks, Albert had progressed well and had discarded several large bags full of books. He had had one setback when he had gone back to the charity shop and said he had changed his mind, but the books had already been sent to a central sorting office. The therapist praised Albert for his progress but said the next session would have to be in his own home.

At the first home-based session, 6 weeks after starting therapy, the first thing the therapist had to gauge was the risk to both Albert and herself. There have been reported incidents where people have been killed or seriously injured due to items falling on the hoarder. Clearly the risk of this occurring increases once items are starting to be moved. Other risks to the therapist include health risks from extreme dirt and squalor, risk of building collapse and risk of being trapped by fire. Any mental health professional *must* ensure their own health and safety as well as that of their patient. If there is a serious risk, then it may be necessary to consider legal enforcement and clearing of the property and there must also be consideration of whether the Mental Health Act is appropriate. It is often necessary for the therapist to have protective overalls and a mask because of dust and dirt. In this case, although the hoarding was severe, there was no immediate danger and Albert agreed not to use the cooker until the kitchen was cleared of fire hazards. First, the therapist gained Albert's permission to take photographs of the different rooms. The house was completely full with piles of items covering almost 80% of all available floor space. The kitchen had books piled up on every work surface and there was a risk of fire from the books being next to the cooker. Albert's bed also was covered with just a small space for him to sleep on the edge of the bed; the bath was piled high with books and Albert had been unable to take a bath for several years; the living room had a small space with one chair and a television and there was a narrow passageway between items to reach this.

Work started on clearing the kitchen, using the same categories of items as before. Again this was very difficult for Albert but he began to feel encouraged as he saw the space around his cooker getting cleared and the work surfaces, which he had not seen for several years, start to appear.

Albert began working with a befriender from his local community mental health team who agreed to come round once a week and help him discard his items, and if they managed to clear as much as they had hoped, they would go for a coffee, having dropped off items at the charity shop. The therapist contacted them every few weeks to ensure progress and to troubleshoot any difficulties. After 15 months from the first appointment, Albert had cleared his house. The local social services had arranged for his flat to be 'deep-cleaned'. Albert was delighted with his new living situation but needed to think about relapse prevention. The therapist and Albert looked at ways he could prevent the same situation recurring. Albert's agreement was:

- 'I will continue to borrow books from the library and attend the reading groups there'
- 'I have purchased an electronic book reader and so will no longer buy paper books'
- 'I will restrict my cash and bank cards when going out and only buy what I have previously decided and take money for those items only'
- 'If I do purchase a new item or new piece of furniture, *something of equivalent size has to be discarded.*'

Treating a person with hoarding problem such as Albert's is a lengthy and painstaking process. Most cases will take many months and a year is not unusual. In these cases, it is unrealistic to expect a therapist to attend weekly for many hours to allow clearing to take place. Consideration should be given to obtaining a 'co-therapist' who may be a mental health worker, a 'befriender' from the local mental health services, a family member or a friend. The co-therapist needs to have the patient's trust and also needs to understand the rules for the treatment:

- moratorium on new items coming into the house
- each item is allocated to the 'discard', 'charity shop' or ' keep' bag
- each item is held for a few seconds (no more that 2 min) for a decision to be made
- items must only be handled once, i.e. no going back on decisions
- once sorted the items are disposed of immediately.

Animal hoarding

A variation on the hoarding theme are individuals who hoard vast numbers of animals. This condition is more common in older women who also frequently have a history of a deprived childhood. Usually, these individuals believe that they are 'rescuing' the animals and that only they can offer them love and proper care. However, they then live in squalor with animals and with the living space covered in faeces (Reinisch, 2009). Indeed, a substantial proportion of people who 'hoard' animals also had dying and dead animals owing to neglect (Frost *et al*, 2011b). Currently, animal hoarding is dealt with by the animal rescue agencies and courts, and there have been no studies concerning psychiatric intervention.

Skin-picking and trichotillomania

These conditions differ from OCD as there is usually no anxiety-producing thought preceding the behaviour. The habit itself causes a pleasurable sense of relief, though this may be followed by remorse and distress. These habits will tend to be worse at times of stress but can occur during daydreaming and absent-mindedness or when concentrating on another task. People with skin-picking or trichotillomania tend to be seen by dermatologists or trichologists rather than in mental health services. The treatment approach of habit reversal can be helpful for these individuals (Teng *et al*, 2006; Flessner & Penzel, 2010).

Cognitive therapy and OCD

Although it may seem logical to try to tackle OCD using cognitive therapy, there is no evidence that it offers any advantage to graded exposure and self-imposed response prevention (Ougrin, 2011; Tyagi *et al*, 2010). Poorly applied cognitive therapy may make some patients with OCD worse. This is because the process of looking for evidence to confirm or refute the obsessions can become incorporated into rituals. Cognitive therapy may turn out to be less cost-efficient, as it requires more training and supervision for the therapist and usually takes more time in therapy.

Theory and practice of cognitive interventions for OCD

An early study into the possible efficacy of cognitive therapy in the treatment of OCD was performed in the Netherlands (Emmelkamp *et al*, 1988). The researchers used rational emotive therapy as they believed that patients with OCD did not sufficiently challenge their obsessive beliefs. Rational emotive therapy was developed by Albert Ellis in the 1960s for a variety of depressive and anxiety disorders and is a confrontative type of therapy where beliefs are actively challenged by the therapist (Ellis, 1962).

In the UK, Rachman proposed that OCD symptoms would be reduced if the patient felt less responsible for any disastrous or harmful outcome (Rachman, 1976). This idea was expanded by Salkovskis, who suggested that the central theme of OCD thinking was an inflated idea of personal responsibility and devised therapy to deal with these beliefs (Salkovskis, 1985). Later he developed the theory and suggested that ideas of overinflated responsibility lead to increased neutralising behaviour, increased selective attention to perceived threat and thus a depressed mood which creates a vicious circle involving feelings of excessive responsibility and guilt (Salkovskis, 1999).

A different foundation for the origins of OCD has been postulated by Menzies and his co-workers. This group worked on their observations that ideas about danger were more highly correlated with compulsive activity than ideas of responsibility, self-efficacy, perfectionism or anticipated anxiety. From this observation, the group developed danger ideation reduction therapy (DIRT) as a treatment for compulsive cleaners and washers. This treatment may be particularly useful for patients with contamination fears who refuse to undertake, or who fail in, exposure therapy (Jones & Menzies, 1998; Krochmalik *et al*, 2001). It differs from previous treatments by not encouraging the patient to confront the feared contaminant. Instead, the therapy is aimed at rationalising and reducing the ideas of danger. Techniques used include:

- cognitive restructuring using rational emotive therapy (Ellis, 1962)
- filmed interviews with people who work in feared situations, e.g. cleaners, asking about any 'precautions' they take and about their general health (despite the lack of 'precautions')
- corrective information about the real risks of 'contamination' as opposed to the deleterious effects of overzealous hand-washing
- attentional focusing whereby patients are taught to focus the mind away from the danger-related intrusive thoughts.

Despite its apparent intellectual attractiveness, there is little work to suggest that cognitive therapy has any advantage over exposure therapy in the treatment of OCD. A small number of trials of rational emotive therapy, DIRT and cognitive therapy targeting heightened sense of responsibility have failed to show that they have any advantage over exposure methods (e.g. Emmelkamp & Beens, 1991; Jones & Menzies, 1998; McLean *et al*, 2001).

Table 7.3 Using cognitive approaches for OCD

Type of problem with ERP treatment	Possible approaches	Notes	Where discussed in this book
Extreme anxiety and high strength of belief in the rationality of the obsessive belief	Psychoeducation, e.g. danger ideation reduction therapy (St Clair *et al*, 2008)		Chapter 7
Severe depression	Beck-style CBT for depression	Most patients with severe OCD have depression and most will respond to intervention aimed at reducing the OCD	Chapter 8
Reluctance to engage in therapy	Motivational interviewing combined with CBT	Some patients have not reached a stage where they want to be treated and leaving the possibility of future referral is all that can be achieved	Chapter 12
Traumatically induced OCD	EMDR combined with CBT		Chapter 15

CBT, cognitive–behavioural therapy; EMDR, eye movement desensitisation and reprocessing; ERP, graded exposure and self-imposed response prevention; OCD, obsessive–compulsive disorder.

Another approach is to use targeted cognitive techniques if ERP is not immediately successful. Thus, cognitive techniques for trauma may be useful in a patient who has experienced childhood sexual abuse and who presents as an adult with OCD and contamination fears. Initial treatment of the trauma memories using cognitive therapy can be followed up with ERP treatment for the obsessive fears. Other examples of where cognitive intervention may be useful in OCD are given in Table 7.3.

It is important to remember that one of the most common reasons for ERP not being successful is that it is not prescribed or performed in a regular, prolonged, predictable manner. For the best results, ERP should be practised three times a day and for sufficient time to allow the anxiety to reduce consistently by at least 50%. ERP can most usefully be applied in the patient's home setting, where the symptoms are usually maximal (Boschen *et al*, 2010; Boschen & Drummond, 2012).

Key learning points

- OCD consists of anxiogenic obsessions which are maintained by anxiolytic compulsions:
  - obsessions may be thoughts, images or impulses
  - compulsions may be motor acts or thoughts.
- Treatment of OCD involves prolonged graded exposure in real life to the feared situation combined with ERP.
- The family may be involved in performing compulsions for the patient or in providing reassurance. The involvement of family members at some stage in therapy is therefore helpful.
- Obsessions with covert compulsions (ruminations) also respond to ERP.
- Hoarding can occur as part of OCD or as a stand-alone disorder, but similar principles apply.
- Cognitive therapy for OCD offers no advantages and some disadvantages over ERP.
- Targeted cognitive techniques can be useful in some patients who fail to respond to ERP.

Suggested measures to use with conditions covered in this chapter

- OCD: Problems and targets, Sheehan Disability Scale (measuring impact on life), YBOCS and the Padua Inventory, all discussed in Chapter 2.
- Hoarding disorder: Problems and targets, Sheehan Disability Scale (measuring impact on life) and Hoarding Rating Scale Interview, also discussed in Chapter 2.

References

American Psychiatric Association (2000) *Diagnostic and Statistical Manual for Psychiatric Disorders* (DSM-IV-TR). APA.

American Psychiatric Association (2013) *Diagnostic and Statistical Manual for Psychiatric Disorders* (DSM-5). APA.

Boschen MJ, Drummond LM (2012) Community treatment of severe, refractory obsessive-compulsive disorder. *Behaviour Research and Therapy*, **50**: 203–9.

Boschen MJ, Drummond LM, Pillay A, *et al* (2010) Predicting outcome of treatment for severe, treatment resistant OCD in inpatient and community settings. *Journal of Behavior Therapy and Experimental Psychiatry*, **41**: 90–5.

Drummond LM, Fineberg NA (2007) Obsessive–compulsive disorders. In *Seminars in General Adult Psychiatry* (2nd edn) (ed G. Stein, G Wilkinson): 270–86. RCPsych Publications.

Ellis A (1962) *Reason and Emotion in Psychotherapy*. Lyle Stuart.

Emmelkamp PM, Beens H (1991) Cognitive therapy with obsessive-compulsive disorder: a comparative evaluation. *Behaviour Research and Therapy*, **29**: 293–300.

Emmelkamp PMG, Visser S, Hoekstra RJ (1988) Cognitive therapy vs exposure in vivo in the treatment of obsessive-compulsives. *Cognitive Therapy and Research*, **12**: 103–14.

Flessner CA, Penzel F (2010) Current treatment practices for children and adults with trichotillomania: consensus among experts. *Cognitive Behavioural Practice*, **17**: 290–300.

Frost RO, Steketee G, Tolin DF (2011a) Comorbidity in hoarding disorder. *Depression and Anxiety*, **28**: 876–84.

Frost RO, Patronek G, Rosenfield E (2011b) A comparison of object and animal hoarding. *Depression and Anxiety*, **28**: 885–91.

Jones MK, Menzies RG (1998) Danger ideation reduction therapy (DIRT) for obsessive-compulsive washers: a controlled trial. *Behaviour Research and Therapy*, **36**: 959–70.

Krochmalik A, Jones MK, Menzies RG (2001) Danger ideation reduction therapy (DIRT) for treatment-resistant compulsive washing. *Behaviour Research and Therapy*, **39**: 897–912.

McLean PD, Whittal ML, Thordarson DS, *et al* (2001) Cognitive versus behavior therapy in the group treatment of obsessive-compulsive disorder. *Journal of Consulting and Clinical Psychology*, **69**: 205–14.

Ougrin D (2011) Efficacy of exposure versus cognitive therapy in anxiety disorders: systematic review and meta-analysis. *BMC Psychiatry*, **11**: 200.

Rachman S (1976) Obsessional-compulsive checking. *Behaviour Research and Therapy*, **14**: 269–77.

Reinisch A (2009) Characteristics of six recent animal hoarding cases in Manitoba. *Canadian Veterinary Journal*, **50**: 1069–73.

Rodriguez CR, Herman D, Alcon J, *et al* (2012) Prevalence of hoarding disorders in individuals at potential risk of eviction in New York City. *Journal of Nervous and Mental Disorders*, **200**: 10.

Salkovskis PM (1985) Obsessional-compulsive problems: a cognitive-behavioural analysis. *Behaviour Research and Therapy*, **25**: 571–83.

Salkovskis PM (1999) Understanding and treating obsessive-compulsive disorder. *Behaviour Research and Therapy*, **37** (suppl 1): S29–52.

Saxena S, Maidment KM (2007) Treatment of compulsive hoarding. *Focus*, **5**: 381–8.

Saxena S, Ayers CR, Maidment KM (2011) Quality of life and functional impairment in compulsive hoarding. *Journal of Psychiatric Research*, **45**: 475–80.

St Clair T, Menzies RG, Jones MK (2008) *Danger Ideation Reduction Therapy (DIRT) for Obsessive Compulsive Washers: A Comprehensive Guide to Treatment*. Australian Academic Press.

Teng EJ, Woods DW, Twohig MP (2006) Habit reversal as a treatment for chronic skin picking: a pilot investigation. *Behavioural Modification*, **30**: 411–22.

Tyagi H, Drummond LM, Fineberg NA (2010) Treatment for obsessive compulsive disorder. *Current Psychiatry Reviews*, **6**: 46–55.

World Health Organization (1992) *Glossary of Mental Disorders and Guide for their Classification*. For use with International Classification of Diseases, 10th revision. WHO.

Further reading

Hyman BM, Pedrick C (2010) *The OCD Workbook* (3rd edn). New Harbinger Publications.

Marks IM (2001) *Living with Fear: Understanding and Coping with Anxiety*. McGraw-Hill.

Depression

Overview

This chapter will examine the theories of depression. It will start by looking at NICE guidance and present some of the interventions for differing degrees of depression. There will be a discussion of some of the early behavioural interventions and their current role in therapy. Beck's cognitive theory of depression will then be discussed. Case examples will be used to demonstrate behavioural activation and activity scheduling as well as cognitive reattribution. There will be a full description of third generation therapies, which may have a role in the treatment of depression, including case examples illustrating mindfulness and acceptance and commitment therapy. The use of CBT and guided mourning for patients experiencing morbid grief will also be demonstrated.

Depression is an extremely common and disabling problem throughout the world. Indeed, depression is ranked as one of the most frequent causes of disability in the world (World Health Organization, 2001).

Based on figures released by NICE, depression accounts for a third of all consultations with the GP in the UK (http://cks.nice.org.uk/depression#!backgroundsub:1). Each year 5% of adults experience an episode of clinical depression. Episodes of depression serious enough to warrant treatment occur in a quarter of women and 10% of men throughout their lives. Prevalence rates of depression are consistently between 1.5 to 2.5 times higher in women than in men.

Depression was the subject of NICE guidance in 2009. In surveys of patients in the UK, patients prefer to receive CBT than medication wherever possible. It has been shown that CBT is as effective as medication in mild, moderate and severe depression. In the more severe forms of depression, combination of drug therapy and CBT seems to improve outcome.

An important aspect of treating depression is to measure the efficacy of any intervention. One way of doing this is to use a self-completion questionnaire such as the BDI (Beck, 1978). This is a 21-item self-rating scale which allows assessment of overall depressive symptoms. Those scoring less than 10 are not depressed, 10 to 19 is mild depression, 20 to 25 moderate depression and 26 and above indicates severe depression. There is also a 13-item shortened version which allows for quick assessment of depression (Beck *et al*, 1974).

Treatment of depression involves various stages. Obviously it is vital to monitor depression throughout treatment and be particularly mindful of any risk factors and suicidality. Full assessment is also needed and this should focus on:

- physical health (many physical conditions can present with low mood, including anaemia, diabetes, etc.)
- psychiatric symptoms (many psychiatric disorders are complicated by low mood; for example, most patients with severe OCD are also depressed but treatment of the OCD resolves the depression (Boschen & Drummond, 2012))
- full risk assessment
- social situation (this can have a profound effect on mood and the prognosis of the intervention).

Treatment of depression

The National Institute for Health and Care Excellence guidance suggests that people with subclinical as well as mild to moderate depression should be offered either:

- computerised CBT
- self-help CBT
- group exercise activity
- behavioural activation therapy.

People with moderate to severe depressive symptoms should be offered either:

- antidepressant drugs
- antidepressant drugs combined with CBT
- CBT.

Individuals who have frequent relapses of depression should be offered CBT followed by mindfulness-based cognitive therapy (MBCT) to try to reduce relapse. This should be combined with continued antidepressant medication for at least 6 months after resolution of the depressive symptoms.

Development of mastery and pleasure activities and behavioural activation therapy

Lewinsohn, one of the early advocates of behavioural treatments for depression, described four types of intervention (Lewinsohn, 1975):

- increasing activity
- reducing unwanted behaviour
- increasing pleasurable activity
- enhancing skills.

One way to achieve these goals is by focusing on mastery and pleasure. The ideas behind the concepts of mastery and pleasure were developed by a number of researchers in the 1970s and were then adopted as part of standard cognitive therapy for depression by Beck (Beck *et al*, 1979).

Seligman (1975) introduced the idea of 'learned helplessness' as a model for depression. This model was developed from experiments using dogs. Initially, dogs were placed in harnesses so that they could not escape, a buzzer was sounded and then they received an electric shock. After several trials it was noticed that even if the dogs were not tethered and were free to leave, they would not try to escape. Seligman called this 'learned helplessness' and suggested it as a model for human depression.

From this model of depression the model of mastery and pleasure was developed. People who are depressed do less and less and so are not receiving the reinforcement that we all receive from doing things for enjoyment (pleasure) or with a sense of achievement (mastery). The more depressed the individual becomes, the less he or she does and a vicious cycle occurs. This can be broken by activity scheduling in which the individual is asked to very gradually increase their activity. The schedule should provide a mix of activities which give a sense of achievement as well as those which are purely pleasurable (Fig 8.1). Someone who is extremely driven and achieved all the time is unlikely to be truly happy any more than an individual who purely engages in pleasurable activities. People are the most content when they have a balance of both types of activity in their lives.

Over recent years there has been increasing interest in third generation CBT. This is a mixture of interventions which tend to be less focused on cognitive techniques (often labelled second generation therapies) and revert back to the earlier behavioural psychotherapy (first generation). One of these third generation CBT treatments is behavioural activation therapy.

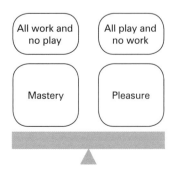

Fig. 8.1   Balance of mastery and pleasure.

115

This treatment is based on the same principles as increasing mastery and pleasure, but also:

- self-monitoring of mood *v.* activities, to demonstrate they are linked
- identification of 'depressed behaviours'
- developing alternative non-depressed behaviours
- addressing avoidance and rumination.

Mastery and pleasure and behavioural activation are demonstrated in Case example 8.1.

Case example 8.1: Mastery and pleasure and behavioural activation

Anne was a 44-year-old housewife with two grown-up children. Over the past 6 months she had been feeling increasingly miserable. She visited her GP, who felt she had mild depression and referred her for psychological treatment.

A full assessment revealed that Anne's mood had deteriorated after her youngest son had left home to go to university. She began to feel 'worthless' and spent increasing time lying around in bed or watching daytime television. In the past she had been busy keeping the household going and in addition she had been an active member of a swimming club, which was an activity she enjoyed. She also regularly socialised with other members of the club, joining them for evening drinks or lunchtime meetings. Since feeling so low, however, she described how she had little energy and so had stopped socialising and attending the club at all.

At this point therapy could have focused either on these negative cognitions (cognitive therapy), or on increasing the fun in Anne's life by activity level changes (behavioural activation). The therapist decided to start with a behavioural activation approach as it would be quicker and easier to implement, less expensive in terms of therapist time (and level of therapist training) and, most importantly, because it was felt that Anne had a mild to moderate condition which would respond to simple interventions.

Anne was asked to complete a diary at home where she would note her activities and also rate her depression and the sense of mastery and pleasure she gained from each of these activities. These three items were scored on a scale from 0 (meaning no mastery or no pleasure, or lowest mood) to 10 (meaning maximum mastery or pleasure, or the best mood) as well as her mood on a scale of 0 to 10. A daily schedule presented in Table 8.1 was obtained for a whole week.

The diary showed that all activities gave Anne little pleasure and no sense of mastery. She had been asked to rate her activities for a week but gave up on the first day at 19.00, saying that there was no point in it. It can be seen that the 'depressive behaviours' were eating three large chocolate bars which made her mood deteriorate further and also ruminating about herself. This was discussed with Anne. She admitted that she did tend to eat large amounts of chocolate when feeling depressed and that, although this temporarily elevated her mood a tiny bit initially, remorse soon set in and left her feeling 'disgusting' for the rest of the day. On discussion, it was agreed that Anne would not keep any chocolate in the house. If she felt she wanted chocolate, she would have to either walk to the local shops to buy some or travel in the car. Buying chocolate and consuming a small bar at a time was rewarding to her but she must not buy more than this and keep any in the house. The role of rumination was also discussed and how thinking about past acts was unproductive and led to low mood. At the end of the session

Table 8.1 Anne's diary at the start of therapy

Day	Time	Activity	Mastery (0–10)	Pleasure (0–10)	Mood (0–10)
Wednesday	8:00	Got up, got dressed, had breakfast	0	0	4
	8:00–10:00	Sat in chair with newspaper but couldn't concentrate	0	0	3
	10:00–12:00	Fell asleep	0	0	2
	12:00	Ate sandwich	0	2	3
	12:05	Ate three large chocolate bars	0	1	0
	13:00–15:30	Watched TV	0	2	1
	15:30–17:00	Sat and thought about my life and how hopeless I am. Shouldn't have eaten three chocolate bars, I am a fat pig!	0	0	0
	17:00–19:00	Watched TV	0	1	0

I am too tired to complete any more of this.

Anne had the following homework tasks:

- to read one page of the newspaper only every day; the page chosen should be the one which was the most interesting to Anne
- to discuss this newspaper story with her husband when he returned from work
- to not keep chocolate in the house
- to walk to the corner shop and purchase one small chocolate bar per day as a 'reward' for sticking to the programme.

She doubted whether she could complete these tasks and failed on the first day to read the page of the newspaper. However, her husband picked a very short article for her to read the next day and she was able to complete this with his encouragement.

Over the next few weeks, it became apparent that depressed activities for Anne included:

- eating sweets and chocolates in large amounts
- sleeping during the day
- ruminating and contemplating her past 'misdemeanours' and failures.

The role of these and the effect on her overall mood was discussed fully with Anne and she was encouraged to replace them with activities that increased her sense of mastery, pleasure and elevated her mood. For example, eating large amounts of sweets and chocolates depressed her mood, whereas sticking to one small bar which she went to the local shops to buy gave her a sense of mastery (being able to walk out of the house) and pleasure (social interaction with shopkeeper and possibly neighbours she might meet as well as the enjoyment from eating something she enjoyed).

After 4 weeks, the therapist talked to Anne about her previous love of swimming.

Anne: 'But the thought of going to a swimming pool fills me with dread.'

Therapist: 'What is the first thought you get if I ask you to plan a trip to the pool?'

Anne: 'I have not got a swimming costume which fits me as I have gained weight!'

It is quite typical for depressed patients to react in this way. Seemingly small difficulties become unsurpassable, and this was dealt with by adopting a behavioural strategy to help her overcome a practical problem.

Anne was given the homework task of buying a swimming costume, followed by going to the swimming pool. Although very reluctant, she agreed to go out to the shops with her daughter who was visiting the following weekend.

The following week Anne returned and said that not only had she bought a costume but she and her daughter had gone swimming. She was pleased with this and explained that, although initially embarrassed by her weight, she had eventually enjoyed it. Using a similar approach Anne was also able to increase her pleasure and mastery of other activities, such as going shopping. At the end of a total of 6 sessions her ratings for mastery and pleasure were significantly improved, as was her depression score. At follow-up 6 months later these scores for a typical day were much better (Table 8.2).

Table 8.2 Anne's diary after 6 months of therapy

Day	Time	Activity	Mastery (0–10)	Pleasure (0–10)	Mood (0–10)
Monday	7:00–8:00	Got up; dressed and had breakfast	0	0	5
	8:00–9:00	Read newspaper	3	3	5
	9:00–10:00	Housework	7	0	4
	10:00–12:00	Swimming and then lunch at pool with friends	7	8	8
	12:00–13:00	Food shopping	3	1	6
	13:00–14:00	Researching family tree on the internet	8	7	8
	14:00–15:00	Walk to local park	3	7	6
	15:00–16:00	Housework	7	0	5
	16:00–17:00	Preparing evening meal	6	2	5
	17:00–18:00	Cut grass and did some weeding and watering in the garden	5	4	6
	18:00–19:00	Telephone calls to family and friends	3	8	7
	19:00–20:00	Dinner with husband	1	8	7
	20:00– 22:00	Conversation with husband	3	7	7
	22:00–midnight	Reading novel	4	7	6
	Midnight	Bed			

Beck's cognitive model of depression

The basis of the theory of depression is that the individual has a distorted or negative view of themselves, the world and the future. This is known as the cognitive triad of depression. The person has negative automatic thoughts (NATs) which result in an immediate change in mood. These NATs arise from deep-seated patterns of beliefs known as schemas (schemata).

All of us develop our view of the world in early life and events which occur shape these. These views and understanding of the world are usually quite primitive and unsophisticated. Because they are developed in early childhood, they have not been subjected to rigorous scrutiny. These patterns of thought are known as schemas. Many of these schemas will be dormant for most of an individual's life. However, a negative activating event can occur and this faulty belief pattern will come to the fore. Negative automatic thoughts then arise from this schema in response to events around the depressed individual (Case example 8.2).

Case example 8.2: Negative automatic thoughts

Sharon (30) had a strong abandonment schema and had spent all her life trying to please others. This schema seemed to develop as a result of Sharon's father leaving her mother when Sharon was 3 years old and then her mother dying when Sharon was 15. Then her boyfriend of 5 years left her suddenly to form a relationship with her close friend. This appeared to be the activating event for her depressive episode.

Sharon went out to the local shops one day and on the way passed a neighbour with her young baby. The woman did not acknowledge her. Sharon's immediate thought was 'she's ignoring me because she doesn't like me; everybody hates me'. If these statements were examined logically, it is obvious that there may be other, more likely explanations for the neighbour ignoring her. The neighbour had a new baby and may have been sleep deprived and preoccupied or she may just not have seen Sharon on the other side of the road.

Cognitive therapy aims to examine the NATs which result in mood change and to help the patient to examine the veracity of these thoughts. Many of the thoughts will be found to have common themes. By examining a number of thoughts it is possible to describe the faulty assumptions that an individual makes. These faulty assumptions are rules which arise from the schema and are held by the individual as 'absolute truths'. They are, however, not logical and are unhelpful. For example, Sharon had a strong abandonment schema. Her faulty assumption which ran through all her NATs was that she was a 'flawed' and unlovable person that everyone would eventually want to leave. Once these faulty assumptions are identified, they can be challenged in the same way as negative automatic thoughts. The advantage of finding faulty assumptions, however, is that they usually underpin most of the NATs.

Thinking errors

Common thinking errors or errors of logic occur in both NATs and faulty assumptions. These are shown in Table 8.3.

Challenging NATs

The basis of CBT for depression and anxiety (and indeed almost all of the treatments described in this book) is known as collaborative empiricism. This means that the therapist does not devise the 'correct' answer but establishes a collaborative relationship with the patient in which the therapist encourages the patient to examine and challenge NATs, examine their beliefs and assess their validity. This collaborative approach is generated by the therapist using Socratic questioning, in which questions are designed for the patient to formulate the answer. For example, when looking at a NAT the patient can be asked:

Table 8.3 Common thinking errors

Thinking error	Desrciption	Example
Overgeneralisation	If one thing is wrong or bad, then everything is wrong or bad	A man attends an interview and does not get the job. He thinks 'I will never get a job, no one will ever take me on'
Magnification or minimisation	Overplaying the importance of negative cues or underplaying the importance of positive cues	A perfectionist school student gets top marks in the class. He thinks 'It's only a small end-of-term examination and does not mean I will do well in the GCSEs'
'All or nothing' thinking	'Black and white' thinking	A woman ruins a special dinner and thinks 'I am a complete failure as a wife and mother'
Selective abstraction and disqualifying the positive	Concentrating on all the negative cues to the detriment of the positive	A man was thinking about his considerable recent successes at work: 'It was all nothing, anyone could have done this better than me'
Arbitrary inference and jumping to conclusions	Conclusions are drawn without weighing up the evidence or considering alternatives	A man with indigestion after a large spicy meal rushes to his doctor thinking 'I must have stomach cancer'
Emotional reasoning		A woman held distressing beliefs based only on her emotions rather than any objective evidence: 'I feel useless, so I cannot be good at anything'

- What is the evidence for this thought?
- Is there any evidence against this thought? (The therapist may need to prompt some replies with additional questions)
- How can we test this out? (Bringing in behavioural experiments)
- Having weighed up the evidence, is there another way of looking at this?

Challenging NATs will be tackled in the next case example (Case example 8.3).

Case example 8.3: Challenging NATs

Freda was 50 years old and worked as an office supervisor. She was married with grown-up children who had moved away from home. Over the past 6 months she had had a severe bout of depression following on from a difficult few years in which her father had died and she had had to move her elderly mother into an old people's home. Freda felt guilty about this but also felt unable to cope with caring for her demanding mother and holding down a responsible job.

In her second session, Freda was extremely depressed and said that this had been caused by an event at work. The previous day she had had a note from her boss asking her to meet with him the following week. Freda immediately felt anxious and depressed. When asked to identify her thoughts she said: 'I have done something wrong. I am a terrible employee, and the boss is probably going to reprimand me for being such a failure.'

Freda was asked for the evidence for this thought and she replied: 'The boss does ask to see people if they are going to be cautioned. I have not been working so well over the past few weeks as I have been very busy and stressed. I am generally slow at work.' She rated her belief in this statement as 95%.

Trying to get Freda to think of evidence against this belief was difficult at first and required the therapist to prompt her with questions such as: 'What do your colleagues think of your work?', 'How fast are you compared with other people?', 'Does the boss ever ask to see anyone for reasons other than to reprimand them?', and 'Are there any other possible reasons the boss may want to see you?'.

Eventually Freda came up with the following evidence against her initial thought:

- 'If I had done something terrible he would ask to see me today/this week.'
- 'My work can't be that bad as I was complimented in last week's board meeting for the quality of my work.'
- 'I am organising a conference next month and it is most likely about that.'

From this evidence, the therapist encouraged Freda to think of a rational response to the original event. This was formulated as: 'I will wait and see why the boss wants to see me. It is likely to be about the big conference I am arranging next month as he did say he wanted to be kept informed about the arrangements and how they are proceeding.' She rated her belief in this rational response as 60%. Her mood improved following this from 2/10 to 5/10.

Clearly it would be very slow if the therapist had to identify every thought and encourage the patient to challenge them in this way. In reality, the therapist needs to do this with a few thoughts and to aim to teach the patient to do this themselves fairly rapidly. The patient needs to do this by keeping a diary and noting down thoughts which lead to a change in mood. Once a number of NATs have been challenged in this way, it is possible using the downward arrow technique to discover the underlying assumptions. If these are challenged, this tackles the basis of the NATs. In addition, the therapist needs to encourage the patient to devise a number of behavioural tests which test out the faulty assumptions and NATs.

Keeping a diary

In the original descriptions of the treatment of depression using CBT, Beck *et al* constructed a six-column diary to be completed by the patient. If such a diary was to be completed by Freda it would look like Table 8.4 (shaded areas represent the six columns described by Beck).

In reality, however, most of the original work on this type of cognitive intervention for depression was done in the USA with private patients who were highly educated, highly motivated and likely to be aware of their thoughts and feelings. This type of diary is usually impossible with NHS patients and it is usually easier to give a simplified diary which can be completed without any risk of failure. Such a diary may look like that in Table 8.5. The diary can then be brought to the session and the full version can be completed during therapy.

Table 8.4 Freda's diary for NATs

Date	Time	Where and what?	Emotion	NAT
13 April	9:00	At work…asked to go and speak to boss next week	Low mood	I have done something wrong

Belief in NAT	Evidence for	Evidence against	Rational response	Belief in rational response
95%	Boss asking to see me Boss does this when something wrong I am generally slow at work	If it was that bad he would ask to see me today/this week I was complimented in last week's board meeting	I will wait and see…this is most likely about the conference I am arranging	60%

NATs, negative automatic thoughts.

Table 8.5 Modified cognitive diary

Date	Time	Where and what?	Emotion	NAT	Belief in NAT, %

NAT, negative automatic thought.

Downward arrow technique to discover faulty assumptions

As already mentioned, once the patient has become used to identifying NATs and challenging them in the way described, it is usually helpful to discover the underlying faulty assumptions behind these thoughts, as they will form the 'themes' of the NATs. By identifying these themes it is usually possible to deal with a whole range of NATs.

The faulty assumptions are accessed by looking at the NATs with the patient and asking the question 'What does that mean?' or 'So what?'. This needs to be done by moving away from the rigid facts and moving more into examining the meaning behind the thought.

In the case of Freda her NAT was 'I have done something wrong' when asked to go and see her boss. The identification of her underlying assumptions was then pursued.

Case example 8.3, continued

Therapist: 'OK, you felt you had done something wrong. What is so bad about that?'

Freda: 'Well you shouldn't make mistakes, it is wrong.'

Therapist: 'Why is it wrong to make mistakes?'

Freda: 'Mistakes show that you are not trying hard enough.'

Therapist: 'What is so bad about that?'

Freda: 'You should always try your best at everything you do.'

Therapist: 'What would it mean if you didn't try your best?'

Freda: 'It would mean you are a worthless person.'

Therapist: 'What is so awful about being a worthless person?'

Freda: 'You cannot be loved or respected by anyone.'

From this conversation, the therapist and Freda were able to identify one of her underlying assumptions to be: 'Making mistakes demonstrates a worthless person who is unlovable and not respected, therefore I must never make mistakes.'

In the dialogue between Freda and her therapist it can be seen that Freda makes a number of statements which feature the word 'should' or 'shouldn't'. This is a common feature when trying to identify underlying assumptions. Because these assumptions are taken as absolute truths and are never questioned by the individual, they often contain rules and instructions to the self featuring the word 'should'. These statements have been called 'tyrannical shoulds'. This idea was initially suggested by the psychoanalyst Karen Horney (1950) and was then developed by Albert Ellis, the founder of rational emotive CBT, into the idea of 'musts' (Ellis, 1994). Both these concepts emphasise the need to look for statements containing these imperative words as they are usually evidence that you are starting to identify the rigidly held, unquestioned core beliefs of the individual.

Behavioural tests

While looking for evidence for and against a particular NAT or an underlying assumption, it is usually helpful to devise a number of behavioural tests to challenge this belief. This was also used in Freda's therapy.

There is often some confusion between behavioural tests and exposure tasks (as discussed in Chapters 6 and 7). Behavioural tests are tasks which are performed to test out a particular belief or hypothesis held by the patient. Exposure tasks are tasks which are designed to produce anxiety and which are performed for sufficient time to allow habituation to occur. Exposure tasks are not performed only once but need to be performed regularly, reliably and for a prolonged time.

To go back to our Case example, Freda and her therapist decided to test whether Freda's NATs were true.

Case example 8.3, continued

The therapist and Freda decided that it would be useful to test whether it was true that people who make mistakes are less loved and respected that those who do not. In order to do this, it was decided that Freda should conduct a survey among her family and friends (behavioural test), asking them:

- 'What do you think of people who never make mistakes?'
- 'What do you think of people who do make mistakes?'
- 'Do you find it easier to respect, like or love someone who never makes a mistake?'

Once Freda completed this survey, she discovered that, contrary to her expectations, most people felt happier and more comfortable with people who were 'human' and did occasionally make mistakes.

Later in therapy, Freda was asked to test out another belief she had, which was that she could not leave the house in casual clothes at the weekend without people looking at her with disdain. Again this was tied into her belief that she needed to be perfect to be loved. She was given two behavioural tests in this case. First, she was asked to go out to the local shopping centre and see how many middle-aged women were wearing casual clothes of jeans or a track suit. The results of this were astounding to Freda, who had been so preoccupied with how she appeared herself, she had not noticed that almost 80% of middle-aged women were wearing casual clothes. The next week she went to the shopping centre wearing jeans and a T-shirt and was asked to particularly focus on people's faces and reactions to her. Again, much to her surprise, few people seemed to notice her at all and most of them were as preoccupied with themselves as she had been!

Normalisation

Many people believe they are 'abnormal' in some way or that the experiences they are having are 'freakish'. It is often useful to try to normalise these experiences. This can be done either by education from the therapist or, often more effectively, by asking the patient to find out this information for themselves, for example be searching the internet (Case example 8.4).

Case example 8.4: Normalisation

A 40-year-old man presented in a very distressed and depressed state. He had recently attended his daughter's school and to his horror had found one of the 15-year-old girls mildly sexually attractive. Filled with remorse, he confessed to his wife, who was similarly horrified. The first job the therapist had to do in this case was to try to normalise this experience. It was explained to him that most men found women and girls of a variety of ages sexually attractive. Mostly, the more sexually mature the girl was, the more likely 'normal' men were to find her attractive. The difference between this and paedophilia is that people with paedophilia do not necessarily favour the more sexually mature girls and even more importantly do not show any restraint and act on their sexual urges. After this had been explained to the man, he was asked to conduct his own internet search to see whether this confirmed what the therapist said. Finally, he was asked to speak to his close male friends and family to discover if they also had similar mild attractions. Performing these three actions effectively reduced some of his guilt and anxiety by normalising his experience. Therapy examining his NATs was then commenced.

Third generation CBT for depressive disorders

These third generation CBT approaches have been developed since the late 1990s. We have already described the evidence for behavioural activation therapy and its efficacy in mild to moderate depression. Third wave therapies which have been used for depression include:

- behavioural activation therapy
- mindfulness-based cognitive therapy (MBCT)
- acceptance and commitment therapy (ACT)
- cognitive behavioural analysis system of psychotherapy
- functional analytic psychotherapy.

A Cochrane review of all studies in third generation CBT therapies compared with standard CBT only found 3 studies with a total of 144 participants that met the eligibility criteria for analysis (Hunot *et al*, 2013). Two of these studies were for ACT and one for behavioural activation. The authors conclude that these therapies appeared to be as effective as standard CBT in the treatment of acute depression but that no other conclusions could be drawn.

Performing a thorough meta-analysis of ACT, DBT, the cognitive behavioural analysis system of psychotherapy, functional analytic psychotherapy (FAP) and integrative behavioural couple therapy, Ost (2008) states: 'The conclusions that can be drawn are that the third wave treatment RCTs used a research methodology that was significantly less stringent than CBT studies; that the mean effect size was moderate for both ACT and DBT, and that none of the third wave therapies fulfilled the criteria for empirically supported treatments'.

Mindfulness-based cognitive therapy

This is a treatment recommended by NICE for the prevention of relapse in moderate to severe depression (National Institute for Health and Clinical Excellence, 2009). It has its roots in meditation techniques from the Far East and Buddhism in particular. As a therapeutic technique, MBCT for chronic and relapsing depression was developed for those patients who cannot maintain the gains after brief time-limited CBT. It originates in Jon Kabat-Zinn's (1990) mindfulness-based stress reduction programme.

Although mindfulness has been used for a variety of psychiatric disorders, the strongest evidence base is for preventing relapse in patients with relapsing depression. This subject has been reviewed by Williams & Kuyken (2012).

Patients with depression and anxiety often focus on the distressing thoughts they experience. In MBCT the patient is instructed in techniques similar to meditation. Using these methods they are encouraged not to 'engage' with the distressing thoughts but to allow these to pass.

In mindfulness, instead of concentrating on changing the content of the NATs, the patient is taught to refocus and to 'distance' themselves from these thoughts. This is done by teaching mindfulness and focusing on the 'here and now'. Practising awareness of how the patient judges and reacts to having NATs can increase the depression, i.e. people may become depressed about the fact they have depressed thoughts rather than seeing these as 'just thoughts'. Identifying this tendency and using mindfulness to distract from these thoughts enables a patient to break the vicious cycle of depressive rumination and to refocus on engagement with life. Full descriptions of mindfulness can be found in Segal *et al* (2002) and in case examples presented below (Case examples 8.5 and 8.6).

Case example 8.5: Recurrent depressive episodes

Sally was a 40-year-old architect who lived with her husband and 4-year-old child. Since she was aged 25 years, she had experienced bouts of depression every 2–3 years. The last episode had been particularly severe and had required her to be hospitalised for strong suicidal thoughts and urges. By the time she was referred to the clinic, she was much improved and rated her depression as 3/10. However, she had still not returned to work and admitted having 'some very dark days'.

Sally was asked to describe the onset of one of her 'dark days'. She had been in the office, one of the juniors had asked her about the details of a housing development and had made the comment that 'I think the first part of this was decided when you were off sick'. After successfully solving the problem, Sally felt herself getting very low. Initially, her thoughts were that she was a 'weak and inadequate person who had depression' and the more she thought about this the more her thoughts escalated. She got a severe headache and after 2 h had to leave the office and return home. She found that her thoughts had now developed and she was panicking that if her negative thoughts could be induced so quickly, she could rapidly descend into very deep depression again. Initially, she had used cognitive challenges for her NATs but she then started to think that just having these thoughts was too much and that she 'could not go on for the rest of my life having these terrible thoughts'.

It was explained to Sally that all people have NATs from time to time. Engaging in these thoughts and escalating them was increasing her problem and resulting in her focusing on her thoughts rather than the things she would want and need to do.

Over the next few weeks, she was taught techniques of mindfulness. This involved teaching her some basic breathing exercises whereby she would concentrate on her breathing and how this made her feel. This was combined with some basic stretches, similar to simple ones used in yoga, to release some of the tension. She was taught to allow her thoughts to come into her mind but, by concentrating on what was actually happening in the world around her, to just note these thoughts rather than engage with them. For example, if she was at the office and experienced some depressive thoughts, she was taught how to 'label' them to herself as depressive and unhelpful and to remember that she had already dealt with them by challenging them in the past. She was to let these thoughts pass and concentrate on what she was doing or what was happening around her. In treating the thoughts in this way and not concentrating on them, she stopped the negative cycle of depressive ruminations from occurring.

Case example 8.6: ACT and mindfulness in chronic low-level depression

George was a 28-year-old man living in a rented shared flat. Since leaving university 5 years earlier, he had not had a permanent job and lived by obtaining occasional bar or seasonal shop work. He had had a low mood since the age of 20 years and, although this fluctuated, he was generally miserable and lacking in motivation and drive. His depression deteriorated 2 years earlier following the breakup of a long-term relationship with a woman that George had been living with since the age of 21 years. His girlfriend said that the main cause of the split was that George was 'going nowhere'. George agreed with this summary of his life but felt unable to 'break out of his negative cycle'. Always a worrier, George would spend several hours in indecision and thinking about everything that had gone wrong during the day and what may go wrong in the future. Previous treatments had included a trial of antidepressants (which George had stopped owing to side-effects) and 12 sessions of CBT. Attempts at behavioural activation had failed because George could not identify any activities he wished to do. It was therefore decided to give him a short trial of ACT.

First, a full risk assessment was performed. George was not, nor had ever been, actively suicidal. Fleeting thoughts of self-harm were more ruminative rather than true plans.

After educating George into the model, he was taught some basic mindfulness techniques, starting with his posture and breathing. The therapist said: 'George, I need you to sit in a comfortable position; some people like to sit on the floor but we will start in our chairs. I want you to sit comfortably with your feel flat on the floor and your back resting against the back of the chair. Please keep your arms comfortably by your side and do not cross them. Now stretch your spine a little – not so that you are stiff and straight but so that you feel very comfortable but also "alert".' This took several minutes to achieve as George was used to sitting hunched up with his head down and his arms and legs crossed. At first he complained that he could not get comfortable but eventually did achieve this. If patients prefer to sit on the floor, then it is advised that they sit 'tailor fashion' with their legs in front of them, bent but not crossed. Some therapists will also advise patients to lie down. After George had made himself comfortable, the therapist continued:

'Now I want us to concentrate on our breathing. Let your eyes close gently and concentrate on thinking about your breathing. Notice how air enters your mouth or nose and feel it as it travels into your lungs. Feel your abdomen stick out as your diaphragm lowers. Now feel the breath coming back up to your nose or mouth as you breathe out. Don't try to change your breathing, just be fully aware of it for a few moments. Feel your abdomen rising and falling. I now would like you to try and breathe in through your nose and out through your mouth and make sure each breath is a full and slow one. Try and feel the relaxation in every part of your body as you breathe out.'

This process is continued with instruction to George to concentrate on his breathing and to notice that gradually with each breath his relaxation deepens. This session was continued for 15 min. Afterwards George reported that he felt very calm and relaxed and much better than he had for a long while. The therapist gave him homework of repeating this 'mindful breathing' for at least 15 min twice a day and to record his mood and stress levels over the week.

The following week, George reported that he felt much more relaxed and had found concentrating on his breathing useful when he was feeling like ruminating about his past failures. He was asked to continue with these techniques and to try to apply them when he was active during the day. Once he was focusing on his breathing, he was also asked to focus on other aspects of the world, such as the colour of the trees and flowers or the gentle rumble of traffic in the local park. The key message was that George must pay attention to the 'here and now' and not start to ruminate on the past which did not achieve anything apart from making him feel miserable. A practice was undertaken when George was asked to sit in a comfortable position and start to ruminate. The therapist then asked him to concentrate on mindful breathing as in the previous session. He was then asked to switch his attention to the sound of the cars on the road outside and the colours in the picture on the wall of the office and to savour and be mindful of them. George was surprised that this technique did distract him from his old patterns of thoughts and allowed him to focus his mind elsewhere. He was instructed that when he started to either ruminate about the past or worry about future events, he was to acknowledge these thoughts but to accept that engaging in them would be unhelpful and move to concentrating on his breathing and then the outside world.

Over the next 3 weeks, George began to be more successful in not engaging with his negative thoughts. He developed the strength to acknowledge these thoughts and let them occur but not then to spend hours ruminating about them. For example, on one occasion his mother telephoned him and told him she was going to the hospital for some tests on her heart the next week. His mother was not unduly worried and had been told this was a precaution as she had recently been experiencing palpitation and irregular heart beat. Normally this information would have meant that George would have sat and ruminated for many hours. He described how he would think about this and would imagine what would happen if his mother died, how his father would cope and about how lonely he would feel. Instead, he was able to hear this news and accept that he would have worrying thoughts coming into his mind but did not allow these to develop into a negative spiral of worries.

George was then asked to practise mindful breathing with the therapist and to think about what he really believed was important in life. What would he want his friends and family to say about him at the end of his life? What did he want to achieve? First, George was flippant saying he wanted 'loads of money and a flash car'. The therapist said:

'That's fine if that is what you want to achieve but let's then look at how you could start to achieve it. What are the ethical values that you deem important? Are there any provisos and things you wouldn't do to achieve this?'

George then admitted that much as he would like to be successful in this way, the most important thing to him was that he could be helpful and supportive to his family and that he passionately believed that there should be more equality in the world and that he would like to help raise money for people in low-income countries. Indeed he admitted that some of his depressive ruminations had been regret that he had been given so much materially, whereas some children were starving in other countries. The therapist then wrote down the two goals of:

- 'Being helpful and supportive to my family'
- 'Helping to raise money for people in low-income countries.'

He was asked to go away this week and, using mindful meditation to clear his mind first, to then sit down and think of his strengths and weaknesses and what he could do to move forward in these life aims. In addition, he was reminded that these were long-term goals and aims that he wanted to achieve and that, although he may be able to make some small steps towards them, he would be working towards these with a series of small steps over many years.

When George came back to the clinic, he had had two major ideas. First, he decided that he would volunteer to accompany his mother to the hospital the following week when she went to see the cardiologist to get her results. He had already telephoned his mother to suggest this. She was delighted, as George had always been so preoccupied with his own worries that he had never volunteered any practical help to others.

Second, he had signed up to run a half marathon in aid of a charity. The race was 6 months away but he had already obtained an online training programme for people who, like him, had not taken regular exercise for a long time and he was committed to completing this. George was praised by the therapist for both of these initiatives. He was asked to make sure he kept his life goals clearly written so that he would remember them whenever he felt despondent or tempted to return to his old ways.

Over the next few months, George had 'ups and downs' but did manage to stick to his basic programme. He volunteered at a charity shop and after 6 months managed to get a badly paid but rewarding job with an international aid agency. He saw this as a 'step on the ladder' to working towards a job that would fully utilise his skills.

Acceptance and commitment therapy (ACT)

Acceptance and commitment therapy has been developed by Steven C. Hayes and Kirk D. Strosahl (2004). The basic tenet of this approach is that most psychological symptoms are a result of people trying to control their unpleasant thoughts, feelings, sensations, urges and memories. In ACT the patient is taught to accept these events for what they are and to concentrate on what they truly believe to be important in life. The key components of ACT are:

- *Living in the here and now*. One of the key tenets of most of the third generation therapies, including mindfulness and DBT. The patient is asked to be in touch with and pay attention to every aspect of the external world in the here and now.
- *Detachment*. This involves the patient 'stepping back' from their unhelpful thoughts, worries and memories. Rather than engaging with them, the patient is taught to acknowledge them and let them pass.
- *Acceptance*. Instead of struggling with worries, thoughts, images and ideas which are painful, the person allows these thoughts 'room' in the mind without engaging with them.
- *Being 'mindful'*. Many third generation therapies involving mindfulness talk about the 'observing self'. This is a concept which is difficult to describe in words but refers to what is generally called the 'mind'. The mind can be divided into two components:
  - the active part, which is constantly thinking and is responsible for thoughts, beliefs, memories, evaluations, etc.
  - the 'observing self', which is the part of the mind that is aware of what an individual is thinking. This is the part which needs to be active in 'mindfulness skills'.
- *Discovering core values*. These are what, deep down, a person wants their life to be about. What are their fundamental beliefs? What do they want to achieve? At the end of the day, what would they like their family and friends to say about them?
- *Acting towards those values*. This involves helping the patient towards achieving these values.

Functional analytic psychotherapy

Functional analytic psychotherapy is a radically behaviourist approach to clinical psychotherapy. It is informed by the work of B. F. Skinner on avoidance. In this therapy, it is postulated that individuals with depression are fearful of situations and relationships. These are addressed by encouraging them to face these fears in the sessions. Although it can be practised alone, this approach is often combined with CBT.

The cognitive behavioural analysis system of psychotherapy is a model of interpersonal and behavioural therapies which has been developed and patented by James P. McCullough (2000, 2006) specifically for the treatment of chronic depression. He describes how he believes in 'disciplined personal involvement' as an alternative to therapist neutrality with patients with chronic depression, explaining how this approach can be used in a contingent manner to successfully modify pathological behaviour.

Abnormal grief and CBT

Grief at a bereavement or other loss is a normal component of the human experience. However, some people experience either greatly prolonged spells of grief or grief which has extreme symptomatology, including extreme depression and suicidal ideation. Exposure therapy for such complicated or prolonged grief was tested in the 1980s by Mawson *et al* using in-patient guided mourning. The theory underpinning guided mourning is that, in abnormal grief reactions, the individual is avoiding coming to terms with the loss fully and is thus avoiding certain cues which make the loss 'seem real'. So, for example, some people keep everything belonging to the deceased person in the same place as they were when the person was alive. Others may avoid cues which remind them of the loss, such as the crematorium. Mawson *et al* (1981) found that the patients who received guided mourning improved more on several measures than control patients who were encouraged to avoid thinking about their loss.

Over the next decade, several clinicians found that, although exposure methods reduced some aspects of abnormal grief, it was also important for the patient to 'move on' in therapy from the loss. Specific cognitive behavioural therapy techniques were introduced to examine some of the guilt feelings as well as encouraging the bereaved person to rebuild their life after their loss (Case example 8.7).

Case example 8.7: Guided mourning and cognitive reattribution

Phyllis, a 70-year-old lady, had been complaining of feeling depressed for the past 7 years, following the death of her elderly mother. Her mother had had Alzheimer's dementia which had been diagnosed 5 years before her death. Phyllis had stopped her work as a nurse to care for her mother once the diagnosis had been made.

Since her bereavement, Phyllis had been experiencing low mood, early morning wakening and a variety of physical complaints. Initially she had thought about returning to work, but felt that she would be unlikely to get a job at the age of 63. Indeed, at first Phyllis had not demonstrated many signs of grief and people had commented on how well she was coping. There was still no grave or monument arranged, even though Phyllis wanted to arrange one. After the cremation, the undertaker had asked her what she wanted done with her mother's ashes and she had told him to scatter them somewhere in the crematorium as she felt confused about what she should do.

In the first session the therapist explained the features of healthy grief and discussed why the current situation was unhelpful for Phyllis. In addition, they reviewed the events prior to her mother's death. She was helped to understand how not facing up to sad feelings at the time of her mother's death was related to her current symptoms. As with patients with a phobia, it is often useful to explain how avoidance can lead to difficulties later on: 'If you fall off a bicycle, the best thing is to get back on right away. The longer you wait, the more difficult it will be for you to ride again. You did not face the sad feelings about your mother at the time, because it was so painful, and that was understandable, but now you can see the importance of facing up to these feelings as soon as possible.'

In the second session Phyllis discussed ways that she might be able to face the loss at this late stage, the problem being that the crematorium meant little to her. As a homework exercise, she was asked to try to think of a way to overcome this problem and decided to arrange a memorial to her mother.

This was to be a rose planted in the garden of remembrance or a seat in the garden of remembrance, with a plaque bearing an inscription to her mother.

First, the issue of guilt was addressed. Phyllis felt she must be a very wicked person to have these angry feelings towards her mother, who had cared for her throughout childhood and had then been very ill and had not meant to interfere with Phyllis' life. Although Phyllis was a highly practical person, she was not well attuned to her thoughts and emotions. The therapist decided to try some role-play first with her. She was asked to role-play a nurse and the therapist would play Phyllis. In this session, Phyllis, who had dealt with bereaved relatives of patients throughout her professional life, was able to give good challenges to all of the NATs and guilt feelings the therapist expressed. She was asked to record her period of low mood and guilt in a diary along with these thoughts. An extra column was included and was headed 'What I would tell someone else having the same thoughts'. By doing this, Phyllis was able to perform cognitive reattribution and to see that her thoughts were, indeed, normal, natural and human.

In addition, Phyllis felt that she had never been able to talk to her mother about certain things and to move on from her death. She was asked to write a letter to her mother, expressing all her gratitude and love towards her, her feelings of anger and frustration, and telling her mother of her dreams for the future. She was also asked to say 'goodbye' to her mother in this letter and to say that she was going to 'move on' with her life.

Phyllis wrote an extensive, moving letter to her mother. She said she wanted to leave this letter symbolically 'with' her mother. To this end, she had arranged to plant a rose bush in the garden of remembrance and had decided she would bury the letter in the soil near to this plant.

Not all patients suffering from grief are as insightful as Phyllis, but it is useful to remember the following phases of treatment, which should be used:

- graded exposure to any avoidance cues
- examination of any unhelpful thoughts and self-blame surrounding the loss using CBT
- encouraging the patient to say 'goodbye' and move on with their life.

Suggested measures to use with conditions covered in this chapter

- Problems and targets (Chapter 2, p. 24), BDI (Beck, 1978), BDI 13-item (Beck et al, 1974), Montgomery Asberg Depression Rating Scale (Montgomery & Asberg, 1979).

References

Beck AT (1978) *Depression Inventory*. Philadelphia Center for Cognitive Therapy.
Beck AT, Rial WY, Rickels K (1974) Short form of depression inventory: cross validation. *Psychological Reports*, **34**: 1184–6.

Key learning points

- Depression is an extremely common problem. Mild to moderate depression can be treated using CBT alone, but more severe depression may require antidepressant drugs, which can be combined with CBT.
- Treatment can involve behavioural activation and activity scheduling to increase opportunities for socially reinforcing activities that can improve mood.
- People who are content have a balance of activities in their lives with a roughly equal amount of mastery and pleasure. In individuals with depression both types of activity are usually at a low level and increasing these can improve mood.
- Beck's cognitive model of depression states that the depressed individual has a distorted or negative view of the world, themselves and the future. This is the cognitive triad.
- Patterns of thoughts are laid down as schema. Many of these remain dormant but can be brought to the fore by an activating event.
- From these schemas, faulty assumptions emerge. These are often illogical and a gross oversimplification.
- NATs arise from the schemas and faulty assumptions. These are thoughts which come into the person's mind and result in their mood deteriorating.
- In cognitive therapy, NATs are challenged using collaborative empiricism and Socratic questioning. Evidence for and against these thoughts is devised and leads to a 'rational response'.
- Once a few NATs have been identified, the downward arrow technique can be used to identify faulty underlying assumptions.
- Underlying assumptions can be challenged by examining evidence and by behavioural tests.
- Normalisation is an educational technique whereby the patient learns that their behaviour is not abnormal.
- Mindfulness-based cognitive therapy is based on the meditation techniques of some Eastern religions. It teaches the patient to let thoughts come and go without necessarily focusing on them. It can be useful for relapsing depressive disorder.
- Acceptance and commitment therapy which has mindfulness as part of its structure can be useful in patients with chronic relapsing depression.
- Other third generation therapies such as functional analytic psychotherapy and the cognitive behavioural analysis system of psychotherapy have also been used to treat chronic depressive disorders.
- Abnormal grief reactions may present with depression. Treatment of abnormal grief can be guided mourning, which is a form of graded exposure. This should be combined with cognitive strategies aimed at assisting the patient in moving on with their life after the grieving process.

Beck AT, Rush JA, Shaw BF, *et al* (1979) *Cognitive Therapy of Depression*. Guilford Press.

Boschen MJ, Drummond LM (2012) Community treatment of severe, refractory obsessive-compulsive disorder. *Behaviour Research and Therapy*, **50**: 203–9.

Ellis A (1994) *Reason and Emotion in Psychotherapy* (revised and updated). Birch Lane.

Hayes SC, Strosahl KD (2004) *A Practical Guide to Acceptance and Commitment Therapy*. Springer.

Horney K (1950) *Neurosis and Human Growth*. WW Norton.

Hunot V, Moore TH, Caldwell DM (2013) 'Third wave' cognitive and behavioural therapies versus other psychological therapies for depression. *Cochrane Database of Systematic Reviews*, **10**: CD008704.

Kabat-Zinn J (1990) *Full Catastrophe Living: Using the Wisdom of Your Body and Mind to Face Stress, Pain, and Illness*. Delacorte Press.

Lewinsohn PM (1975) Behavioral study and treatment of depression. In *Progress in Behavior Modification, Vol. 1* (eds RM Eisler, PM Miller). Academic Press.

Mawson D, Marks IM, Ramm L, *et al* (1981) Guided mourning for morbid grief: a controlled study. *British Journal of Psychiatry*, **138**: 185–93.

McCullough JP (2000) *Treatment for Chronic Depression: Cognitive Behavioral Analysis System of Psychotherapy*. Guilford Press.

McCullough JP (2006) *Treating Chronic Depression with Disciplined Personal Involvement: Cognitive Behavioral Analysis System of Psychotherapy*. Springer.

Montgomery SA, Asberg M (1979) A new depression scale designed to be sensitive to change. *British Journal of Psychiatry*, **134**: 382–9.

National Institute for Health and Clinical Excellence (2009) *Depression: Treatment and Management of Depression in Adults, Including Adults with Chronic Physical Health Problems* (Clinical Guideline CG90). NICE.

Ost LG (2008) Efficacy of the third wave of behavioral therapies: a systematic review and meta-analysis. *Behaviour Research and Therapy*, **46**: 296–321.

Segal ZV, Teasdale JD, Williams J (2002) *Mindfulness-Based Cognitive Therapy for Depression*. Guilford Press.

Seligman MEP (1975) *On Depression, Development and Death*. WH Freeman.

Williams JM, Kuyken W (2012) Mindfulness-based cognitive therapy: a promising new approach to preventing depressive relapse. *British Journal of Psychiatry*, **200**: 359–60.

World Health Organization (2001) *Mental Health: A Call for Action by World Health Ministers*. WHO.

Recommended treatment manuals and other reading

Beck AT, Rush JA, Shaw BF, *et al* (1979) *Cognitive Therapy of Depression*. Guilford Press.

Crane R (2009) *Mindfulness-Based Cognitive Therapy*. Routledge.

Ekers D, Richards D, McMillan D, *et al* (2011) Behavioural activation delivered by the non-specialist: phase II randomised controlled trial. *British Journal of Psychiatry*, **198**: 66–72.

Flaxman PE, Blackledge JT, Bond PW (2011) *Acceptance and Commitment Therapy*. Routledge.

*Gilbert P (2009) *Overcoming Depression: A Self-Help Guide Using Cognitive Behavioural Techniques*. Constable & Robinson.

*Greenberger D, Padesky CA (1995) *Mind over Mood: Change How You Feel by Changing the Way You Think*. Guilford Press.

Kanter JW, Busch AM, Rusch LC (2009) *Behavioural Activation*. Routledge.

Williams M, Teasdale J, Segal Z, *et al* (2007) *The Mindful Way Through Depression*. Guilford Press.

*Suitable to recommend to patients.

Generalised anxiety disorder and panic

Overview

Effecting change in lifestyle and behaviour including encouraging healthy diet, regular exercise and avoiding the usage of stimulants and depressants will be demonstrated as well as the effect this may have on anxiety symptoms. The use of anxiety management training will be demonstrated and cognitive challenges will be introduced in clinical case examples including the use of behavioural avoidance tests. The difference between behavioural avoidance tests and graded exposure will be discussed. Clark's cognitive model of panic will be explored. Finally, there will be a discussion about the use of cognitive therapy for patients in different situations, including those at end of life as well as the role of mindfulness techniques for anxiety.

Anxiety is a universal phenomenon. All of us experience anxiety in response to dangers or threats in the environment. Too high or too low anxiety levels hinder performance at tasks and there is an optimal level of anxiety to aid performance. This phenomenon is known as the Yerkes–Dodson law (Yerkes & Dodson, 1908), illustrated in Fig. 9.1.

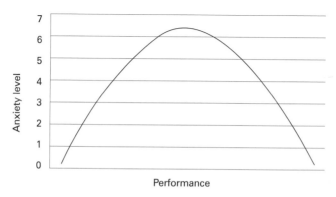

Fig. 9.1   Yerkes–Dodson law – the optimal level of anxiety to aid performance.

People also vary in the anxiety they experience and in their background level of anxiety (known as trait anxiety). Some individuals are very 'laid-back' with low trait anxiety and some people are very 'highly strung' with high background levels of anxiety. The situations and stimuli that increase anxiety (known as state anxiety) also vary from person to person. It can thus be seen that there is not any one level of anxiety that can be described as universally abnormal as it depends on the person's inherent nature as well as their current circumstances. A useful definition of pathological anxiety is 'anxiety which is either more severe or more frequent than the individual can tolerate or is used to'.

Anxiety is a state which can mimic a range of conditions, involving all systems of the body; some of these are listed in Table 9.1. These symptoms can be seen to be a function of an imbalance between the sympathetic and parasympathetic autonomic nervous system, a predominance of the sympathetic nervous system or increase in muscular tension as the individual prepares for 'fight or flight'.

Psychological experiences of anxiety are often described as:

- foreboding
- loss of control
- feeling as if about to die.

Differential diagnosis of anxiety disorders

Some physical disorders can present with apparent symptoms of anxiety. To prevent potentially treatable physical causes being overlooked, it is always advisable to think of the following possible causes (this list is not exhaustive):

- mitral valve prolapse
- 'normal' extrasystoles and palpitation
- postural orthostatic tachycardic syndrome (this is a condition of autonomic dysfunction or failure which is frequently misdiagnosed as generalised anxiety and panic)
- anaemia (can cause palpitation as well as headache and muscle pain)

Table 9.1 Possible symptoms of anxiety

Body system	Examples of symptom
Cardiovascular	Palpitation, tightness in chest, flushing
Respiratory	Breathlessness, tightness in chest
Genito-urinary	Urinary frequency, incontinence
Gastrointestinal	Diarrhoea, incontinence, dyspepsia, nausea
Central nervous	Headache, light-headedness
Musculoskeletal	Muscle pains and tension

- paroxysmal atrial tachycardia
- thyrotoxicosis
- poorly controlled diabetes
- adrenal tumours
- carcinoid syndrome
- Zollinger–Ellison syndrome (hypoglycaemia leading to increased sympathetic outflow).

In addition the following lifestyle factors can also lead to anxiety symptoms:

- excessive caffeine intake
- excessive use of nicotine
- excessive use of alcohol (withdrawal in the form of a 'hangover' is partially characterised by increased sympathetic outflow)
- drug misuse (cannabis excess generally leads to increased vagal output; amphetamines to increased sympathetic output)
- withdrawal from benzodiazepine medication
- irregular meals leading to hypoglycaemia
- reactive hypoglycaemia
- insufficient regular exercise
- excessive tiredness.

Anxiety can also occur as a symptom in almost any psychiatric disorder, including most commonly depression and psychosis. In most cases, anxiety is a symptom and thus treatment should be aimed at the underlying condition, for instance treatment of the psychotic illness with antipsychotic drugs or treatment of the depression or anxiety/depression with antidepressant drugs in the first instance.

Diagnosis of anxiety disorders

Anxiety disorders can be divided into:

- phobic anxiety
- OCD (although this is no longer categorised as an anxiety disorder, it does still frequently present with the major symptom of anxiety)
- generalised anxiety disorder
- panic disorder.

In DSM-5 (American Psychiatric Association, 2013) anxiety disorders are included under the heading of mood disorders. Similar proposals are made for ICD-11 (Clark & Watson, 2006). This is because of the noted interlinking of anxiety and depression. Whereas in DSM-IV and ICD-10 panic disorder took diagnostic precedence over other disorders such as agoraphobia, in DSM-5 these are separated and so agoraphobia may or may not be comorbid with panic disorder. It is likely that ICD-11 will follow similar classification to DSM-5.

Generalised anxiety disorder and panic

Many patients with generalised anxiety disorder may also experience panic. In general, the approaches to both conditions are similar, though there are additional strategies which can be useful in panic and these will be described later in the chapter.

With many patients with generalised anxiety disorder there will be a need to consider both cognitive and behavioural strategies to overcome the problem. In some situations, simple interventions examining the patient's lifestyle can radically reduce the symptoms without the need to resort to more intensive treatments. Even if it is clear that the individual's behaviour is having a definite impact on their symptoms, it is often difficult to effect change. This is where collaborative empiricism and Socratic questioning are useful. See Case example 9.1.

Case example 9.1: Poor lifestyle leading to generalised anxiety

Richard, a 32-year-old unmarried merchant banker, was referred to the clinic with a 1-year history of severe panic attacks. These could happen at any time of the day or night and consisted of palpitations, sweating and a feeling of impending doom. They occurred approximately once a month and would last for 2–3 days. During an episode, panic symptoms would last for approximately 30 min and occur 4–6 times a day. Richard could not think of a precipitant for these symptoms.

A full history was taken of the problem, including some examination of Richard's lifestyle. He woke at 7.00 and left the house 20 min later, having had no breakfast. A busy morning at work would also involve him drinking at least 3 cups of espresso. In addition, Richard smoked approximately 15 cigarettes a day. Lunch consisted of either a sandwich or frequently a bar of chocolate if he was busy. During the afternoon he would again have 5–6 cups of espresso before finishing work at 18:30 or 19:00. Then he often met friends to eat out in a restaurant, consuming up to half a bottle of wine before returning home to bed after midnight. Richard took little exercise and his only hobbies were eating out or visiting the pub to drink. Although he was not overweight, he noticeably lacked tone, had poor posture, and appeared much older than his years.

Richard was asked what he thought about his lifestyle. He said he realised it was 'appalling' but found it extremely difficult to change. Several times he had decided to quit smoking and stop drinking at the same time but had always gone back to both within a few days.

The therapist started by educating Richard about healthy lifestyles. Smoking greatly increased his risk of heart disease, stroke and cancer, and stopping smoking would be the single most important step Richard could make in his bid to improve his health. Smoking a cigarette causes a temporary increase in blood sugar which returns to normal after half an hour. These changes, and particularly the reduction in blood sugar when combined with Richard's poor diet, might well contribute to his having bouts of hypoglycemia, which could trigger palpitation, nausea, malaise and panic. In addition, nicotine is a stimulant drug which increases the sympathetic outflow and makes panic more likely.

Richard currently drank half a bottle of red wine every day. It was explained to him that he was consuming in the region of 49 units of alcohol a week. The maximum safe limit of alcohol for men up to the age of 60 years is 21 units (half this amount beyond age 60 years). In addition, there should be at least 2–3 alcohol free days a week and the maximum number of drinks per session should be 4–5. Continuing to drink at the excessive level that Richard was consuming was endangering his liver, heart and cardiovascular system and placing him at increased risk of many serious conditions, including ischaemic heart disease, stroke and cancer. In addition, alcohol interferes with glucose metabolism. After the alcohol is metabolised by the body, the blood sugar frequently drops the next day. The effect is that Richard was likely to be hypoglycaemic, and this was increased by his not eating breakfast and by his smoking. This hypoglycaemia may trigger the symptoms resulting in panic.

Other factors which were likely to contribute to Richard's symptoms were:

- irregular meals leading to erratic blood sugar levels
- eating high-sugar foods on an empty stomach, which may lead to hyperglycaemia followed by hypoglycaemia
- high caffeine intake (caffeine is a stimulant and thus can precipitate anxiety and panic)
- lack of exercise and working long hours in a sedentary job.

Richard's resting pulse rate was 98 beats per minute. This demonstrated his lack of fitness and made it more likely that he would experience palpitation.

Clearly no one could expect Richard to revolutionise his entire lifestyle immediately. The therapist, therefore, asked him what he would feel able to tackle initially. Richard was sceptical that his lifestyle had any effect on his symptoms at all but eventually agreed to test this out. He was adamant he was not ready to tackle his most serious problems of tobacco and alcohol misuse but agreed to examine his diet.

He agreed to eat three meals a day consisting of the following foods: breakfast – porridge with one banana and glass of orange juice; lunch – round of sandwiches and a piece of fruit; dinner – in restaurant. Richard agreed to eat at least two portions of vegetables at this last meal. In addition, he agreed to stop drinking espresso and to change to the decaffeinated variety or to drink tea, which contains less caffeine. The therapist warned Richard that when people stopped or reduced their caffeine intake, many would suffer from withdrawal symptoms. These usually consisted of a headache, which generally started 24–48 h after the reduction in caffeine, and could be accompanied by sweating and tremulousness. These symptoms should reduce after approximately 24 h and were evidence of caffeine dependence. Richard was asked to record his success with these changes and to record the time and situation of any 'panic' episodes.

At the end of the first week, Richard reported that he was feeling much better than before. He had experienced a mild headache after reducing his intake of fresh coffee, but this had settled quickly. Nearly all his 'funny turns' were happening in the morning, and he felt that he would like to reduce his alcohol intake to below the recommended limit of 21 units. A full drinking history was taken from Richard and the therapist suggested ways in which he could pace and slow his drinking as well as advising him on low-alcohol and alcohol-free beverages. Richard felt that he could reduce his alcohol intake best by travelling to the restaurant or pub in his car as he would never drink and drive. He could do this by refusing lifts from others and volunteering to take others in his car (over the past few years, he felt that he 'owed' most of his friends a large number of car journeys).

When Richard returned 2 weeks later, he had been remarkably successful in reducing his alcohol intake and did not require any of the specific interventions for reducing excessive alcohol consumption (these will be described in Chapter 12). The therapist praised him for his rapid and excellent progress. He was only complaining of 'funny turns' once or twice a week. Richard was then asked if he wished to concentrate on consolidating his gains for a while or start to introduce another behavioural change. He felt that he did not wish to reduce his smoking at this time, but enquired about exercise. It was explained to him that it was extremely important for him to find a form of exercise which he could enjoy and perform regularly and not something which would be a penance. Regular exercise would not only increase his general fitness and reduce his heart rate and tendency to palpitations, but also give him another interest apart from work. Indeed, regular aerobic exercise has been shown to have a beneficial effect on people with true anxiety symptoms (Sciolino & Holmes, 2012).

Richard felt that he would hate jogging or running. After some discussion with the therapist, it was revealed that while at school, Richard had been a member of the school swimming team. He had not swum for several years and had not thought about restarting as he realised that at his age he was too old to take part in true competitive swimming. The therapist suggested that he might like to think of other alternatives and should visit the local baths and find out about life-saving classes, long-distance swimming clubs and veteran swimming clubs for adults. Richard agreed to do this and committed to the goal of going swimming at least once a week.

Over the next few weeks, Richard became increasingly enthusiastic about his rediscovered hobby of swimming. He had joined a club for people aged over 30 years which met twice a week and organised galas with races for different age groups. He had also managed to reduce his smoking and was planning to stop as he felt it had a deleterious effect on his swimming performance. The incidence of 'panic' episodes was now negligible and this improvement was maintained at one year follow-up.

Sleep hygiene

Many people with anxiety disorders complain of difficulty sleeping. This lack of sleep makes the individual more prone to symptoms of anxiety and depression. Indeed, poor sleep is a widespread complaint among the general population and is more common in older people. General practitioners are often asked by their patients to prescribe hypnotic drugs. The main category of these drugs are benzodiazepines, which should be used for a maximum of 6 weeks. Benzodiazepines can cause both tolerance and dependency and, particularly in elderly people, can result in confusion, drowsiness and falls (a particular worry in this patient group). The quality of sleep achieved with these drugs is not as deep or as refreshing as 'natural' sleep. Sleep deprivation may precipitate positive symptoms of schizophrenia and other psychotic disorders (see Chapter 13).

Sleep hygiene measures are a group of techniques which can help to treat insomnia, thereby reducing benzodiazepine prescription and also making people who feel unwell due to lack of sleep feel better again. The principles of sleep hygiene are discussed below.

Psychoeducation

Many patients do not realise that, in general, we need less sleep as we get older. Whereas most people recognise that children need progressively less sleep as they get older, many are not aware that elderly people need less sleep than young adults. In general, younger people will have a tendency to be 'owls' and be able to stay up late and like to sleep in late in the morning, but the normal diurnal variation tends to change as we age and previous 'owls' become 'larks', feeling sleepy early and being unable to sleep in the morning.

To be able to sleep well, people need to engage in physical as well as mental activity. Many people today do not engage in even minimal exercise. Exercise during the day, particularly outside, is good at assisting sleep at night. In general, most people will benefit from walking 10000 steps a day (approximately 4–5 miles) plus three episodes of moderate aerobic activity of at least 30 min each per week.

Alcohol is often thought to help people to sleep but in reality it is similar to benzodiazepines in its effect, causing people to sleep lightly and fitfully and to awaken feeling unrefreshed.

Drinks containing caffeine should be avoided for the last 4 hours before bedtime as they can have a dramatic effect on the ability to sleep. Caffeine can be found in coffee, tea and many proprietary drinks including 'colas' and 'energy' drinks.

Preparation for bedtime

For the last 2 hours before bedtime, it is advisable not to drink any fluid to prevent the urge to have to get up in the night to pass urine. If the individual really feels the need of a drink then either warm milk or a malt-based drink can assist the feeling of sleepiness.

Time should be spent relaxing in low light, maybe with a reading lamp and a relaxing book. People with difficulty sleeping should avoid working using the computer (or other electronic devices) or watching television for 2 hours before bedtime (Figueiro *et al*, 2011), as it has been found that the blue light they emit supresses the production of melatonin necessary to induce sleep.

Some people find that a warm bath helps them to relax.

Making the bedroom a place for sleep

The bedroom should be a place for sleeping and no other activity. There should not be any television, computer or other device in the bedroom. Nor should the patient read in bed. The idea is to ensure that the bedroom becomes the place associated with sleep and not other activities.

It is important that the bedroom is dark and as quiet as possible. Darkness encourages the secretion of melatonin, which helps induce natural sleep.

141

Coping with sleeplessness

The patient should be encouraged to lay in bed relaxing and with eyes closed for 30 min. If sleep has not occurred by that time, then they should get up and return to sitting quietly in a darkened room elsewhere. Once they feel sleepy again, they should return to bed and try again. There may be multiple episodes on the first night with the patient going to bed and then getting up. This will tend to get less as the programme continues.

Regularising daily patterns of behaviour

Many people with poor nocturnal sleep dose or nap at other times of the day. It is very important that this does not happen, as these naps reduce the tendency to sleep at night. The patient will often complain that they will feel too sleepy if they do this, but that is the main objective: to go to bed tired and have a good night of sleep!

Exposure treatments for non-phobic anxiety

The idea that exposure can be used for non-phobic anxiety is, at first sight, somewhat surprising. There are, however, three ways in which this may be useful:

- avoiding avoidance
- hyperventilation provocation
- prediction testing (behavioural tests).

Avoiding avoidance

Although people with generalised anxiety do not, by definition, have clear phobic anxiety, many do have more subtle avoidance strategies which can affect their symptoms.

For example, a 54-year-old man had had a heart attack 3 years before. He had received a stent procedure to unblock one of his coronary arteries, had improved his diet, was now exercising regularly and had lost weight so that his body mass index (BMI) was within normal range. However, he presented with extreme fear that he would have another heart attack. He was constantly monitoring his pulse rate and was introspective and concerned by any bodily symptoms. Further delving into his history revealed that he avoided intercourse with his wife – this was because his initial symptoms began when having intercourse and he feared bringing on another attack. Treatment involved him facing up to the feared activity and when he had done so he made a rapid recovery.

A 25-year-woman with anxiety symptoms claimed she worked from home as she preferred to do so and wished to avoid spending money commuting. However, careful questioning revealed that she had once had an episode of panic while on an underground train and since then had tried to work exclusively from home. Again, treatment involved some graded exposure.

Hyperventilation provocation

This technique was first used by Joseph Wolpe in 1958 when he asked patients to inhale a mixture of 65% carbon dioxide and 35% oxygen. This induced shortness of breath, flushing, paraesthesia, light-headedness and dizziness which he noted to be similar to panic.

Many patients start to breathe rapidly and shallowly when they become anxious. This causes the same symptoms noted by Wolpe. Patients can be taught to breathe deeper and slower by placing their hand below their diaphragm on their abdomen and noting how this should go out on inhalation and go in on expiration. They are advised to count slowly to 5 for an in-breath; 5 when they hold their breath and 5 for an out-breath.

In the 1980s, David Clark developed a cognitive model of panic. He utilised hyperventilation as a way of inducing panic and would then use this behavioural test as a challenge to the NATs (Clark, 1986). Clark's model for panic will be discussed later in this chapter (p. 149).

Hyperventilation can also be used as a form of exposure. Many anxious patients are so frightened by the idea of panic and the symptoms they experience that they avoid any situations which may provoke this. By encouraging them to hyperventilate and induce symptoms, they can learn to control these panic episodes.

To induce these symptoms, it is usually necessary to hyperventilate for up to 2 min. Most patients have difficulty in performing over-breathing to a sufficient extent to reproduce symptoms if just asked to do so. For this reason, it is better for the therapist to perform the exercise along with the patient. The resultant symptoms and signs produced in the therapist can be an additional useful learning experience for the patient. Any therapist should remember that this technique does produce a number of unpleasant symptoms and it is advisable for the therapist not to drive for at least 30 min after performing this exercise. Getting the patient to over-breathe is useful in two ways: it helps put symptoms in perspective ('Well, I survived that, so perhaps that real thing is not going to kill me after all') and also is good practice in exposure to feared symptoms and their consequences.

As well as giving the patient an experience of how hyperventilation may provoke symptoms, it is also useful to teach controlled breathing so that the patient learns to control the panic symptoms. These breathing techniques were described fully in the case example of Adrian (Case example 6.2, pp. 80–82).

There are some medical conditions where hard hyperventilation may be contraindicated, such as recent myocardial infarction and some forms of obstructive airways disease. In these cases the therapist may demonstrate the effect of voluntary hyperventilation on self and then tell the patient what effect it had. It is also a sound practice to use modelling in this way with any patient reluctant to use this technique.

Relaxation

Relaxation and stress reduction exercises can be useful if a patient is experiencing constantly high levels of anxiety. There are many forms of relaxation available in audio form online and a version which suits the patient can be used and taught by the therapist. A few patients, however, do find it very difficult to relax and any encouragement to do so can result in further tension as they 'try very hard to relax'. In these cases mindfulness, a form of relaxation which encourages relaxation by meditation, may be useful.

It is also wise to remember that relaxation has only a very limited role in helping anxiety and should rarely, if ever, be used alone. For example, most people can be taught to relax at home. However, if after being taught relaxation, the person is taken for the first time into a light aircraft and told to jump with a parachute, they are likely to experience anxiety. Any amount of relaxation training will not change this in most cases. Thus, although relaxation may be helpful for general stress and tension, it is not helpful for situational anxiety.

Anxiety-management training

Anxiety-management training programmes or stress reduction programmes vary in their content but generally consist of:

- education of the patient about their symptoms and normalisation of anxiety symptoms
- teaching the person how to identify the maintaining factors and examining how to eliminate these (the most common maintaining factors are anticipatory anxiety, fear of fear, avoidance and loss of self-confidence)
- teaching coping skills for the maintaining factors, for example distraction and relaxation for anticipatory thoughts, exposure for fear of fear and avoidance, relaxation skills for fear of fear, and assertiveness training for loss of self-confidence and social anxiety
- reinforcing self-statements often in the form of cue cards to remind the person: to pay more attention to their surroundings than their internal experiences; that anxiety is temporary and will pass; or of their coping strategies.

Such a programme is presented in Case example 9.2.

Case example 9.2: Anxiety-management training

James, an extremely anxious 55-year-old man, had a large number of physical complaints. He became breathless for no apparent reason, had sensations of 'pins and needles' in both arms and a feeling of discomfort in his abdomen, which he described as 'like butterflies in the stomach'. His doctor could not find any organic cause for the symptoms which seemed to arise 'out of the blue'. They started a year earlier at the time that his brother, who was 2 years his senior, had suffered a heart attack. His brother had now made a complete recovery.

Education and normalisation

A session was spent allowing James to talk about the symptoms and how and why they occur. It was pointed out that when he becomes anxious he breathes too fast and it was explained that this lowers the carbon dioxide levels in his blood too much and is the cause of the 'pins and needles'.

Similarly, he was given an explanation for the abdominal discomfort: 'When you feel tense you become aware of sensations from gut contractions that you would not otherwise experience – it is a normal physiological reaction that you are pathologically aware of due to your overarousal.'

Teaching coping skills

To begin with, James was taught to monitor his breathing and to practise controlled breathing when he began to feel anxious. He was asked to place his hand on his solar plexus and to take a deep breath in and feel his abdomen swell for the count of 5. Then he was told to hold his breath and then exhale, both again for the count of 5.

He also found it useful to have a cue card which reminded him what was happening to him when in a state of anxiety:

- 'Breathing too fast is something I do when I get anxious'
- 'Breathing too fast removes the carbon dioxide from my blood and then I get the pins and needles'
- 'Butterflies in my stomach are due to anxiety'
- 'If I just calm down and wait, these anxiety symptoms will go away'.

Each of these statements was devised following discussions between James and his therapist. Each one was only written on the card after James had agreed that it was a meaningful statement that was relevant to his difficulty. He was given the homework task of reading the card each evening and carrying it around in his pocket. Whenever he experienced a symptom, he was to pull out his card and read it to himself.

Coping with the feeling of being overwhelmed

At times, utter panic would cause James to tremble such that he could not even hold the card still enough to read it. To deal with these attacks he was taught relaxation techniques.

Reinforcing self-statements

The main aim of anxiety management training is to give the patient the competence to cope with anxiety. Initially, the therapist gives social reinforcement and encouragement. The patient also needs to learn to 'not be hard on themselves' and to be able to acknowledge their progress. This can be done by encouraging the patient throughout therapy to examine their success and to take the credit for overcoming their anxiety. Again, cue cards with positive self-statements can be a useful reminder. In James's case he had a cue card which said 'I have done really well to face up to the panic and anxiety and have proved I can overcome them'.

Cognitive therapy for generalised anxiety disorder

Beck & Emery's (1985) cognitive model of anxiety is very similar to Beck's cognitive model for depression (Chapter 8, pp. 119–125). Schemas are laid down in early life and based on experiences at that time. However, because they are formed while very young, they are not necessarily logical and are not subjected to scrutiny by the individual. From these schemas arise a number of assumptions which are 'rules' held to be absolute truths by the individual and not questioned. From these underlying assumptions, NATs arise in response to situations and result in an immediate change in mood. Just as with depression, most schema are dormant unless activated by an activating (usually negative) event.

In performing cognitive therapy for anxiety there are two main differences to depression:

- NATs may not be accessible to the patient when they are not anxious – thus there may be a greater need for behavioural tests or imagined exposure to access the NAT
- with panic, Clark's model of cognitive therapy for panic disorder can be applied.

There is often confusion between exposure tasks and behavioural tests (experiments). An exposure task is a piece of behaviour whereby the individual faces up to their feared situation for a prescribed length of time. The task is selected for the hierarchy of exposure tasks and is performed repeatedly in accordance with the behavioural programme. Thus for exposure tasks to be effective, they should be graded in accordance with anxiety, performed predictably and regularly (ideally at least 3 times a day) and of sufficient duration for habituation to occur. Behavioural tests however are behaviours which are performed to test out what happens in a given situation. Therefore, a patient who is fearful of fainting in a supermarket may agree to perform a behavioural task where they visit the supermarket to 'see what happens'. This behavioural task is thus only performed once and does not have the predictability, regularity or duration of regular exposure tasks.

The belief that thinking of something will make it more likely to happen is known as magical thinking and is fairly frequent in patients with OCD. There are a number of tests which can be used to get the patient to challenge this belief. Of course it is very threatening to start by asking them to think of horrible things befalling their nearest and dearest and so this can be done in a more graded fashion. To start with, to test the belief that thinking a thought is the same as doing a deed, sometimes known as thought-action fusion, it may be an idea to suggest that the patient think of the numbers which will win the lottery and that the therapist will buy a ticket. Over the next week, the patient is asked to think of the 'winning' numbers repeatedly. In reality, it is rarely necessary to do this as the individual can see that this is unlikely to be successful. Second, it is often easier for the patient to think about a horrible disaster happening to the therapist, for example that the therapist dies a horrible death in a car crash. Once the patient has done this, it may be possible to encourage them to take more risks with their own family. See the story of Trish, where treatment for generalised anxiety disorder is explored (Case example 9.3).

Case example 9.3: Treatment of generalised anxiety disorder

Trish, 36, had been anxious all her life. However, following the death of her father 2 years earlier she had become much more anxious about making a mistake and being a bad mother. She had given up her work as a receptionist 5 years earlier when she had had her first baby and currently was a housewife looking after her two children, Gwen (5) and Lucy (3).

Her whole day was one of constant worrying, according to Trish. She would worry that the children did not eat enough breakfast, that she did not pay sufficient attention to them, whether or not she should have sent them to nursery. When she went out with the children, she would worry about the roads and was very careful when buying food to check all the 'sell by' dates to ensure the food was wholesome. This problem had become so bad that her husband was becoming angry at her worrying and felt it was having a negative impact on all of their lives.

After a full assessment of Trish and education about her condition, the following formulation was given to her:

'You have always been a very anxious and nervous person but, until recently, this has not interfered with your life. You were always very close to your father and described him as your "rock", as he was a very phlegmatic and rational man. After he died suddenly and prematurely, you began to be more anxious about a variety of issues. Gradually, you started reducing your activity which also left you with more time to worry. So the more anxious you become, the less you do and thus the more time you have to worry and to become anxious. This vicious circle seems to maintain the problems.'

First, Trish was taught some relaxation techniques because it was noted that this may be a useful skill for her as she had always been an anxious person. The therapist asked her to sit in a chair in a comfortable position. Starting at the toes, the therapist asked her to contract the muscles for the count of 5 and then to exhale and relax the muscles. Once these were relaxed, the therapist moved progressively up the body to the feet, legs, abdomen, arms, hands, and on to the neck, face and head. This session was recorded on Trish's telephone so that she could try listening to it twice daily.

It was very difficult for Trish to remember any thoughts which came into her head, so she was asked to record the day, time and content of thoughts which resulted in anxiety before the next session. This was recorded in a diary, the first page of which is shown in Table. 9.2. The rest of the diary was very similar. Trish was asked to pick a thought which was causing her current anxiety and she chose the fear that Gwen might have meningitis.

First, the therapist wanted to establish how much Trish knew about meningitis. She said she was too fearful to even check on the internet but she was aware that her children had been vaccinated against one type of meningitis in infancy. A friend had mentioned that a child at school had also recently been treated for leukaemia. The therapist explained to Trish that in the UK, most children get vaccinated against meningococcal type C and haemophilus influenzae type B. Children that are very young or those who have other illnesses are particularly susceptible to illnesses such as infection by haemophilus influenzae type B.

Table 9.2 Trish's diary

Date	Time	Where and what?	Emotion	NAT	Belief in NAT
1 July	10:00	At home saw a police car in the road	Anxiety	'Something terrible has happened to Jeff (husband) and the police are coming to tell me'	92%
1 July	12:00	Out in the park with Gwen and Lucy (children) and it started to rain heavily	Anxiety	'The children could catch pneumonia and die'	95%
1 July	16:00	Telephone call from friend who told me that a child at Gwen's school had been diagnosed with meningitis	Anxiety	'Gwen will catch meningitis and die and it will spread to Lucy too'	100%

NAT, negative automatic thought.

Trish: 'But there is a chance that Gwen could get meningitis.'

Therapist: 'Yes, there is always a risk that any child could catch a range of diseases, but let's try and establish the likelihood of it occurring in this case.'

Trish: 'Well I think the child was in the older class and they don't mix much with the younger ones. However, there could be germs floating around.'

Therapist: 'What do you think the risk is of a child who has been vaccinated catching the disease this way?'

Trish: 'Probably quite small... 10%?'

Therapist: 'I would think you would find it is much lower than this, but let's pretend that Gwen was infected by the meningitis germ. What would happen then?'

Trish: 'Well she would die!!!' At this point Trish became very shaky and anxious.

Therapist: 'Hang on a minute, let's look at this. What is the first sign of illness?'

Trish: 'She would get a temperature and would look unwell.'

Therapist: 'Do you know what happened to the other child?'

Trish: 'Well, my friend said they had taken her to hospital and she was being treated by antibiotics and seemed to be responding.'

The therapist then explored this further and encouraged Trish to really examine the probabilities of her daughter catching meningitis and dying when she had been vaccinated and generally was a fit and healthy child. At the end of the session, Trish said that her belief that Gwen would catch meningitis and die had reduced from 100 to 30%. Her belief that Lucy would also catch it reduced from 100 to 15%, as she felt Lucy could be given a course of antibiotics before she developed any symptoms. Although these figures are clearly still inflated from the real probabilities, it shows how, within a short time, anxious people can be taught to re-evaluate their negative automatic thoughts and resultant beliefs.

It became clear that many of the anxiety-provoking thoughts Trish experienced focused around harm occurring to her family. Using the downward arrow technique (described in Chapter 8, p. 123), several underlying assumptions emerged:

- 'I must always be vigilant of any danger to keep my family safe'
- 'Thinking about harm happening to one of my family makes it more likely to happen'.

These two assumptions were then challenged:

Therapist: 'Let's look at the evidence for the belief that you need to be vigilant to keep your family safe. What evidence do you have for that?'

Trish: 'Well, they are all OK so far, although I am concerned that Gwen is also starting to show anxiety. The other day, she did ask me if I was sure Lucy would be safe at nursery.'

Therapist: 'OK, so it sounds as if you think that she may be picking up on your fear and becoming anxious herself.'

Trish: 'Yes, and I really don't want her to go though the same thing that I have and have a restricted life.'

Therapist: 'OK, can we think of any way to test out whether remaining vigilant at all times means that your family is more likely to be safe?'

Trish: 'Well, I am meeting up with several friends who have children and I think I could ask them how vigilant they are.'

Over the next few weeks, Trish started to pay more attention to the precautions (and lack of precautions) other mothers took with their children. Previously, she had been so preoccupied with her catastrophic thoughts that she had paid scant attention to anyone else. It became clear to Trish that some mothers were more careful than others but that her fears were clearly more excessive than in the vast majority of parents. Discussing with the therapist, she began to realise that being excessively cautious with her children was more likely to lead to them becoming fearful and not enjoying life to the full. Trish realised that she did not need to be constantly vigilant to keep her family safe, nor should she be neglectful, but that there was a 'happy medium' whereby she could be alert to real dangers without restricting her children at all times. Eventually, Trish she started to feel she might be able to start to work again part time while the children were at nursery, which would give her less time to worry.

Panic

Clark devised his model of panic in 1986. He states that the individuals who experience panic attacks do so because of a tendency to interpret a range of bodily sensations in a catastrophic fashion. This interpretation leads to a further increase in bodily sensations and a vicious circle ensues. In other words, it is not the symptoms themselves but how they are interpreted that is the problem. Many people with anxiety disorders are more aware than the general population of any bodily symptoms and are more likely to misinterpret these symptoms. Clark's model is demonstrated in Case example 9.4 and another factor contributing to panic attacks, hyperventilation, is discussed in Case example 9.5.

Case example 9.4: Panic and fear of cardiac arrest

Frank is 42 years old and was experiencing panic with palpitation. Every time he experienced palpitation he would think 'my heart is beating really fast, no one can go on like this, it will stop soon and I will die'. Owing to these beliefs Frank had stopped all exercise and always took a lift rather than walking up stairs. Before his symptoms started 2 years earlier, he had been an active sportsman. Clearly it is a bad idea to get someone who has avoided all exercise to suddenly start exercising excessively. However, a behavioural test was set whereby Frank agreed to test his beliefs by measuring the therapist's resting pulse rate and their pulse after the therapist had run up five flights of stairs. Frank was amazed by this as he discovered that the therapist's heart rate after the exercise was higher than his had ever been. The formulation of his problem and a diagram like then one in Fig. 9.2 was given to Frank.

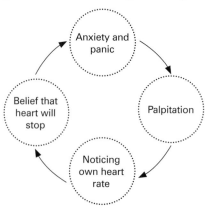

Fig. 9.2 Vicious cycle of anxiety and panic for Frank.

Following a check from his GP that he was fit to participate in exercise, Frank was asked to start introducing exercise into his life by doing some walking/running 3 days per week. He was to start by running for 30 s followed by walking for 2 min and to repeat this for up to 20 min. Gradually, he was asked to increase the time running and reduce the time of the walking intervals. Following any periods of running he was to record his heart rate. Frank discovered that his heart rate went very high to begin with but reduced as he became fitter. He stopped panicking about the speed of his heart and the panic episodes diminished.

Case example 9.5: Hyperventilation and panic attacks

Jamie was a 19-year-old student who had begun to have panic attacks since moving to university and following a once-off experimentation with drugs. He had had a bad experience and had found himself alone in his student room and became convinced he would die. Since then, panic episodes occurred approximately once a week. On closer assessment, it was clear that he also hyperventilated. His formulation is shown in Fig. 9.3.

In this case, following a full assessment and education about the role of hyperventilation in producing panic, Jamie was taught breathing exercises. The therapist helped him with this and both took rapid breaths for 30 seconds. Jamie was then asked to describe how he felt. He said 'It's terrible, I'm going to die! I can't breathe, my head is fuzzy…please help me, I need to go to hospital!'. Jamie was encouraged to start his controlled breathing exercises. At first he had difficulty in doing this, but as the therapist continued to speak calmly and quietly to him, he started to control his breathing rate. The therapist then asked him about his NATs and the belief he was going to suffocate and die. He was asked to look for the evidence for and against this belief.

'Evidence to support my belief I will suffocate and die:
- I feel as if I can't get a breath
- I feel light-headed and fuzzy
- I'm not sure if I can stop these feelings without help.

Evidence against this belief:
- I can induce these symptoms by over-breathing and so it seems rational that I can reverse them too
- Breathing slowly and deeply makes me feel better.'

After examining this evidence, Jamie's belief that he was going to die during a panic reduced from 100 to 45%. This exercise was practised another two times during sessions with the therapist. In between sessions, Jamie was asked to search the internet for descriptions of the symptoms of hyperventilation and descriptions of panic, and how the two interrelate. This research and also the continued practice of hyperventilation encouraged

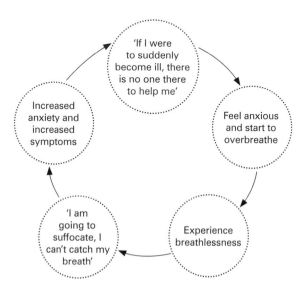

Fig. 9.3 Jamie's formulation for panic attacks.

Jamie to believe he may not die and that his symptoms may be related to panic. Once this was established, he was asked to practise hyperventilation-provocation on his own daily so that he could practise controlling the symptoms.

Jamie managed to do the hyperventilation and discovered how quickly his symptoms abated when he practised controlled breathing. His belief that his symptoms were due to panic and anxiety and not evidence of a fatal illness was now 95%.

CBT for life-altering and life-shortening diagnoses

Cognitive–behavioural therapy can be adapted for a variety of medical conditions. Techniques such as problem-solving, distraction and mindfulness may help to ease the problems of chronic illnesses such as rheumatoid arthritis.

This type of therapy has also been used to address the anxiety often found in patients with terminal cancer. In such cases there needs to be some adaptation from the usual CBT for generalised anxiety and depression as some of the patient's fears concerning their life-shortening illness are realistic. However, many cancer patients have other worries too and these can be addressed by CBT.

Greer *et al* (2010) described a four-module CBT package which could be effectively used with terminally ill patients:

1 *Psychoeducation and goal-setting* (approx. 1 session)
2 *Relaxation training* (approx. 1 session as also involves psychoeducation about stress and stress reduction). Sometimes mindfulness can be useful.
3 *Coping with fears* (approx. 3 sessions):
    • identifying NATs and worries and challenging these
    • dealing with realistic worries using problem-solving skills.
4 *Activity planning and pacing.* Having advanced cancer will leave patients feeling drained and helping them to realistically pace themselves using activity scheduling can be useful.

Mindfulness and generalised anxiety

The use of mindfulness-based therapies in reducing anxiety has been evaluated in a meta-analytical study (Hofmann *et al*, 2010). This study examined reported trials in patients with generalised anxiety, terminal illness, chronic pain and depression. Overall, it was found that mindfulness was useful for generalised anxiety, reducing anxiety in terminal illness and in chronic pain. However, despite numerous published studies, most did not use intention-to-treat analysis. Also, many were comparing mindfulness against a placebo treatment and thus it is not possible to compare it with more standard CBT techniques.

Key learning points

- Anxiety is a universal phenomenon, a survival advantage for a species.
- There is an optimal level of anxiety to aid performance (Yerkes–Dodson law).
- Anxiety can produce symptoms affecting most systems of the body. These symptoms are due to increased sympathetic outflow, imbalance between the parasympathetic and sympathetic systems or increased muscular tension.
- Anxiety can be a symptom of any psychiatric disorder or a stand-alone disorder.
- Physical illness can mimic anxiety and poor lifestyle can exacerbate it.
- Behavioural interventions (e.g. exposure treatments of avoiding avoidance and hyperventilation to induce panic) can be useful, as can relaxation training.
- Anxiety management training usually comprises: education and normalisation, examination and rectification of maintaining factors, reinforcing self-statements.
- Cognitive therapy for generalised anxiety is based on the work of Aaron T. Beck. It is similar to the intervention used in depression.
- There are two potential differences between the cognitive therapy for anxiety and therapy for depression. First, the patient may only be aware of the NATs when placed in a fear-provoking situation, and second, specific work may be needed to address panic.
- Cognitive therapy for generalised anxiety means identifying NATs, challenging them (often by using a behavioural test) and arriving at a rational response.
- The downward arrow technique can be used to identify underlying assumptions which can also be challenged.
- Clark's cognitive model of panic suggests that benign physical symptoms are interpreted as being dangerous, which increases the anxiety. This increase in anxiety causes more physical symptoms and a vicious circle of fear ensues.
- CBT can be adapted for those with life-changing and life-limiting diagnoses.
- Mindfulness may be useful as a means of allowing the patient to relax without engaging in worrying thoughts.

Suggested measures to use with conditions covered in this chapter

- Problems and targets, Fear Questionnaire (includes a measure of general anxiety), Hamilton Anxiety Scale (all three scales discussed in Chapter 2) and Beck Anxiety Inventory (Beck *et al*, 1988).

References

American Psychiatric Association (2013) *Diagnostic and Statistical Manual for Psychiatric Disorders (DSM-5)*. APA.

Beck AT, Emery G (1985) *Anxiety Disorders and Phobias: A Cognitive Perspective*. Basic Books.

Beck AT, Epstein N, Brown G, *et al* (1988) An inventory for measuring clinical anxiety: psychometric properties. *Journal of Consulting and Clinical Psychology*, **56**: 893–7.

Clark DM (1986) A cognitive approach to panic. *Behaviour Research and Therapy*, **24**: 461–70.

Clark LA, Watson D (2006) Distress and fear disorders: an alternative empirically based taxonomy of the 'mood' and 'anxiety' disorders. *British Journal of Psychiatry*, **189**: 481–3.

Figueiro MG, Wood B, Plitnick B, et al (2011) The impact of light from computer monitors on melatonin levels in college students. *Neuroendocrinology Letters*, **32**: 158–63.

Greer JA, Park ER, Prigerson HG, *et al* (2010) Tailoring cognitive-behavioral therapy to treat anxiety comorbid with advanced cancer. *Journal of Cognitive Psychotherapy*, **24**: 294–313.

Hofmann SG, Sawyer AT, Witt AA, *et al* (2010) The effect of mindfulness-based therapy on anxiety and depression: a meta-analytic review. *Journal of Consulting and Clinical Psychology*, **78**: 169–83.

Sciolino NR, Holmes PV (2012) Exercise offers anxiolytic potential: a role for stress and brain noradrenergic-galaninergic mechanisms. *Neuroscience and Biobehavioural Reviews*, **36**: 1965–84.

Wolpe J (1958) *Psychotherapy by Reciprocal Inhibition*. Stanford University Press.

Yerkes RM, Dodson JD (1908) The relation of strength stimulus to rapidity of habit-formation. *Journal of Comparative Neurology and Psychology*, **18**: 459–82.

Recommended treatment manuals and other reading

Butler G, Fennell M, Hackman A (2010) *Cognitive-Behavioral Therapy for Anxiety Disorders: Mastering Clinical Challenges*. Guilford Press.

Clark DA, Beck AT (2010) *Cognitive Therapy and Anxiety Disorders*. Guilford Press.

*Greenberger D, Padesky CA (1995) *Mind Over Mood: Change How You Feel by Changing the Way You Think*. Guilford Press.

Moorey S, Greer S (2012) *Oxford Guide to CBT for People with Cancer (Oxford Guides to Cognitive Behavioural Therapy)*. Oxford University Press.

Wells A (1997) *Cognitive Therapy of Anxiety Disorders: A Practical Manual and Conceptual Guide*. John Wiley and Sons.

*Suitable to recommend to patients.

Body dysmorphic disorder and the somatic symptom and related disorders

Overview

This chapter will examine the treatment of BDD and health anxiety (hypochondriasis). Body dysmorphic disorder has recently been reclassified by the American Psychiatric Association as part of the obsessive–compulsive spectrum disorders. The various theories and developments of cognitive strategies used in combination with behavioural change in the treatment of BDD will be discussed. Health anxiety, which also has many similarities with OCD, will then be explored. The use of cognitive interventions in combination with ERP will be discussed and illustrated using case examples. The possible role of techniques such as mindfulness to reduce anxiety will be explored.

Body dysmorphic disorder

Until 2013, BDD had been categorised as a somatoform disorder along with health anxiety, somatisation and pain disorders. In DSM-5 (American Psychiatric Association, 2013) it has been moved into the category of obsessive–compulsive and related disorders. One other difference in DSM-5 is that insight is no longer a prerequisite for the diagnosis of OCD but is also categorised on a continuum from complete insight to total lack of insight.

Body dysmorphic disorder is defined as a preoccupation about an imagined or trivial defect. This preoccupation causes clinically significant distress or impairment in social, occupational or other important areas of functioning (American Psychiatric Association, 2013). A study of 200 individuals with BDD (Phillips *et al*, 2005) identified chief concerns people had, presented here in Table 10.1. It can be seen from the table that many people have more than one concern. In addition, there does seem to be some gender difference in the area of the body most likely to be complained about (details available from the author on request).

It is a surprisingly common condition with an estimated point prevalence of 0.7–2.4% in the general population, although the majority of individuals

Table 10.1   Chief concerns in people presenting with body dysmorphic disorder

Body part causing the most concern	Proportion of patients	Comments
Skin	80.0%	e.g. feeling it was uneven or blotchy
Hair	57.5%	e.g. too thin
Nose	39.0%	e.g. too large or protuberant
Stomach	32.0%	e.g. too large or protuberant
Teeth	29.5%	e.g. uneven, discoloured
Weight	29.0%	e.g. too fat or too thin
Breasts	26.0%	e.g. too small
Buttocks	21.5%	e.g. too large
Eyes	21.5%	e.g. too small, 'piggy' eyes
Thighs	20.0%	e.g. too fat
Eyebrows	19.5%	e.g. uneven on each side of face
Overall appearance of face	19.0%	e.g. 'I look like a monkey'
Small body build	18.0%	
Legs	18.0%	e.g. too fat
Face (size or shape)	16.0%	e.g. 'I have a huge face, like a cartoon character'
Chin	14.5%	e.g. too protuberant
Lips	14.5%	e.g. too thin or too protuberant
Arms	13.5%	e.g. 'scrawny arms'
Hips	12.5%	e.g. too large
Cheeks	10.5%	e.g. 'fat cheeks like a pig'
Ears	10.5%	e.g. 'my ears stick out, I look like the football cup'

Source: Phillips *et al* (2005).

do not seek psychiatric or psychological intervention (see reviews by Phillips, 2009 and Bjornsson *et al*, 2010). It generally starts in adolescence and progresses from there. Epidemiological studies have found an almost equal gender incidence but with a slight predominance of women (Bjornsson *et al*, 2010). Most patients attend dermatology and cosmetic surgery clinics and request treatment for their imagined defect; there tend to be few patients with BDD seen in psychiatric clinics.

Until recently, BDD was often subsumed under the heading of OCD. Indeed, it is often, but not always, comorbid with OCD. Early studies on the treatment of BDD concentrated on using graded exposure with response prevention (e.g. Marks & Mishan, 1988).

Cognitive–behavioural model of BDD

Body dysmorphic disorder is similar to OCD in that there is an anxiogenic intrusive thought which is then maintained by a number of anxiolytic behaviours. In this case the anxiogenic thought is the idea about the person's perceived bodily flaw, which then leads to a number of anxiolytic behaviours such as:

- checking appearance in the mirror
- camouflaging the perceived abnormality with make-up, posture, clothing or a hat
- seeking reassurance from relatives and friends
- skin-picking to try to get rid of the flaw (and consequently making the appearance much worse)
- checking the imagined 'abnormality' by touching the affected area
- seeking medical reassurance and cosmetic surgery by consulting dermatologists, cosmetic dentists, orthodontists and cosmetic surgeons.

It can thus be seen that BDD has a number of similarities with OCD and also health anxiety. In addition, it often leads patients to avoid social situations and thus is often comorbid with social anxiety disorder.

A model for the maintenance of BDD is shown in Fig. 10.1.

In addition to the anxiolytic safety behaviours described, patients will often spend considerable amounts of time comparing themselves to models in magazines and people on the street. Indeed, it was found that almost half of individuals with BDD spent at least 3 hours a day involved in checking behaviours, which they found hard to resist (Phillips *et al*, 1998).

The cognitive–behavioural model of BDD shown in Fig. 10.2 uses the example of a 24-year-old man who was convinced his penis was too small and who kept asking for a penoplasty. Multiple doctors had told him that they could see nothing wrong with his penis.

It should be noted that BDD, like OCD, has a considerable social impact and patients with BDD are much less likely to be married or cohabiting

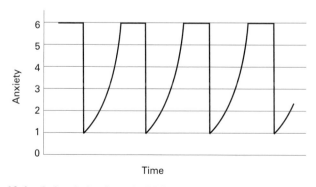

Fig. 10.1   Safety behaviours in BDD maintain the beliefs.

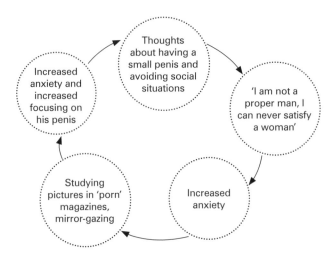

Fig. 10.2 Cognitive model for a man with BDD concerned with the size of his penis.

and to be employed than the general population. The rate of suicide is also high, with almost 25% of patients with BDD having attempted suicide and 80% admitting to suicidal thoughts (Phillips, 2009). The first case history shows how debilitating BDD can be (Case example 10.1).

Case example 10.1: BDD concerning face

Trudy was a 30-year-old woman who lived with her parents. She had developed an extreme concern about her face at the age of 13 years. At that time she had recently moved to a new school and had been subject to bullying by a small group of girls. These girls had teased her because, having moved from another part of the country, she had a different accent to them. Trudy became so fearful of this bullying that she eventually dropped out of school and was home tutored by her mother. At this time she began to become preoccupied with her appearance. She believed that her facial skin was red and blotchy to the extent that she believed herself to be 'deformed'. In reality she did have a slight tendency to mild eczema in one area of her right cheek but this was barely noticeable to everyone apart from Trudy. In addition, she believed her face to be too long and was convinced she looked like 'an ugly horse'. Her face was somewhat long but was well within normal limits. Indeed, on first meeting with Trudy, one of the most striking features was that she was extremely attractive.

Despite her problems, she managed to gain reasonably good qualifications and 4 years ago completed an online degree in web design. Since that time she had done some work from home on freelance projects. Although she had had some success in her academic life, the rest of Trudy's life was extremely restricted. She would only go out when wearing very thick make-up to try and hide her skin and polo-neck tops as she believed these made her face look shorter. The only reason she left the house was for appointments that needed to take place outside such as dental appointments. Everything else took place in her own home. Any socialisation took place online and Trudy had never been out with friends. She would speak to friends from her home city on the telephone and online. These friends often commented that they had never seen a photograph of her and asked her to post one online but she would always refuse.

Assessment of Trudy was difficult. She did arrive at the clinic but was wearing full make-up, a thick polo-neck sweater and a baseball cap which she pulled down over her eyes. Her parents accompanied her and it was notable that she had the appearance of a teenager despite her age. When asked a question, Trudy would always look towards her mother to see whether she would answer the question for her. A full description of the CBT model for BDD was given to the family. It was explained that treatment would involve three components:

- cognitive therapy to examine some of the unhelpful beliefs and thoughts
- graded exposure to spending more time outside the home
- response prevention in the form of elimination of the 'safety behaviours'.

Because Trudy was unable to travel to the clinic on her own, it was agreed that treatment would be started at her home but that it would be geared towards getting her to be able to travel on public transport to the session. During the first session, Trudy was asked to look at herself in the mirror and describe what she saw. She said 'I see an ugly woman with a long face and the most terrible skin…like leprosy or something'. In reality, she had two or three tiny red papules on a small area of her right cheek. The therapist asked whether she could take a photograph on her phone to use in therapy. Trudy reluctantly agreed on the understanding that this would only be seen by the therapist and herself unless she specifically gave permission for anyone else to see it. Following this, the therapist persuaded Trudy to remove her make-up. This was extremely difficult for Trudy but she eventually agreed. Even more reluctantly, the therapist persuaded Trudy to let her photograph her again. The therapist then put both photographs on to Trudy's computer and asked her to describe what she saw. Initially, it was very hard for Trudy but eventually she admitted that the extreme covering of her face in make-up made her spots more noticeable. This had been a long session of 3 hours and the therapist gave Trudy the task of not wearing make-up at all at home until she was seen again the following week. She was also asked to write a list of all her safety behaviours.

At the next session, Trudy was not wearing any make-up or a baseball cap. She had found this difficult but had managed and had been out in the garden throughout the week. When asked about going outside, Trudy said she felt she might be able to go with the therapist to the underground train station. Before this the therapist encouraged Trudy to put lipstick on the therapist's face to ensure that they both looked 'deformed'. In reality, of course, the therapist's 'rash' looked much more noticeable than any of the minor blemishes on Trudy's face. Trudy's prediction about going out without make-up was that 'everyone will stare at me and will then turn away in horror'. The therapist therefore asked Trudy to pay particular attention to everyone who walked past them and to see whether they paid any attention.

Trudy was extremely anxious as she walked to the underground station. The therapist urged her to watch all the people that passed them and take note of their reactions to them. When they arrived at the station, the therapist went to the desk and asked for an underground map. Trudy was asked to watch the reaction of the rail worker carefully for any signs of horror or surprise when confronted with the therapist's 'rash'. They also went into a newsagent's and a sweet shop and again Trudy was asked to note any reactions. She was amazed that not only did most people seem to pay them no attention at all, but that even when the therapist directly spoke to individuals, they seemed to have no reaction to her 'rash'.

Following on from this session, Trudy was asked to go out daily for a walk to the local shops without wearing make-up and to record her journeys in a diary as well as her anxiety levels and any thoughts which came into her mind and raised her anxiety. At the next visit, the therapist looked at this diary. Mostly Trudy had done very well, but she had experienced a rise in anxiety when seeing a newsagent which had a cartoon of a celebrity. This celebrity was being accused of 'looking like a horse'. Trudy felt this also applied to her. The therapist asked Trudy to examine these thoughts and what they meant. Trudy said: 'She is ugly because she looks like a horse. I also look like a horse and so I am ugly.'

Therapist: 'What evidence do you have for being ugly?'

Trudy: 'Well, I must be. No one has ever said it but I just *know* it.'

After some persuasion, it was agreed that the therapist could show the two pictures on her telephone to a number of staff and therapists working in the clinic and would record their reactions for Trudy the next week. The remainder of the session was spent repeating the exercise of the previous week but with Trudy wearing a normal t-shirt without a polo neck. Once again, Trudy was asked to record any negative reactions. This went smoothly, although there was an anxious moment when a tourist asked Trudy for directions. Trudy looked extremely anxious but was able to answer and also to note that the man had not looked at her strangely nor 'as if she were a freak'. She was asked to continue going out at least once a day wearing no make-up, baseball cap or polo necks and the next week she agreed to travel with the therapist on a crowded underground train. This was particularly difficult for Trudy as, when walking, she could pass people fairly quickly. Her fear on the trains was the proximity of so many stationary people. It was agreed that she would create a 'rash' on the therapist's face next week to see what happened.

The following week, the therapist started by showing Trudy the reaction to her photograph. The therapist had asked eight members of staff and all except one had rated her as more attractive without make-up. Comments had ranged from 'a very attractive woman' to 'she looks very anxious'. No one had remarked on either her rash or the length of her face. These reactions had been written down by the people asked and so the therapist left these with Trudy for her to examine. Trudy was concerned that maybe the therapist had 'doctored' the reactions in some way but the therapist was able to truthfully promise her that she had presented all the material she had. They then left to travel on the train having created a 'rash' on the therapist's face. Once again, Trudy was surprised at how most people were preoccupied with their own business and paid very little attention to anyone else.

Treatment then progressed with Trudy attending the clinic and travelling on her own. She managed to post a photograph of herself on her social network page and was gratified by the positive comments she received. Progress was not always in one direction, however, and she found it much more difficult when she had a 'break-out' of her rash. With encouragement, however, she managed to achieve increased social interaction and freedom. Six months after treatment, she contacted the therapist to say she had managed to find a job and was working as a web designer in an office.

The case history of Trudy demonstrates how graded exposure with response prevention (removing the safely behaviours) and cognitive reattribution can be successful in treating even long-standing problems.

Many patients, however, do not present at the psychiatric clinic willingly but may be referred by others. The next case history (Case example 10.2) describes such a situation.

Case example 10.2: Deeply entrenched BDD

Ryan was 41 years old when he was referred to the clinic by his GP, who was reluctant to refer Ryan for more surgery without a psychiatric opinion. Since his teens, Ryan was convinced that his nose was too big. At the age of 35 he had received a rhinoplasty on the NHS because of the distress he experienced due to his nose. Initially, he felt better and gained more confidence but then he began to worry that his nose was still rather large. He returned to the surgeon who told him that he would not recommend further reduction. Ryan then went to see several NHS doctors, all of whom told him there was nothing wrong with his nose. Consequently he became convinced that if he could afford to visit a cosmetic surgeon privately, he could obtain the 'perfect' nose. However, he had asked the GP to send him for one final opinion before he used his life's savings to have surgery. The GP refused to refer him, unless Ryan agreed to a psychiatric assessment.

When he arrived for the appointment, Ryan was very unenthusiastic and did not want to engage with the therapist at all. He kept on saying 'If I just have the surgery I'll be OK'. The therapist suggested to him that he was unlikely to get further surgery just now and there was no evidence that the last surgery had helped. Cosmetic surgery is an imprecise science which depends on the individual's concepts of aesthetics and thus anyone seeking a 'perfect' nose is likely to be disappointed. Ryan felt this was wrong and that he definitely needed surgery. The therapist suggested that there were two possible explanations for the way he was feeling:

- he had an extremely large nose which was ugly as he believed and was the cause of comment for everyone who saw him; the only way to rectify this situation would be for Ryan to have surgery
- it was the way Ryan felt about his nose which caused the problem and that this fed into a vicious circle (Fig. 10.3).

Ryan listened to the therapist's theory but said he still believed that the first interpretation was correct and that only surgery would correct it. He did, however, agree to have five sessions of CBT 'if only to convince my doctor that I really do need surgery'. The therapist agreed to this. Before Ryan left, the therapist conducted a full mental state examination on Ryan. He appeared depressed and miserable and the therapist was concerned about his low mood. Ryan admitted his mood had been low recently but felt this was purely due to his not receiving surgery. Although he admitted to suicidal thoughts, he denied any plans but felt he might attempt suicide if he did not ultimately get the surgery he felt he needed. The therapist suggested that his symptoms of depression might be helped by treatment with a serotonin reuptake inhibiting drug (which is also an evidence-based treatment for BDD), but Ryan was adamant that he would not take the medication. Before the next session, Ryan was asked to think of other men who had large noses and come back with a list.

The following week Ryan arrived with a list of people with larger noses, including the French film actor Gerard Depardieu and other successful

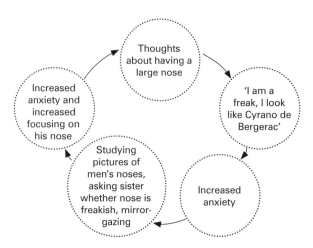

Fig. 10.3 Cognitive–behavioural model for Ryan's concerns regarding his nose.

politicians and actors. The therapist asked Ryan what he noticed about these men. He replied, 'I know what you are going to say, yes they all have big noses and yes, they have all had successful careers and success with women, but that is different to me as my nose is much worse!' The therapist asked Ryan to bring some photographs of men he felt were attractive to the next session. For the remainder of this session, Ryan agreed to walk along the high street with the therapist to observe how many people stared at Ryan's nose. The result of this was that contrary to Ryan's prediction, no one stared at his nose.

The next week the therapist measured the length and breadth of Ryan's nose and also the length and breadth of his face. Ryan agreed that the nose should be in proportion with the face. From these figures was calculated the width and length ratio for his nose. Similar measurements were taken from the photographs which Ryan had brought. It was soon discovered that Ryan's nose was average in both its length and width. Ryan, however, dismissed this by saying that 'mine still looks much larger'. For homework this week, the therapist asked Ryan not to look in the mirror for more than 5 min three times a day and only to check his hair. In addition, he was asked to not telephone his sister for reassurance about his nose. Ryan did not feel that either of these requests was reasonable. A compromise was therefore reached whereby he would seek reassurance and mirror-gaze as much as he liked on one day and record his anxiety throughout the day. On the second day he was to carry out the programme as suggested by the therapist and record his anxiety. For the rest of the week he could do whichever he felt was the most useful.

When Ryan returned the next week, his records did show that he felt better when he did not mirror-gaze or seek reassurance. However, he had gone back to the mirror-gazing and telephoning his sister for reassurance as he felt that doing the programme was 'just trying to forget my problem'. The therapist then asked Ryan to go around the hospital grounds with him and conduct a survey asking people what they thought about Ryan's nose. Ryan was fairly shy about this to begin with but did agree. Most people were complimentary about his nose, which was described as 'chiselled' and 'a fine Roman nose' and others were neither complimentary nor critical and said 'just looks normal'. At the end of this, the therapist asked Ryan what he concluded from the exercise and he said 'It does seem that the problem is more my thoughts about my nose rather than my nose *per se*'. From this point onwards Ryan worked well in therapy, though he still did not wish to continue beyond five sessions. He agreed to reduce the time he spent in front of the mirror and to stop asking his sister for reassurance about his nose. He had decided to put his request to see a cosmetic surgeon 'on hold' for a while, but said that whereas he was happy to try and 'live with my nose' for the next few months, he would seek surgery if he deteriorated again.

Ryan's case history shows how many patients can be ambivalent about psychiatric and psychological intervention. Drug treatment can be a very useful adjunct to psychological therapy but many patients are unhappy to take medications.

Health anxiety (hypochondriasis)

Patients with health anxiety use a disproportionate amount of medical time both in primary and secondary care. Even when it is clear that there is no medical or surgical diagnosis, the treating physician's fear of a negligence claim often means such patients have recurrent and unnecessary investigations. Unnecessary physical investigations result in risks to the patient, considerable cost to the health service and frustration to general physicians and surgeons. These patients are usually highly distressed, do experience multiple physical symptoms and feel that the investigations are incorrect and a serious physical diagnosis is being overlooked. Referral to mental health services is usually actively resisted and many patients view such referral with hostility, as they feel this is tantamount to saying they are fabricating symptoms.

Warwick & Salkovskis (1990) developed a cognitive–behavioural model for health anxiety. In this model, it is suggested that the patients are extremely sensitive to any bodily sensations. They then misinterpret these innocuous sensations as evidence of serious disease. This thought results in anxiety and anxiety itself can increase the number of physical symptoms experienced. The individuals will tend to seek medical reassurance, engage in bodily checking, pay increased attention to physical symptoms, engage in avoidance of certain situations, pay attention to any information related to their feared illness, and develop a number of safety behaviours (Fig. 10.4).

In addition, it was suggested that people who are prone to health anxiety have underlying assumptions related to health and illness which makes them more susceptible to worry about any physical symptoms.

This model was tested in a controlled trial by Warwick *et al* (1996) with some success. It can be seen that health anxiety is somewhat similar to OCD in that a number of worrying thoughts come into the person's mind and these cause high anxiety. To try to relieve the anxiety, the person engages in a number of anxiolytic behaviours such as seeking reassurance, bodily checking, internet checking of symptoms and signs of the feared disease, avoidance and other safety behaviours Because high anxiety is

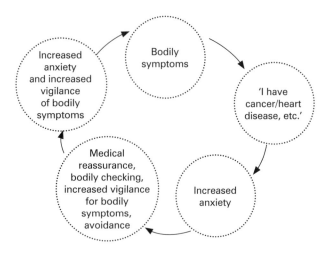

Fig. 10.4 Vicious cycle of anxiety in health anxiety.

very unpleasant, the reduction in the anxiety caused by these anxiolytic behaviours is like a reward and thus the anxiety reduction reinforces the checking behaviours. Just as in OCD, these anxiolytic 'rituals' are inefficient as, although they may reduce anxiety, the effect is small and short-lived and so the person finds they have the desire to repeat the anxiolytic behaviour after a short while. The pattern here is the same as in BDD (Fig. 10.2) and it is illustrated in Case example 10.3.

Case example 10.3: Maintaining factors in health anxiety

Ash was a 25-year-old man who was referred for assessment by the gastroenterology team. He was extremely reluctant to see a psychiatrist but was eventually persuaded by being told that many patients benefit from seeing the psychiatrist irrespective of their diagnosis as any emotion can have an effect on the bowel.

The history showed that Ash was the only child of quite elderly parents and had been a much-wanted child as it had taken his parents many attempts at *in vitro* fertilisation to conceive him. Consequently, he had been quite 'molly-coddled' as a young child and was always described as 'sickly', requiring considerable time away from school, although no serious pathology had ever been found.

At the age of 18 years, Ash had moved away from home to attend university. He developed some abdominal pains and went to the student health centre. He was told that this was most likely due to his poor diet since leaving home. Ash, however, was not happy with this and started searching the internet. He convinced himself that he suffered from a form of ulcerative colitis and that he would die from the complication of carcinoma unless this was dealt with. After several visits to the health centre, they eventually sent him to the hospital to see a gastroenterologist. The consultant at the clinic performed a sigmoidoscopy on Ash and reassured him there was nothing wrong. Initially Ash was relieved but over the next few days he was plagued by thoughts such as: 'Doctors can get things wrong ... what if he missed the pathological area';

'I only had sigmoidoscopy and that can only examine the lower bowel. Maybe the upper bowl is affected'; 'Maybe he's only telling me there's nothing wrong because he thinks I'm really ill and the prognosis is hopeless'. These thoughts meant that Ash asked for an urgent return visit to the clinic and eventually was given a colonoscopy. Each new test reduced his anxiety for a while but then the catastrophic thoughts would creep back in.

Eventually, the local clinic refused to see him. By this time, Ash was so crippled by his anxieties that he was no longer attending to his studies. He returned home, where his parents were very concerned about his weight loss. Ash had started to restrict his diet to that advised for people with ulcerative colitis and thus was avoiding most sources of insoluble fibre (e.g. bran, whole foods, sweetcorn) and also any dairy produce, including milk, cheese and cream. As well as trying to avoid physical activity in case it upset his bowel, Ash took a variety of tablets from health food shops, consisting of a range of vitamin and mineral supplements and also herbal medicines supposed to act on the bowel.

Over the next few years, Ash ended up having more and more investigations and going to see a multiplicity of NHS and private gastroenterologists. Every time he was discharged from a clinic, his anxiety would rocket and he would seek out another physician and surgeon. At the time of referral to the psychiatric clinic, Ash had a body mass index (BMI) of only 16 and spent most of his days lying in bed. He was pale and unwell and spent his time searching for a cure for his 'ulcerative colitis'. His parents were extremely anxious and really did believe Ash had a serious medical condition. His mother said 'Look at the state of him, he's undernourished and can barely get out of bed...there must be something seriously wrong with him that the doctors haven't found.' The family had spent over £10000, which they could barely afford, to try to get a diagnosis for Ash.

The case history of Ash demonstrates how medical practitioners unwittingly exacerbate the symptoms of health anxiety and hypochondriasis. Most patients will attend their GP or hospital clinic and happily accept the outcome of relevant tests. However, medicine is not an exact science and there are hardly any situations when a doctor can honestly say he or she is 100% certain. If a patient returns and becomes insistent, then the doctor, mindful of the potential for medico-legal allegations and negligence claims if a diagnosis is overlooked, will often concede to the patient's demands and order further tests. As can be seen from Ash's history, this can form a vicious cycle with a downward spiral of the patient.

In treating patients with health anxiety the first thing the psychiatrist needs to do is to establish with the patient that there will be no more medical tests or seeking of reassurance for the duration of psychological treatment. This is easier said than done. Patients with health anxiety really believe they have a serious physical illness which may threaten their lives and so it will seem as if the therapist is asking them to take a big risk. One way of approaching this is to present two scenarios to the patient. This can be demonstrated in the story of the treatment of Ash.

Case example 10.3, continued

Ash was very unwilling at first to agree to stop consulting doctors about his bowels. He felt this would be 'dangerous' and that his symptoms might progress and worsen. The therapist said:

'I understand your concern about your bowels but if we look at this, you have been seeking a diagnosis for over 7 years now. I am asking you to agree to no further investigations for the next 4 months while we start to look at alternative answers. I am going to propose to you that there are two possible explanations for you situation.

First, your current belief is that you have a serious bowel condition such as ulcerative colitis and that this will result in a life-threatening situation. All the doctors and specialists who have seen you have managed to miss this diagnosis but if you keep on seeing more specialists and having more tests, you will eventually obtain a diagnosis of inflammatory bowel disease.

My theory is that you do indeed suffer from a variety of bowel symptoms. These symptoms may well have been precipitated originally by a poor diet when you left home. However, once you became anxious that you had a serious bowel disease, your anxiety increased. Chronic and high anxiety can cause various symptoms which you describe, such as colicky pain, intermittent diarrhoea and constipation, and a feeling of nausea. Every time you go and see a specialist, you feel better for a day or two and then start to worry they may have overlooked the diagnosis and your anxiety and symptoms get worse. In addition, your restricted diet has made you severely underweight. This diet may well be contributing to your bowel symptoms and also being malnourished means you will have low energy, lack of drive and a feeling of malaise. This in turn leads you to spend increasing time in bed. Remaining in bed makes you weaker and also has a deleterious effect on your physical symptoms.'

Ash did not think the therapist's theory was correct but, persuaded by his parents, agreed to give it a try. He said he would not consult any bowel specialist for the next 6 weeks. The therapist gave him a chart to take away (Fig. 10.5). Ash also promised to stop the herbal medicine but decided to remain on the vitamin supplements.

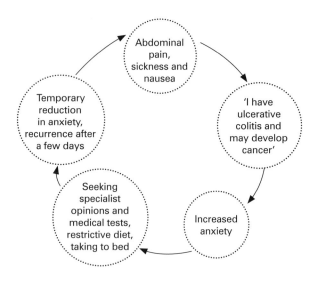

Fig. 10.5 Vicious cycle of Ash's symptoms.

In therapy the first thing was to try to modify some of Ash's beliefs about his symptoms. He was asked to search the internet to read about some of the symptoms caused by anxiety and to see whether any of these matched the ones he had. Over the next few sessions, the emphasis was placed on examining Ash's symptoms and thoughts and by working with Ash using collaborative empiricism, trying to discover whether there were any alternative explanations for his symptoms other than serious bowel disease. At the end of several sessions, Ash conceded that his belief that his symptoms were caused by anxiety had increased from 0 to 40%. He was asked if he would be willing to try expanding the repertoire of his diet. After a long discussion, Ash agreed to include dairy produce in his diet for a week to see whether this caused his symptoms to improve or deteriorate.

Ash managed to incorporate dairy produce without ill effect and was successfully challenging many of his NATs concerning serious bowel disease. He was already spending less time in bed but the therapist worked with him to look at introducing graded exercise to gradually increase his physical activity. He found that as he grew stronger and was eating a better diet, his symptoms were less prominent. After several weeks, he agreed to eat wholemeal and foods rich in fibre. Once a full and varied diet was established, he agreed to stop his vitamin and mineral supplements.

Although Ash was progressing much quicker than anticipated, it was felt important to examine some of his underlying assumptions and core beliefs to see whether these could be challenged and thereby decrease his chance of relapse. Using the downward arrow technique a core belief was obtained (Fig. 10.6).

From this downward arrow it can be seen that Ash had always considered himself to be a weak and sickly person who was prone to illness. When he was asked to think of the evidence for this he said: 'I had lots of time off school as a child'; 'I was not able to take part in contact sports at school because I was weak'. Closer examination of these statements demonstrated that Ash had indeed had time off school as a child but this was mainly for minor coughs and colds. He had never had more serious illnesses. Indeed, he began to see that many of his classmates may have gone into school with similar symptoms to him but that his mother preferred him to stay at home. His parents had been very worried about contact sports as a cousin had been badly injured playing rugby. Ash was thus given a note of excuse by his mother. Consequently, Ash had never participated in much sport and had never tried to improve and strengthen his body.

Following on from this, Ash decided to try to take up judo. He enrolled in a local class and to his surprise not only enjoyed the sport but was reasonably good at it.

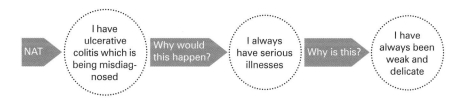

Fig. 10.6 Example of downward arrow technique to find Ash's underlying assumption. NAT, negative automatic thought.

Not all patients are as easy as Ash to either engage in therapy or get to stick with it. Actually getting the patient to at least consider an alternative explanation for their symptoms can take several sessions. There are several key things to remember in treating these problematic patients.

1   *Assessment and engagement of the patient.* It takes a long time to assess a really reluctant patient with health anxiety, so always ensure there is sufficient time to fully listen to them. As well as gaining medical reassurance form health practitioners, many such patients watch medical programmes on television and read alarming stories in magazines and newspapers, where the conditions are often sensationalised and perceived shortcomings in the healthcare providers are highlighted. In addition, patients will often search the internet and may have detailed knowledge about a range of medical conditions. Whereas much of this information is correct, most patients do not realise that symptoms are not all that it takes to make a diagnosis. Most symptoms can be found in both serious and benign conditions.

2   *Always acknowledge that the patient's symptoms are real.* Many of these patients have been told it is 'all in their mind'. This does not fit with their very real experience of symptoms. The mind and body are closely interlinked. Patients with health anxiety experience real bodily symptoms and sensations. Compared with the general population, they pay increased attention to them. This increased bodily vigilance leads to anxiety and exacerbation of the physical symptoms.

3   *Formulation.* Always use specific examples that the patient gives you. It can also be useful to sometimes give the patient's formulation as well as your own (as demonstrated in the case history of Ash).

4   *Self-monitoring.* It is helpful for patients to self-monitor their symptoms in a diary. This diary should include: Where? What symptoms? Thoughts? Emotion (and level of anxiety if this is the emotion experienced on a 0–10 scale)? Action taken?

5   *Identification and challenging of NATs.* It is important that the therapist fully examines all of the patient's beliefs and explanations, however irrational they may seem (e.g. a 30-year-old woman would hold her head whenever she experienced headache as she believed this would prevent her from having a stroke; the evidence for this belief was examined by getting her to research whether stroke units employed this technique to reduce strokes or not).

6   *Modification of any maintaining factors.* This includes stopping medical reassurance and other reassurance from friends and family.

7   *ERP* in cases where the patient is checking excessively.

8   *Relapse prevention:*
     a   identifying and challenging core beliefs and underlying assumptions

b   advice about recognising symptoms of health anxiety when they occur and discussion on prevention strategies to stop these symptoms getting 'out of hand'.

The use of mindfulness in health anxiety

Mindfulness has been used to try to help some individuals with health anxiety by attempting to shift their focus of attention away from their physical symptoms and catastrophic thoughts. A recent study examined the possibility of teaching individuals to use mindfulness via a computer program. This course involved 10 sessions which could be studied at a rate suitable to the individual patient but over a minimum of 4 weeks. The online course consisted of guided meditation videos and automated emails, with elements of mindfulness-based stress reduction and mindfulness-based cognitive therapy. At the end of the study the group who had received computerised intervention had results comparable to those who received face-to-face mindfulness training or other interventions such as cognitive–behavioural therapy for stress (Krushe *et al*, 2013).

Key learning points

- Both BDD and health anxiety have strong similarities with OCD and both may be comorbid with OCD.
- In both conditions there are worrying thoughts or ideas which cause anxiety and lead to reassurance-seeking, checking, avoidance and other anxiolytic behaviours.
- In both conditions, patients are frequently reluctant to seek psychiatric help as they believe they have a physical disorder and require a physical medical or surgical intervention.
- In the case of the reluctant patient, it can often be helpful to present them with two hypotheses: their current hypothesis and the one the therapist believes.
- Treatment involves engaging the patient, education, stopping the anxiolytic behaviours, exposure to anxiogenic thoughts and situations, and cognitive therapy aimed at reducing NATs.

Suggested measures to use with conditions covered in this chapter

- BDD: Problems and Targets, Sheehan Disability Scale (measuring impact on life), Yale–Brown Obsessive Compulsive Scale – BDD version (Phillips *et al*, 1997); also vital to measure depression in BDD, e.g. BDI (Beck, 1978); all measures discussed in Chapter 2.
- Health anxiety: Problems and Targets, Sheehan Disability Scale, Health Anxiety Inventory (Salkovskis *et al*, 2002).

References

American Psychiatric Association (2013) *Diagnostic and Statistical Manual for Psychiatric Disorders* (DSM-5). APA.

Beck AT (1978) *Depression Inventory*. Philadelphia Center for Cognitive Therapy.

Bjornsson AS, Didie ER, Phillips KA (2010) Body dysmorphic disorder. *Dialogues in Clinical Neuroscience*, **12**: 221–32.

Krusche A, Cyhlarova E, Williams JM (2013) Mindfulness online: an evaluation of the feasibility of a web-based mindfulness course for stress, anxiety and depression. *BMJ Open*, **29**: 3.

Marks I, Mishan J (1988) Dysmorphophobic avoidance with disturbed bodily perception: a pilot study of exposure therapy. *British Journal of Psychiatry*, **152**: 674–8.

Phillips KA (2009) *Understanding Body Dysmorphic Disorder: an Essential Guide*. Oxford University Press.

Phillips KA, Hollander E, Rasmussen SA, *et al* (1997) A severity rating scale for body dysmorphic disorder: development, reliability, and validity of a modified version of the Yale-Brown Obsessive Compulsive Scale. *Psychopharmacology Bulletin*, **33**: 17–22.

Phillips KA, Gunderson CG, Mallya G, *et al* (1998) A comparison study of body dysmorphic disorder and obsessive–compulsive disorder. *Journal of Clinical Psychiatry*, **59**: 568–75.

Phillips KA, Menard W, Fay C, *et al* (2005) Demographic characteristics, phenomenology, comorbidity, and family history in 200 individuals with body dysmorphic disorder. *Psychosomatics*, **46**: 317–25.

Salkovskis PM, Rimes KA, Warwick HM, (2002) The Health Anxiety Inventory: development and validation of scales for the measurement of health anxiety and hypochondriasis. *Psychological Medicine*, **32**: 843–53.

Warwick HMC, Salkovskis PM (1990) Hypochondriasis. *Behaviour Research and Therapy*, **28**: 105–17.

Warwick HM, Clark DM, Cobb AM, *et al* (1996) A controlled trial of cognitive–behavioural treatment of hypochondriasis. *British Journal of Psychiatry*, **169**: 189–95.

Recommended treatment manuals and other reading

*Northumberland, Tyne and Wear NHS Foundation Trust (2010) *Health Anxiety: A Self Help Guide*. Available at http://www.nhs.uk/conditions/hypochondria/Documents/Health%20Anxiety%20A4%20%202010.pdf.

*Phillips KA (2005) *The Broken Mirror*. Oxford University Press.

Phillips KA (2009) *Understanding Body Dysmorphic Disorder: An Essential Guide*. Oxford University Press.

Tyrer H (2013) *Tackling Health Anxiety: A CBT Handbook*. RCPsych Publications.

*Suitable to recommend to patients.

Eating disorders

Overview

This chapter will explore the whole range of eating disorders, starting with the most widespread problem of obesity and possible treatment approaches for this serious and costly condition. Patients with psychiatric disorders tend to die earlier and have greater physical health morbidity than the general population. Many of the drugs routinely prescribed in mental health practice contribute to obesity, yet the problem of obesity has often been ignored by mental health providers. However, we are now beginning to realise the health implications of this. Behavioural and cognitive treatments for all types of eating disorders will be examined. Case examples of treatments for obesity, bulimia and anorexia nervosa will be presented. These will include clinical cases which encourage examination of addictive and obsessive personality traits in these disorders.

Eating disorders are a major problem in industrialised societies. These range from obesity, with its effects on mortality and morbidity and a huge cost to the NHS, to anorexia and bulimia, which appear to be on the increase and in the case of anorexia is starting in increasingly younger children, particularly girls.

Obesity

Obesity has been called the scourge of industrialised society. An abundance of plentiful cheap food and a sedentary lifestyle has meant that the number of obese and overweight people is increasing every year. Indeed, the prevalence of obesity in England has more than tripled in the past 25 years and the 2010 Health Survey for England (Office for National Statistics, 2011) found that:

- 63% of adults (aged 16 or over) were overweight or obese
- 30% of children (aged 2–15 years) were overweight or obese
- 26% of all adults and 16% of all children were obese.

The most common way to judge whether an individual is overweight or not is to use the BMI which is obtained by dividing the weight (in kilograms) by height (in meters squared (kg/m^2)). This method has some limitations as athletes and people who engage in many hours of sports a week can have a high BMI despite having normal fat composition. Also some ethnic groups have slightly different BMI values for health. However, in general the classification in Table 11.1 is accurate.

Being overweight and obese increases the rate of:

- type II diabetes
- certain forms of cancer (e.g. bowel cancer)
- hypertension, a major cause of heart disease and stroke.

Mental health and obesity

It has long been recognised that patients with severe, enduring mental health problems, such as schizophrenia, tend to die considerably younger than the general population. This excess mortality has only a very small component linked to suicide, with obesity, smoking, lack of exercise and alcohol misuse thought to be mainly responsible as well as the late diagnosis of physical conditions in these patients (Laursen *et al*, 2012). Indeed, weight gain during in-patient stay and the frequency of weight problems has also been reported among patients with refractory OCD (Drummond *et al*, 2012), bipolar disorder (Winham *et al*, 2013) and depressive disorder (Luppino *et al*, 2010). These associations between mental health issues and obesity may be due to the mental health condition or related to treatment with drugs such as dopamine-blocking agents and selective serotonin reuptake inhibitors (Lopresti & Drummond, 2013). Irrespective of the mechanisms, it seems important that we work with patients to prevent and cure obesity.

Treatment of obesity

Attempts were made to treat obesity throughout the 20th century, but it was found that diet and exercise were generally insufficient to maintain

Table 11.1 BMI categories for adults (over 16 years)

BMI	Category
<15	Seriously underweight, at danger of sudden death
15–19.99	Underweight
20–24.99	Normal
25–29.99	Overweight
30–39.99	Obese
40+	Morbidly obese

BMI, body mass index.

long-term weight loss. Psychological treatments including psychodynamic psychotherapy were also unhelpful. The 1960s saw the development of behavioural treatment packages (e.g. Stuart, 1967). Although these appeared more successful, it must be noted that encouraging a patient to diet may produce short-term weight loss, but with every diet invented, it has always been the case that people tend to regain weight once they stop dieting. Usually, they not only regain the weight they have lost but also tend to gain further weight. The most successful weight-loss programmes combine healthy eating with an increase in activity which can be maintained over the long term for the rest of the patient's life (Case example 11.1). The principles of the behavioural treatments can, however, be used in such a regime. There are four key elements of behavioural treatments for obesity:

1   *Description of behaviour to be controlled:* patients are asked to keep daily diaries of amount of food, time and circumstances of eating
2   *Modification and control of the discriminatory stimuli governing eating:* patients are asked to limit their eating to one room, to use distinctive table settings and to make eating a 'pure' experience unaccompanied by other activities, e.g. reading, watching television, etc.
3   *Development of techniques to control the act of eating:* e.g. counting each mouthful of food and replacing utensils after each mouthful, always leaving some food on the plate at the end of a meal
4   *Prompt reinforcement of behaviours which delay or control eating.*

Case example 11.1: Use of behavioural interventions to promote a healthier lifestyle

Joyce was a 35-year-old housewife with two young children. She had been overweight during her teens but had lost weight when she had started work as a telephonist and had maintained a normal weight until the birth of her eldest child 10 years earlier. After the birth she had stopped working. She had gained 2 stone in weight during pregnancy but believed that this would reduce with breastfeeding. Her weight did not reduce and she tried several strict dieting regimes, during which she would lose a few pounds and then binge and regain the weight. Her younger daughter was born 5 years earlier and at the end of pregnancy, Joyce was 5 stone above her ideal weight. Again, she would diet for a few days with good intentions and then a minor crisis in the home or boredom would lead her to break the diet. Once she had eaten 'forbidden' food she would feel a failure and eat anything that was readily accessible to try and comfort herself. Joining a slimming group had not helped and she had even been to a private slimming clinic to ask about surgical techniques.

At the first session, the therapist performed a full behavioural assessment of the problem, ascertaining that Joyce would eat well-balanced meals of normal size three times a day and that her 'binges' would occur at other times. She would feel the urge to eat if she was miserable or bored. The food chosen was whatever was readily available and had ranged from a packet of biscuits, to the children's Easter eggs, to a pound box of chocolates bought as a present for a friend and eaten in frustration at a bus stop when the bus failed to arrive on time. This eating was normally so rapid that Joyce hardly tasted the food and was generally performed with her standing or walking. Following a 'binge' she would feel guilty, a failure and disgusted with herself.

Her husband was a supportive and loving man, but he had started treating her weight loss attempts as a joke and told her that she would always be 'big and cuddly'.

The therapist asked Joyce to eat normally over the next 2 weeks but to note down in a diary every food that she consumed. As well as recording the quantity and type of food she ate, she was asked to note the time, place and circumstances as well as her mood before and after eating. It was emphasised that she was not to diet, but to eat absolutely normally.

Joyce arrived at the second session looking very pleased with herself as she had lost 4 lb in weight by just monitoring her food intake. The diary demonstrated that sadness and boredom were likely to result in 'binge' eating. Joyce was then instructed about some other measures she was to introduce. Her knowledge of nutrition was good due to her extensive reading about diet. She was asked not to diet, but to eat three well-balanced nutritious meals a day. At no time was she to starve herself or feel hungry. If she was hungry at other times she could eat a 'snack' and should keep nutritious 'snacks' like tomatoes and low-fat yoghurts in her refrigerator at all times. The only restriction on her was that she should only eat in the dining room, sitting at the table and using a red place setting and serviette. Whenever practical, the food should be eaten with a knife and fork. While eating, she was to concentrate on what she was doing, was not to read, listen to the radio or watch television. Between each mouthful, she was to place her utensils on the plate. Solid food should be chewed at least 15 times for each mouthful. She was only to eat enough to satisfy her hunger and should leave some food on her plate at the end of a meal or snack.

As well as controlling her general eating patterns, certain 'problem' situations were identified by Joyce and the therapist. Certain foods led to her eating in excess. Biscuits and sweets were a particular problem. Joyce agreed that the safest thing for her to do was not to buy them, even for the children. Instead, she would give them fruit as treats. If her mother gave sweets to the children, Joyce was to keep them in a large tin with a notice on it which read: 'These are not for you, Joyce, they are for Graeme and Sophie. Stop, think and do something to occupy yourself!'

Waiting for the bus to go to the shops was another difficult time as the bus stop was near a sweet shop and the boredom of waiting frequently led Joyce to buy sweets. She decided that the best way would be for her to walk to the shops which were only a few stops away and catch the bus back.

At times when she felt miserable or bored in the house Joyce compiled a list of alternative pleasurable activities she could do. These included:

- having a bubble bath
- washing and setting hair
- manicuring nails
- reading a chapter of a book
- taking the dog for a walk in the park
- riding her 'trim cycle' for 10 min.

It was emphasised to Joyce that she needed to increase her exercise slowly to at least 3 hours a week. This exercise should make her slightly breathless. Joyce remembered that a few years ago she used to walk the dog for 30 min every morning and had enjoyed this. She had stopped doing this when the children came along and her husband took the dog out instead. She decided that she would start taking the dog herself and ask her husband to ensure the children got ready to go out.

A ban was put on her weighing herself, as weight loss is slow and prone to fluctuations, and Joyce had become disheartened in the past when she thought she was not proceeding fast enough. It was also important that Joyce should reward herself for sticking to her programme. She decided that she would save sufficient money from not buying sweets and chocolates for herself and by walking to the shops to be able to buy herself a new lipstick and nail polish at the end of the week. Further suggestions for 'rewards' at the end of subsequent weeks were also made.

At the end of the session, all of the rules of the programme as well as the lists of problems and strategies were written down and given to her. She was also asked to continue keeping her food diary, and to also note times of temptation and the strategies she had employed.

Over the following 2 months, Joyce was seen weekly to monitor her progress with the behavioural programme, to 'troubleshoot' any difficulties and to receive reinforcement and encouragement from the therapist. At the end of this time she had lost 2 stone in weight and had gained much confidence. It was therefore decided to reduce the visits to the clinic to monthly sessions.

One year later, Joyce had reached her target weight, having lost over 5 stone. As the regime had not involved any strict rules of dieting, it was relatively easy for her to gradually increase her food intake to maintain this weight, and not to revert to her old eating habits. Joyce was asked to gradually increase her portions of nutritious food until her weight (measured fortnightly) was stable. It was explained to her that this was the most difficult time of the programme, as research has shown that whereas many people can lose weight, most people regain weight again once they 'relax' their rules. For this reason, it was arranged that Joyce should visit the clinic for the usual 1-, 3- and 6-month follow-up and thereafter continue to attend every 6 months to help increase her incentive to keep her weight stable. In addition, Joyce had joined a slimming club in her area, and was keen to continue attending this as a further motivating factor to maintain weight loss.

Two years later, Joyce remained at her ideal weight. She was an animated and busy person who had recently retrained and returned to work. In addition, she was an active member of a squash and tennis club. Both Joyce and her husband were delighted with her success, and she reported that her marriage and general health had greatly improved.

Anorexia nervosa

In many ways the opposite of obesity, anorexia nervosa also appears to have been on the increase over the past few decades and appears to be linked to the promotion of an extremely thin 'ideal' body image, mostly for girls and women. In anorexia nervosa the individual strives to achieve an extremely low body weight by severe food restriction with or without:

- exercise
- self-induced vomiting
- purging with laxatives
- misuse of other anorectic drugs.

The prevalence of anorexia in the UK is 19 per 100000 of the population per year for women and 2 per 100000 per year for men (National Institute for Health and Clinical Excellence, 2004). The peak age of onset is around puberty. Recently there is evidence of increasing incidence in children as young as 8 or 9 years presenting with symptoms (Halmi, 2009). Anorexia seems to be linked to cultures which place high value on thinness and thus has been noted to increase in cultures that become 'Westernised' (DiNicola, 1990).

Anorexia has a higher mortality than any other mental disorder, with death most commonly being due to the effects of starvation on the heart or suicide. Self-starvation and extremely low weight affects all systems of the body, but some of the most serious complications are acute kidney failure, liver damage and heart failure, whereas long-term complications include infertility and osteoporosis.

Treatment of anorexia nervosa

Any treatment for anorexia nervosa needs to have the following stages:

- immediate treatment
  - attention to immediate physical needs and any necessary medical intervention
  - weight gain programme (which is usually based on behavioural principles)
- longer-term treatment: examination of the precipitating and perpetuating factors for the eating disorder; there is evidence for the use of family therapy in adolescents, but other commonly used therapies include:
  - CBT
  - motivational enhancement therapy
  - interpersonal therapy
  - short-term psychodynamic intervention.

Treatment for younger children and adolescents usually focuses on family therapy (Case example 11.2), whereas for older teenagers and adults it usually involves both behavioural and cognitive–behavioural interventions.

Case example 11.2: Treating anorexia nervosa

Lucia was referred to the clinic with a 5-year-history of weight loss due to severe restriction in her dietary intake, self-induced vomiting (approximately once a week when she felt 'very fat') and excessive exercising. This problem had started shortly after her parents divorced. Lucia, who was the elder of two sisters, had always been a 'daddy's girl' and found it particularly difficult when her father moved out of their city and relocated to live with his new partner. She now only tended to see her father during school holidays. Like many people with anorexia, Lucia was a bright girl who was attending a private girls' school with high academic expectations. She was currently studying for her A-levels in biology, history and geography and hoped to go on to read history at a good university. Lucia had taken a year off school because of ill health and was not due back for another 6 months. This ill health had consisted of recurrent infections, which were extensively investigated and she was discovered to have anaemia with low iron and also low B_{12} and folate. She had never menstruated and her mother had assumed she was 'just a late developer'. Initially, she was investigated for possible coeliac disease and then a diagnosis of anorexia nervosa was made. Her mother had not realised the extent of Lucia's food restriction as she was very busy herself running her own business.

Lucia was accompanied to the clinic by her mother. The first thing that was notable was how young Lucia appeared, looking more like a 12-year-old than a girl of her age. When asked a question, she would immediately look to her mother to answer and the first hurdle was to encourage Lucia to speak for herself. At a height of 1.68 m (5 ft 6 in) Lucia weighed 47 kg (7 st 5 lb) and this meant her BMI was 16.5. Lucia, however, was initially reluctant to be weighed as she said she was 'so very fat'. When presented with the fact that she was in fact seriously underweight, she denied this and claimed to have 'light bones'.

The first thing was to educate Lucia and her mother of the dangers of anorexia. It was explained how it could lead to a number of deficiencies, including a calcium deficiency which could contribute towards 'brittle bones' or osteoporosis. In addition, the lack of menstruation could result in long-term fertility problems. Unless treated, anorexia tends to be chronic and can be deteriorating. Very low weight can result in sudden death due to organ failure. At this point, Lucia's mother started to cry, whereas she previously had seemed almost dismissive of her daughter's problem. She said she had not realised how dangerous a situation had arisen and felt she needed to keep a closer eye on the situation at home. It was explained that Lucia was not at an extremely low weight and thus there was a good prognosis. The first thing that needed to happen was for everyone to agree to participate in treatment and to look to the future. Because Lucia was not at an extremely low weight, she did not need emergency medical intervention. If her weight had been lower or there had been medical complications, it would have been necessary to ensure that she was seen by a specialist eating disorder service.

Lucia's mother agreed and Lucia reluctantly agreed too, but insisted 'I don't want to get fat, I won't go over 48 kg (7 st 10 lb)'. The therapist explained that the important thing was to introduce a healthy diet into Lucia's life. This should contain all the vitamins and minerals that she needed to maintain health and start menstruation. The target weight would be to give Lucia a BMI of 18 (which is within the low end of normal for a girl of her age). This weight was 50 kg (7 st 12 lb) but the therapist emphasised that the important thing was not to start arguing over weight but to concentrate on healthy eating. In order to do this, it was explained that Lucia would need to have three healthy, well-balanced meals and two snacks per day. In addition, she should drink 0.5–1 l (1–2 pints) of milk a day. This could be semi-skimmed if preferred. A diet plan was devised with Lucia and her mother that took into account Lucia's food preferences (Table 11.2).

Lucia's mother agreed that she would arrange to work from home for the next month so that she could monitor Lucia's progress. It was agreed that the family would sit together for meals (when her sister was home in the evening) and that Lucia would not eat alone. She would remain with her mother for at least an hour after the meal to reduce the risk of self-induced vomiting. During this time, rather than the mother play the role of custodian, positive

Table 11.2 Diet plan for Lucia

Meal	Content	Notes
Breakfast	• 1 cup (125 ml) of cereal with 1 cup (125 ml) of milk • 1 glass orange juice • 2 slices wholemeal toast with butter and marmalade, jam or Marmite • Tea or coffee with milk	Milk comes from the total allowance
Mid-morning snack	• Piece of fruit or a biscuit with tea or coffee with milk	
Lunch	• Fish, meat or Quorn approximately the size of Lucia's palm or piece of cheese (size of a matchbox) • Salad of 3 cups of 3 items of different colours (e.g. 1 cup tomatoes, 1 cup spring onions and 1 cup watercress) • 2 slices of bread with butter • 1 cup of milk pudding or 1 slice cake	Milk comes from the total allowance
Mid-afternoon snack	• 2 plain biscuits, tea or coffee with milk	
Dinner	• Fish, meat or Quorn approximately the size of Lucia's palm • 2 cups of different vegetables • 1 cup of potatoes, rice, pasta or noodles • Dessert of cake, milky pudding, etc.	
Before bed	• Mug of hot chocolate or malted drink	Milk comes from the total allowance

and enjoyable activities could be arranged. It was agreed that up to twice a day they would take their dog out for a walk, but this was to be for no more than 30 min and was to be at the speed that her mother dictated (previously Lucia had been 'power walking' for up to 10 miles a day in an attempt to control her weight). On other days they might spend time going to the local swimming pool for a 30 min swim (in exchange for one of the walks), sit and talk or go shopping. Lucia's progress would be monitored by her in a food diary, which would also contain information about any self-induced vomiting or over-exercising.

One of the important items was that Lucia was asked not to weigh herself but to wait until she returned to the clinic. This is because people with eating disorders can get preoccupied with weighing themselves. Weight may vary by as much as 1 kg from day to day depending on hydration and contents of the bowels.

It was also important that Lucia should be 'rewarded' for sticking to the programme. The first 'reward' was, of course, spending more time with her mother, which was something Lucia wanted. Second, they agreed that if she stuck to the programme for the whole week, the family would go out to the cinema. Any refusal to eat the diet, self-induced vomiting or extra exercise would delay this cinema trip by 1 day.

Over the next month, Lucia progressed reasonably well. After the first week, her mother reported that she had induced vomiting once but not since that time. Lucia's weight had increased to 49 kg (7 st 10 lb) and it was felt that it was time to give Lucia more responsibility for her own programme. Her mother was to return to work, but the whole family would still sit down to eat breakfast and dinner together. Lucia was to attend the clinic weekly to examine her thoughts which led to her eating disorder. She was to continue keeping a food diary and to record any vomiting and over-exercising (limited to 30 min per day).

To start examining Lucia's NATs, the therapist asked her about the previous day when Lucia reported that she had a very strong urge to make herself sick. The therapist asked her what went though her head.

Lucia: 'I just felt fat and bloated and disgusting.'

Therapist: 'Why was that?'

Lucia: 'I had just eaten my evening meal when I had had spaghetti carbonara and I looked at my chest and realised my breasts were getting larger.'

Therapist: 'What is so bad about that?'

Lucia: 'Oh! I don't want to look like a glamour model or anything, I have always been flat-chested.'

Therapist: 'A glamour model?'

Lucia: 'OK maybe that's an exaggeration… but I really don't want to develop a chest. I've never had to wear a bra.'

Therapist: 'Most girls of your age have been wearing a bra for the past 5–7 years, why do you not want to?'

Lucia: 'I really don't want to have men staring at me.'

Therapist: 'Why would receiving appreciative looks from men be such a bad thing?'

As the interaction continued, it became clear that Lucia hated anything which made her look like a grown woman, preferring instead to stay looking like a child. Growing up meant to Lucia that she needed to take responsibility for herself and she did not feel ready for this. Also, she hoped that one day her father might return to live with the family again and that they'd be 'one big happy family again'. A formulation was then constructed (Fig. 11.1).

Lucia was asked to think of the pros and cons of staying as a child and not moving on with her life. Working collaboratively, Lucia and the therapist came up with a list (Table 11.3).

It was decided that the first thing that needed tackling was the expectation on Lucia's part that if she remained child-like her father might come back to the family and everything would be as it had been before. She was set the homework of thinking of the evidence for and against this idea.

The next session was opened by Lucia saying 'I know that Dad won't really come back but I really would like him to!' Over the week she had looked at the evidence as requested and had realised that her father would not come back to them as he now had a settled life and a new baby with his new partner. Lucia had realised how jealous she was of this new partner. The therapist asked 'If you accept that Dad won't come back if you remain a child, what would the next step be?' Lucia said her Dad had invited her to go and stay with his new family but Lucia had not taken up the invitation. On discussion with the therapist, she said that she had never really met her step-mother as she had just demonised her as 'the woman who took Dad away'. She now

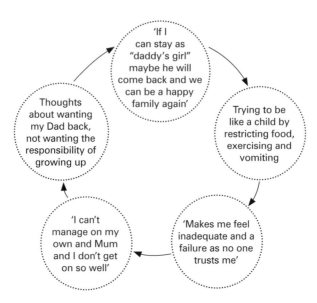

Fig. 11.1 Some of the maintaining thoughts for Lucia's anorexia.

Table 11.3 Pros and cons of growing up for Lucia

Advantages of growing up	Disadvantages of growing up
'Mum won't be constantly nagging me'	'I need to take responsibility for myself'
'I can go and do what I want and like'	'Dad may come back to us'
'I can leave home and study at university'	'Everything could be as it was when I was
'I can go out with friends'	young and we were happy'
'I may eventually have a home and a family	'People will look after me'
of my own'	

realised that her mother and father had had problems for many years and this is why her father had tended to spend so much time with her rather than with her mother. She also understood that to start to grow into an adult, she should take up her father's invitation and try to gain a relationship on an adult footing with her father and step-mother.

Thereafter followed several sessions in which Lucia tested out the idea of being more 'adult' and the advantages and disadvantages of this. Her weight only crept up very gradually but she did not at any point lose weight. She denied any vomiting or excessive exercise. She started experimenting with wearing make-up and clothes more appropriate for a teenager. An added benefit to this was that her mother and sister became interested in going out with her and trying new styles. After 5 months Lucia felt ready to return to school and to resume her A-level studies. At 48 kg (7 st 10 lb) she was still underweight but was healthier and continuing to slowly gain weight. She was wearing a bra and recently reported that she had had her first period. Therapy had been concentrating on her maturation and also examining how she felt about her changing body and any NATs related to this. Therapy continued after she returned to school but was reduced to once a month. Any sign of relapse meant she would have to have more sessions (which Lucia did not want as she felt it made her 'different' from the other students).

This case history emphasises another aspect of anorexia nervosa which is that it can take many months to treat. Despite this, many people can recover. A small but significant number of individuals have a chronic and relapsing condition; a small number have chronic anorexia. The risk of suicide as well as sudden death in anorexia mean it has the highest mortality rate of any psychiatric condition. Suicide is, of course, more of a risk in the more chronic conditions, but a full risk assessment is always essential.

Bulimia nervosa

Bulimia nervosa is more common than anorexia nervosa and tends to occur in an older age group, with most individuals presenting in adult life and an average age of onset in late teens. In this condition there is an attempt to control weight by severe food restriction, followed by binging where huge amounts of food can be consumed. There are often 'forbidden foods' which are avoided at all costs and then consumed in huge quantities during a binge. Foods which are used in a binge tend to be energy-dense foods such as chocolate, sweets, biscuits, cakes, bread and even cheese. In addition to restriction of food intake there are often other attempts to control weight, including laxative misuse and self-induced vomiting. As with other eating disorders, bulimia nervosa can often be associated with depression and low mood, poor self-esteem and alcohol misuse. One variant of bulimia nervosa has been labelled multi-impulsive bulimia nervosa as the patient may misuse alcohol and drugs and be involved in other impulsive behaviours such as violent or other illegal behaviour (Lacey, 1993). This subgroup of 'sensation-seeking' patients with bulimia have been found to be more likely to have suffered childhood sexual abuse (Groleau et al, 2012).

Treatment of bulimia nervosa

Treatment of bulimia is similar to that described in anorexia nervosa but without the need for refeeding and weight gain. Instead, as hunger and restriction of the type and quantity of food eaten are one of the main causes of binge eating, it is important to establish a regular eating pattern to reduce the risk of binge-eating and to identify any cues which precipitate binges and modify them. Almost two-thirds of patients with bulimia who undertake CBT show a good response to treatment (Case example 11.3).

Case example 11.3: Bulimia nervosa

Hilary was a 30-year-old single woman who worked as a solicitor in a large legal firm. When she was seen at the clinic, she weighed 60 kg (9 st 7 lb) and was 1.73 m (5 ft 8 in) tall, which meant she had a normal BMI of 20.

181

However, she gave a long history of difficulty with controlling her food intake. As a child she had been mildly overweight and had been teased about it. In her teens, she decided to control her weight and went on a strict calorie-controlled diet of 1000 kcal per day and lost weight. After she stopped this diet, she found she was regaining weight and so she continued with a series of extreme 'fad' diets and a roller-coaster of weight gain and loss. Following a degree at university, Hilary went on to law school to do a conversion course. She found this pressurised and began to restrict her diet completely. After a short while, she developed an urge to binge. These binges occurred 2–3 times a week and were after a particularly stressful day. A binge would start by Hilary going to the local late-night store and buying 5–6 packets of chocolate digestive biscuits (which she vehemently refused to eat at other times for fear of provoking a binge), 2–3 loaves of bread and a 0.5 kg slab of cheese. She would then go home and sit in the kitchen and consume these foods rapidly and without really tasting them. While eating the food she felt relieved but almost as if she was 'in a trance'. Following the binge she was filled with disgust and self-loathing and would immediately force herself to vomit. In addition, she would swallow large amounts of a senna-based laxative. Describing herself, Hilary felt she was a 'disgusting creature' who had no self-control and would one day become a 'huge, amoeba-like, fat slob'.

After a full assessment, the therapist talked to Hilary about how her calorie restriction led to the eating binges. These binges were also fuelled by her self-loathing and low self-esteem. Treatment would involve:

- regularisation of her diet
- identifying precipitating factors for a binge and modifying any stimuli which may precede the binge
- identification of NATs and underlying assumptions and modification of them.

First, Hilary was asked to stick to a regular eating pattern consisting of three meals and two snacks a day. This is similar to the eating regime introduced for Lucia (Case example 11.2), but whereas Lucia's regime was designed for her to gain weight, the one for Hilary was designed to maintain a healthy weight and consisted of 2000 kcal. It was emphasised that it was important for her to maintain healthy eating and to have at least 0.5 l (1 pint) of milk a day as well as eating five portions of different fruit and vegetables, protein twice a day and at least three portions of complex carbohydrates which would help to maintain her blood sugar levels and make a binge less likely. A comprehensive day plan was produced by Hilary together with the therapist (Table 11.4).

The idea of this diet plan was for Hilary to remain feeling satiated throughout the day and without any dips in her blood sugar level. Alcohol is generally a very bad idea as it can weaken resolve and provoke a binge as well as raising blood sugar followed by a 'slump'. Hilary felt she would be unable to tell friends she did not want to drink and so the therapist agreed that she could have two small glasses of wine twice a week. With red wine, which Hilary tended to drink, this would be approximately 5 units of alcohol (which is within the recommended 'safe' level of a maximum of 14 units for women 18 to 60 years of age; half of this level for people over 60 years). The therapist asked Hilary to record her progress as well as any urges to binge and the details of these in a diary (Table 11.5).

When Hilary returned the next week, she had stuck to her diet, had had two urges to binge but had not succumbed. The therapist praised her for

Table 11.4 Daily eating plan for Hilary

Day	Breakfast	Mid-morning	Lunch	Mid-afternoon	Supper
Monday	Porridge made with milk and fresh fruit	Apple	Ham salad followed by fruit yogurt	Small chocolate biscuit	Chicken breast with broccoli, carrots and new potatoes, individual-size trifle, milk drink before bed
Tuesday	Muesli with banana and milk	2 plums	Cheese salad and fruit jelly	2 digestive biscuits	Homemade Thai prawn curry with spinach and rice, mango slices
Wednesday	Porridge made with milk and fresh fruit	Pear	Macaroni cheese and side salad in local cafe	1 chocolate digestive biscuit	Tuna and sweetcorn bake with new potatoes, fruit yoghurt, milk drink before bed
Thursday	Muesli with banana and milk	Apple	Beef salad followed by banana	2 digestive biscuits	Homemade cauliflower cheese with carrots and potatoes, individual-size chocolate mousse, milk drink before bed
Friday	Wholemeal cereal and fresh fruit	Banana	Prawn and avocado wholemeal sandwich, fruit jelly	2 digestive biscuits	Dinner with friends, 1 glass of wine (125 ml), milk drink before bed
Saturday	2 boiled eggs and 2 slices of wholemeal toast	Glass of milk	Cheese ploughman's lunch	2 digestive biscuits	Dinner with friends, 1 glass of wine (125 ml)
Sunday	Grilled mushrooms, bacon and tomato, 2 slices of wholemeal toast	Glass of milk	Boiled egg salad, fruit yogurt	2 digestive biscuits	Salmon fillet with watercress and potatoes, fruit salad, milk drink before bed

Table 11.5 Thought diary for Hilary

Date, time and place	What was happening	Your thoughts	Urge to binge (0 lowest, 10 highest)	Outcome (i.e. did you binge or not and what did you do?)

183

this. The times when she had been tempted to binge were when she was at work and started comparing herself with colleagues in the office. In the first case, one of the senior partners had praised her colleague for some work she did. Hilary thought: 'Stephanie is very good…and also very slim and beautiful. I am useless and a fat frump in comparison.' In the second case, one of the senior partners asked a colleague to take on a case. Hilary thought: 'He's asked Brian because he knows I'm rubbish and would make a mess of it all.'

The therapist asked Hilary to think of the evidence for and against these statements. In the case of the first example, she was asked to focus on the evidence for her being a 'fat frump'. With prompting from the therapist she came up with two lists.

Evidence for being a 'fat frump':
- 'I sometimes feel fat and frumpy'
- 'I do binge eat'.

Evidence against:
- 'My weight is at the low end of normal'
- 'Several friends commented on how much they admire my figure'
- 'On Monday Jane said that I was the best-dressed woman in the office'.

Using this evidence, Hilary produced the rational response of 'Stephanie is very slim and beautiful but I am slim and stylish'.

'Evidence' was also obtained for the second NAT.

Evidence for being useless:
- 'Brian was asked to do this work'
- 'I could have done the work'.

Evidence against:
- 'I have recently been assigned two complex cases'
- 'Brian has just finished a case and would have had some slack time'
- 'I was praised for my work by the senior partner not long ago'
- 'At my appraisal, my work was rated A+'.

This produced the rational response that 'Brian was asked to do this work because he had time to devote to it'.

As a solicitor, Hilary found this searching for evidence fairly easy and progressed well with challenging her NATs. After three sessions, the therapist decided to examine the underlying assumptions behind these negative thoughts. The main theme of her thoughts was that she was 'useless'. Using the downward arrow technique, the therapist discovered that Hilary's underlying assumption was that she was useless and hopeless and would always be inferior to others. This assumption was then challenged and some evidence was obtained to this effect.

Evidence for Hilary's belief that she is useless and hopeless:
- 'I often feel as if I am useless and hopeless'
- 'I was teased at school'
- 'I have bulimia and I binge eat'.

Evidence against:
- 'I gained good A-levels'
- 'I gained a 2:1 degree at university'
- 'I passed my law exams with good marks'
- 'At my appraisal, my work was rated A+'.

Hilary began to understand that her emotions and feeling as if she were useless or hopeless or fat and frumpy were not based in reality but were part of her feelings, probably related to her experience of being bullied in the past. Her life had now moved on and she was a successful career woman. Once Hilary had realised this, her progress was dramatic and swift and she stopped all binge eating.

Hilary's case history demonstrates the use of dietary regulation and cognitive reattribution in bulimia nervosa. With some patients, it is also possible to alter the stimuli that provoke a binge. For example, alcohol can lower the resolve and make a binge more likely. Others may keep 'binge-on' foods in the house and this means that a binge can occur easily, whereas it would be better not to keep these foods near at hand.

Eating disorders not otherwise specified (EDNOS) and binge eating disorder

Many individuals with abnormal eating patterns do not fulfil diagnostic criteria for anorexia or bulimia nervosa but are still potentially damaging their health by poor diet. They are classified as having EDNOS (World Health Organization, 1992). In DSM-5 there is a new category of binge eating disorder as well as EDNOS (American Psychiatric Association, 2013). Treatments described in this chapter can be used in both these cases, depending on the problem presented.

Key learning points

- Obesity is a rapidly increasing problem in high-income countries and causes a major challenge to UK health services. Healthy eating and exercise plans can be implemented with the help of behavioural techniques for some obese people to good effect.
- Anorexia is another increasing problem in the UK. It has a high mortality rate. Although mostly affecting women and girls, an increasing number of men and boys are also affected. Treatment involves behavioural intervention followed by cognitive reattribution of the thoughts concerning food, weight and self-image.
- Bulimia nervosa is more common than anorexia and features a slightly older age group. Again, women are mostly affected but doctors are seeing an increasing number of men with the problem. Suicide rates are high. Most people with bulimia require dietary advice and behavioural intervention as well as cognitive reattribution. They tend to have low self-esteem, which can be tackled using cognitive therapy.
- Many patients with eating disorders do not meet strict criteria for either anorexia or bulimia. These disorders have been categorised as eating disorders not otherwise specified in ICD-10 and in DSM-5 are in a new category of binge eating disorder as well as EDNOS.

Suggested measures to use with conditions covered in this chapter

- Problems and Targets, weight measurement (once weekly), direct observation *in vivo* and Yale–Brown–Cornell Eating Disorders Scale self-report questionnaire (Bellace *et al*, 2012) if associated with binge eating.
- Anorexia nervosa and bulimia nervosa: Problems and Targets, Sheehan Disability Scale (measuring impact on life), weight measurement (once weekly), direct observation *in vivo*, Yale–Brown–Cornell Eating Disorders Scale self-report questionnaire.

References

American Psychiatric Association (2013) *Diagnostic and Statistical Manual for Psychiatric Disorders* (DSM-5). APA.

Bellace DL, Tesser R, Berthod S (2012) The Yale–Brown–Cornell eating disorders scale self-report questionnaire: a new, efficient tool for clinicians and researchers. *International Journal of Eating Disorders*, **45**: 856–60.

DiNicola V (1990) Anorexia multiforme: self-starvation in historical and cultural context. Part II: Anorexia nervosa as a culture-reactive syndrome. *Transcultural Psychiatry*, **27**: 245–86.

Drummond LM, Boschen MJ, Cullimore J (2012) Physical complications of severe, chronic obsessive-compulsive disorder: a comparison with general psychiatric inpatients. *General Hospital Psychiatry*, **34**: 618–25.

Groleau P, Steiger H, Joober R, *et al* (2012) Dopamine-system genes, childhood abuse, and clinical manifestations in women with Bulimia-spectrum disorders. *Journal of Psychiatric Research*, **46**: 1139–45.

Halmi KA (2009) Anorexia nervosa: an increasing problem in children and adolescents. *Dialogues in Clinical Neuroscience*, **11**: 100–3.

Lacey JH (1993) Self-damaging and addictive behaviour in bulimia nervosa: a catchment area study. *British Journal of Psychiatry*, **163**: 190–4.

Laursen TM, Munk-Olsen T, Vestergaard M (2012) Life expectancy and cardiovascular mortality in persons with schizophrenia. *Current Opinion in Psychiatry*, **25**: 83–8.

Lopresti AL, Drummond PD (2013) Obesity and psychiatric disorders: commonalities in dysregulated biological pathways and their implications for treatment. *Progress in Neuropsychopharmacology and Biological Psychiatry*, **45**: 92–9.

Luppino FS, de Wit LM, Bouvy PF, *et al* (2010) Overweight, obesity, and depression: a systematic review and meta-analysis of longitudinal studies. *Archives of General Psychiatry*, **67**: 220–9.

National Institute for Health and Clinical Excellence (2004) *Eating Disorders, Core Interventions in the Treatment and Management of Anorexia Nervosa, Bulimia Nervosa, and Related Eating Disorders* (Clinical Guideline CG9). British Psychological Society & Royal College of Psychiatrists.

Office for National Statistics (2011) *Health Survey for England – 2010: Trend Tables*. Health and Social Care Information Centre.

Stuart RB (1967) Behavioral control of overeating. *Behaviour Research and Therapy*, **1**: 357–65.

Winham SJ, Cuellar-Barboza AB, Oliveros A, *et al* (2013) Genome-wide association study of bipolar disorder accounting for effect of body mass index identifies a new risk allele in TCF7L2. *Molecular Psychiatry*, **doi**: 10.1038/mp.2013.159. [Epub ahead of print]

World Health Organization (1992) *Glossary of Mental Disorders and Guide for their Classification for Use with International Classification of Diseases, 10th revision*. WHO.

Recommended treatment manuals and other reading

*Brownell KD (2000) *The LEARN Programme for Weight Management* (10th edn). American Health Publishers.

Cooper Z, Fairburn CG, Hawker DM (2003) *Cognitive-Behavioural Treatment of Obesity: A Clinician's Guide*. Guilford Press.

Fairburn CG (2008) *Cognitive Behavior Therapy and Eating Disorders*. Guilford Press.

*Fairburn CG (2013) *Overcoming Binge Eating: The Proven Program to Learn Why You Binge and How You Can Stop* (2nd edn). Guilford Press.

*Freeman C (2009) *Overcoming Anorexia Nervosa: A Self-help Guide using Cognitive–Behavioural Techniques*. Constable & Robinson.

Latner JD, Wilson GT (2007) (eds) *Self-Help Approaches for Obesity and Eating Disorders: Research and Practice*. Guilford Press.

*Suitable to recommend to patients.

Addictive behaviour

Overview

Alcohol misuse is a major cause of ill health internationally. Harm reduction and treatment programmes are an important part of our health service. Many patients find it extremely difficult to maintain willpower to stop using alcohol, but techniques such as motivational interviewing can help to increase compliance. In this chapter, the application of motivational interviewing, coping skills training and relapse training will be described in the treatment of alcohol misuse. There will also be a discussion about the use of such strategies with other substance misuse. Comorbidity of substance misuse will be explored. Smoking is also a major cause of mortality and morbidity throughout the world and CBT for smoking cessation will be discussed as will the application of CBT in the case history of a problem gambler. Finally, the controversial concept of sexual addiction will be raised.

Alcohol

Alcohol misuse is creating a huge burden to the NHS. Over recent decades there has been an increase in binge drinking as well as an increase in regular drinking in all sectors of society. Whereas historically alcohol misuse was more common in men, nowadays increasing numbers of women are drinking to excess. Binge drinking is mainly a problem among the younger age groups, but an increasing number of middle-aged and elderly people are consuming dangerous levels of alcohol in their own homes and without realising the perils they face (Royal College of Psychiatrists, 2011).

The main problem with alcohol is that it is not only a highly addictive but also a legal drug. Many people thus feel it must be 'harmless' and anyone suggesting a reduction in alcohol consumption is a 'killjoy'. There is thus a social pressure for people to drink alcohol and toleration of excessive consumption until severe addiction occurs. Some of the deleterious effects of alcohol are:

- liver damage (which may eventually lead to cirrhosis)
- pancreatitis (and ultimately pancreatic cancer)
- brain damage
- cardiovascular effects with increased risks of strokes and heart attacks
- increased rate of cancer
- increased risk of accidents
- increase in violent behaviour
- worsening of many psychiatric disorders, including depression.

Alcohol is converted in the body to sugars and it is also a cause of obesity as these sugars provide no nutritional benefit to the body. The recommended maximum consumption of alcohol in the UK is different for men and women: 21 units of alcohol per week for men, no more than 4 units in any one day, and at least 2 alcohol-free days a week; and 14 units per week for women, no more than 3 units in any one day, and at least 2 alcohol-free days a week. A group of experts suggest that people over the age of 65 should reduce consumption to half this amount, owing to less efficient processing of alcohol and potential interaction with prescribed drugs (Royal College of Psychiatrists, 2011).

One unit of alcohol consists of:

- half a pint of ordinary strength beer, lager or cider (3–4% alcohol by volume)
- a small pub measure of spirits (25 ml; 40% alcohol by volume)
- a standard pub measure of fortified wine such as sherry or port (50 ml; 20% alcohol by volume).

One-and-a-half units of alcohol is:

- a small glass of ordinary strength wine (125 ml; 12% alcohol by volume)
- a standard pub measure of spirits (35 ml; 40% alcohol by volume).

Therefore, a 30-year-old woman drinking a large glass (175 ml) of wine per night every night would be drinking between 14 and 21 units of alcohol a week with no alcohol rest days and would be endangering her health.

The strength of any alcoholic drink is measured as alcohol by volume (ABV). Thus a spirit such as whisky is 40% ABV, whereas table wine is 12–15% ABV. The number of units of alcohol in any drink can be calculated by the following formula:

The recommendation from NHS Choices is that pregnant women or

$$\frac{\text{Strength (ABV)} \times \text{volume (ml)}}{1000} = \text{units}$$

women trying to conceive should not drink alcohol at all. If they do choose to drink, to minimise the risk to the baby, they should not drink more than 1–2 units of alcohol once or twice a week and should not get drunk (www.nhs.uk/chq/Pages/2270.aspx?CategoryID=54#close).

Other addictive drugs

The approach to treating alcohol or other addictive drugs is similar. The differences are that, whereas alcohol is a legal drug, other agents are not. Drug users are therefore more likely to come into contact with crime to obtain the drugs or to be involved in criminal activity if they have a severe drug habit they need to fund. Some drugs are like alcohol and induce considerable tolerance and the potential for addiction readily, whereas others do not. Bearing in mind these factors, which may affect the necessary medical interventions and the route of referral (either voluntary or compulsory via the justice system), the basics of treatment are identical.

Treatment of alcohol and drug misuse

Many people seem unaware of the health facts about alcohol stated earlier. If a patient is drinking slightly more than the recommended levels, education may be sufficient to alter this pattern. It may also be useful to examine some of the cues to drinking with the patient and work out some strategies and alternative behaviours. For example, the patient may have developed the habit of having a glass of wine every night to 'unwind' after work. Discussion about this and working out alternative strategies can be useful. They may find that going for a brisk walk, going swimming, reading a newspaper or making a telephone call to a loved one is equally as 'unwinding' but considerably better for health! Encouragement to keep a diary and record this can be useful in tracking progress.

For more extreme misuse the following interventions can be useful:

- motivational interviewing (to engage the patient)
- coping skills training
- relapse prevention training.

Motivational interviewing

Motivational interviewing (Miller & Rollnick, 2002) is a form of engaging a patient in therapy which encourages them to develop their readiness to change. Many people with alcohol and drug problems do not see their addiction as a problem in the way the outside world may do. They may have many ways of justifying their behaviour. Any therapy with an ambivalent patient can be difficult. There are qualifications and courses describing motivational interviewing in full, which are beyond the scope of this book. However, it is useful for any therapist embarking on therapy with this patient group to be aware of the principles and apply them as much as possible.

Express empathy

This involves trying to see the world through the patient's eyes. Patients with addiction problems often think the 'world is against them'. The therapist must have a non-judgemental stance and listen to the patient, acknowledging their difficulties and troubles.

Develop discrepancy

Using Socratic questioning, the therapist should try to let the patient see the discrepancies between their future goals and current behaviour. Examining the pros and cons of their behaviour can be useful in developing this in a similar way to challenging NATs.

Roll with resistance

This involves not reacting to resistance in the patient but letting it pass. No resistance is challenged and instead the therapist encourages the patient to explain their resistance further. Therefore there is no reinforcement of their argumentative stance and no confrontation between therapist and patient. The therapist accepts a resistance to change as a natural way for a person to react.

Support self-efficacy

This means accepting the patient's decision, even if when fully informed of the consequences of this decision, they choose not to change. In addition, the therapist encourages the patient to devise their own solutions to the problems they have defined.

It can be seen that these principles are generally being used by any good CBT therapist who is engaged in pragmatic empiricism with the patient. It is, however, particularly useful to bear these four points in mind when faced with a patient who resists therapy. Let us see how those principles can be applied in practice (Case example 12.1).

Case example 12.1: A long history of heavy drinking

Neil, a 40-year-old accountant, was a married man with a history of relatively heavy drinking since his university days. Over the past 5 years he had settled into a pattern of heavy drinking. Although apparently able to function at work, his wife with their two young children had recently separated from him as she felt that he had 'no time and no interest in us'. The referral to the clinic had occurred because Neil had recently attended his GP and was found to have some widespread liver damage.

The start of the interview was difficult. Neil made it plain that he did not believe he had an alcohol problem, that he felt people were 'over-reacting' and that he drank no more than 'anyone who wasn't a do-gooding teetotaller'. The therapist used the principles of motivational interviewing and listened to his reservations, expressing empathy concerning his shock at being referred to a psychiatric clinic. The therapist then looked at what he had been told was necessary for his future health and any ways in which his life might be better if he was drinking a little less. Neil then admitted that he wished his wife and children had not left and although expressing the view that 'they'll be back, it's just her hormones', he did become slightly tearful. The therapist used Socratic questioning to get Neil to examine whether or not drinking as he was doing was helpful to his long-term aims (*developing discrepancy*).

Throughout the assessment Neil was periodically argumentative and felt he was 'being picked on' by his wife and his GP. He expressed the view that he felt coming to the psychiatric clinic was 'just ridiculous' as 'what need do I have of a shrink?' The therapist did not 'rise to the bait' of any of his provocative statements but encouraged him to come back to examine where he wished to go from here (*roll with resistance*). In encouraging Neil to come up with his own solutions, the therapist was using the principle of *encouraging self-efficacy*.

Eventually, the following pattern of drinking emerged:

6.30	Wake up and get ready for work
7.30	Train into the city
8.00–13.00	In the office
13.00	Lunch with clients (half a bottle of red wine and a brandy to finish)
15.00–17.30	In the office
17.30–19.30	After-work drink with colleagues (usually drink half a bottle of wine)
19.30	Train home
20.00	Dinner with a large glass of wine
20.30–23.00	Watch television and may drink another glass of wine
23.30	Bed

Looking at this pattern, it could be seen that Neil was drinking 1.5 bottles of wine and 1 brandy on most days. At the weekends he admitted to drinking more. As he drank red wine, this was approximately 15% ABV most days. His average unit of alcohol consumed was calculated:

15 (% ABV) x 1000 (ml of wine) = 15 000
15 000 /1000 = 15 units per day from red wine
plus 1 standard measure of brandy = 1.5 units
Total per day = 16.5 units
Total per week >115.5 units

Clearly Neil was drinking huge amounts of alcohol and it was necessary to ensure he was physically safe to proceed with any treatment. Neil denied any craving before lunchtime and did not drink during the day. He denied any shakes or nausea in the morning and said he was able to clean his teeth without retching. However, it was felt wise not to risk an abrupt cessation when drinking at this level. He was asked to visit his GP and to start an alcohol-withdrawal regime using chlordiazepoxide, which would be prescribed on a reducing dose over the 7–10 days. The therapist expressed concern that Neil was living alone and also that he should not be working while undergoing detoxification.

Neil agreed to be signed off work by his GP, who would record this as 'liver problems' on his sickness certificate. He said he would stay with his sister for the next fortnight to ensure his physical safety. It must always be remembered that people who are dependent on alcohol can have a number of serious and potentially life-threatening complications if they stop the alcohol abruptly. These include seizures as well as the risk of the potentially fatal delirium tremens. The GP also prescribed a multivitamin including vitamin B_1 (thiamine), as although it was felt that Neil was eating well, it was important to ensure he was not short of thiamine which could lead to brain damage (and in the most severe cases Wernicke's encephalopathy and Korsakoff syndrome). The therapist also asked Neil to record in his diary any times when he felt more tempted to drink. Neil was sure that he only drank 'to be sociable' with everyone but then did admit that he was frequently the person urging everyone else to accompany him for a drink and then urging people to drink more. It was explained that people who drink heavily will usually do this for a particular reason such as feeling isolated and lonely, anxious or depressed and then use alcohol to deal with this emotion.

When Neil was seen the next week, he had stuck to his detoxification programme and was feeling reasonably well. He had identified times when he had had a very strong urge to drink. These had been two specific occasions. First, his sister had asked him to accompany her to her daughter's school play. Neil had immediately felt that he would need a drink. Second, he had been told that his wife was going to bring the children round to see him that evening and he had felt a strong urge to drink.

The therapist felt there was the need to move on to some coping skills training with Neil. In many cases, people who have a history of heavy drinking can also be prescribed a drug such as acamprosate which reduces alcohol cravings. Neil was adamant he would not use such an agent and that he wished to 'do it alone'.

Coping skills and relapse prevention training

These techniques have been fully described by Kadden (2001).

Relaxation skills

Many people who misuse alcohol and drugs have difficulty relaxing without using them. They can be taught relaxation exercises and also need to learn to enjoy other ways of relaxing without the use of psychoactive substances.

Finding new pleasurable activities

Heavy drinkers and drug users have usually restricted their repertoire of pleasurable activities that most people enjoy. They need to be encouraged to take up previously enjoyed or new activities. For Neil, he rediscovered his love of cinema and also began enjoying spending more time with his children.

Decision-making

Many people with addiction problems have difficulty in making decisions and sticking by these decisions. They can practise a technique whereby the therapist asks the patient to identify all the evidence in favour and against a particular decision. The patient is then asked to put a numerical value on each of these points. After adding up the values, an answer can be reached. If this answer does not seem correct, then it can be changed immediately, but once a decision has been made, it is important to stress that it should not be changed unless more evidence comes to light that alters the situation. Many patients not only have difficulty making the initial decision, but fluctuate and brood on it afterwards, which results in emotional stress and distress (which can lead to alcohol/drug misuse).

Problem-solving

Again, this requires the therapist to encourage the patient to 'brain-storm' all potential answers to a situation and then give a numerical value to the practicality and acceptability of the answers. Just as in the decision-making process, excess brooding once a decision has been made should be avoided.

Planning for the unexpected

Unexpected events can cause difficulties for patients. The approach here is similar to that for problem-solving but the situation is more immediate. Discussion about this can be an important part of relapse prevention.

Social skills

Neil had some social anxiety but generally good social skills. Some people with substance addiction have had the problem since adolescence or for such a long time that they have either 'forgotten' or have never developed appropriate adult social skills. In these cases, social skills training (as described in Chapter 4) should be provided.

Declining invitations to drink/take drugs

This is a vital part of any relapse prevention regime. The patient needs to be able to handle old friends and acquaintances who will try and attract them back to their old behaviour. In this case role-playing with the therapist in a variety of hypothetical situations can be invaluable.

Refusing requests

Many people with addiction problems have assertiveness problems and have difficulty in stating their opinion for fear of being 'rude'. They can then become resentful, which can lead them to misuse alcohol or drugs. Assertiveness training can be used in these situations (as described in Chapter 4).

Dealing with intimate relationships

Addiction has a negative impact on people's relationships with significant others. In some cases the relationship is damaged beyond repair, but in others relationship therapy can be useful (as described in Chapter 5).

Some people with addiction have problems expressing emotion and this can lead to them misusing psychoactive substances. This can be tackled by helping the individual to express their feeling and examining the NATs which may inhibit them from doing this.

Case example 12.1, continued

Using the approach of collaborative empiricism, the therapist and Neil started to examine his triggers for drinking excessively (antecedents) and also what he hoped to achieve from drinking (desired consequences; Fig. 12.1a) as well as what happened in reality (true consequences; Fig. 12.1b). By examining his thoughts and feelings further, a model of Neil's drinking behaviour was developed (Fig. 12.2). It was clear from this model that two approaches were necessary:

- examine the NATs and underlying assumptions leading to feelings of inadequacy

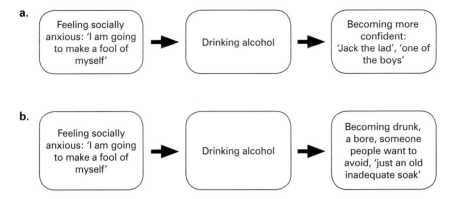

Fig. 12.1 Antecedents and consequences of Neil's drinking: a. what Neil *hopes* is true; b. what Neil *knows* is true.

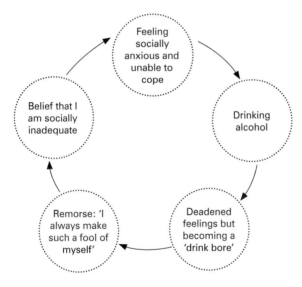

Fig. 12.2 The vicious cycle of drinking behaviour.

• develop alternative strategies to drinking which would help Neil when faced with the urge to drink.

Neil was keen to stress that he needed to return to work very shortly. This meant there was an immediate need to ensure he had some strategies for dealing with situations where he would normally drink. He was adamant that he would not join an organisation such as Alcoholics Anonymous (AA) as he was still ambivalent about accepting his drinking problem and had an idea that it would be full of 'down and outs'. It was explained to him that AA had different groups which encompassed all sectors of society and that there would be a group full of successful business people like him. This did not persuade him, although he agreed to 'look into it'.

The therapist and Neil then looked at the immediate problem of how he was going to deal with taking clients to lunch and not drinking. Neil decided that he would say that he was currently having extensive medical tests at the hospital and that he was unable to drink while these were going on. He felt this would be easy with lunch clients but was more concerned about how he would deal with work colleagues who would expect him to go out to the pub. The therapist and Neil practised some role-play with the therapist pretending to be Neil and Neil playing the role of a work colleague and *vice versa*. It was also necessary to come up with some activities which would substitute for the time Neil spent in the pub. Neil and the therapist worked on the following timetable of after-work activities:

- Monday: cinema
- Tuesday: go to leisure centre to see if there are any activities I would like to try
- Wednesday: concert
- Thursday: volunteer to take children for evening
- Friday: visit parents
- Saturday: stay with sister
- Sunday: stay with sister

He was asked again to record any urges to drink and any NATs which occurred over this time.

When Neil arrived the following week, he had stuck to his plans and was feeling very proud of his achievement in working for a week without any alcohol. His wife had been pleasantly surprised at his offer to take the children and had been surprised at his sobriety. Similarly, his parents had appreciated his visit and his mother had commented that he was 'less snappy and argumentative than usual'. Not all of the week had been plain sailing, however, and Neal had had two serious urges to drink.

On the first occasion, he had met with an old colleague who had come into the office and had tried to encourage him to go out with him. Neil had agreed to go to the wine bar but had explained that he was not able to drink. The friend had been relentlessly insistent but Neil had managed to resist. The therapist praised him for this and explained about how certain stimuli in the outside world, not just emotions, can become associated with drinking. Neil could relate to this as he remembered when he gave up smoking 10 years earlier, it was always more difficult when he had a coffee or an alcoholic drink as these were always times when he had had a cigarette. The principles of stimulus control techniques and management were discussed with Neil (similar to Joyce, Case example 11.1, pp. 173–175). At first Neil could not think of any obvious cues, apart from the emotional ones of anxiety, which preceded drinking. Then he thought that certain places where he particularly liked to drink may be associated and it might be better to go to other bars or restaurants to break the pattern.

The second occasion when Neil had felt the urge to drink was when he had been in the shops with his sister on the Saturday morning. While there, he met an old school friend who acknowledged him but then said he was sorry and had to rush off. Neil immediately had the thought, 'He's running away because he thinks I'm useless and boring.' He immediately felt that he would like a drink. The therapist and Neil then began to examine this thought. Neil was asked to think of evidence for and against the thought. Using this technique (e.g. Chapter 11), he was able to see that there were other explanations such as the man really did have an urgent appointment and was late on his way there.

Over the next few sessions, Neil's underlying social anxiety and poor self-esteem became clear. These were addressed by using the downward arrow technique (Chapter 8) to understand Neil's underlying assumptions. These were on the theme that he was not as attractive and capable as other men and that he always felt much more attractive and capable when he was drunk. He could recognise that drinking did not improve him in these respects. The ideas that he was not as attractive or capable as others were also challenged by looking for evidence to support and refute these statements. He was about to be given a behavioural test of his capability as he was due his appraisal at work. In this the boss noted that whereas his performance had been patchy over the first part of the year, he had improved recently and was now a highly valued employee. This improvement coincided with Neil stopping drinking. Before discharge, it was important to work with Neil on some relapse prevention strategies.

Relapse prevention and the overlap with coping skills

Relapse prevention skills are very similar to coping skills and are ways of pre-empting triggers to drinking in the future. The key areas to consider for both coping skills training and relapse prevention are:

- managing thoughts and cravings
  - this had been discussed with Neil over the course of therapy
- managing negative thinking
  - again this had been the focus of work with Neil; another important aspect of this is helping patients to handle criticism from others without becoming intoxicated – this can be approached using a cognitive approach combined with problem-solving
- anger management
  - this had not been an issue for Neil; some patients will drink when angry and need help to recognise the warning signs that they are becoming angry and identify more productive ways to dissipate this anger.

Comorbidity of alcohol and other drug misuse

Patients with a variety of anxiety and mood disorders may present with alcohol or other substance misuse. The range of conditions include schizophrenia, bipolar and other psychotic disorders as well as anxiety disorders (particularly social anxiety), depressive, obsessive–compulsive and body dysmorphic disorders. In the case of the psychotic disorders, it can be difficult to assess whether the psychotic symptoms are caused or exacerbated by the substance misuse or unrelated to it. However, the efficacy of antidepressants and antipsychotic drugs is compromised by alcohol and other drugs and thus it is important to manage the substance misuse in parallel with the treatment of the underlying condition. In the case of anxiety disorders, obsessive–compulsive and body dysmorphic disorders, not only does alcohol interfere with the efficacy of drug treatment but it also makes any treatment involving exposure very difficult. CBT in general and exposure methods in particular are stressful treatments. Abstaining from alcohol and other drugs is similarly stressful. It is generally unhelpful to expect a patient to go through two simultaneously stressful treatments. In these cases, it is generally advisable for the individual to be helped to conquer their addictive problems first. Once they have been abstinent for 2–3 months, they can be assessed for further treatment. Although this is difficult, it helps the patient to fully evaluate what they hope to gain from treatment and how they will cope in their life.

Stopping smoking

Smoking is a major cause of death and morbidity in both high-income and low- and middle-income countries. In the UK, an estimated 10 million people smoke (approximately one-sixth of the population) and smoking is more prevalent in young adults. Throughout the high-income countries, smoking is more prevalent in lower socioeconomic groups and it has been shown to be a major factor in health inequalities between rich and poor. Approximately half of all smokers will die of a condition related to their smoking (Action on Smoking and Health, 2013). Smoking rates are much higher among people with mental health problems than among the general population (Mc Neill, 2004). People with mental health problems are known to die earlier and have more physical illnesses than the general population and smoking seems to be a major contributor to this. Smoking is also important because it interacts with many other drugs, including, most importantly for many psychiatric patients, antipsychotic agents. This interaction means that patients who smoke are likely to require higher antipsychotic doses, which can cause additional physical health risks.

Proven treatment to aid people stopping smoking include:

- nicotine replacement: can be administered as gum, lozenge, tablet, spray, inhalator or as electronic 'cigarettes'
- bupropion: a selective inhibitor of the neuronal reuptake of noradrenaline and dopamine (theoretically there were concerns that this might interfere with the antipsychotic action of drugs for schizophrenia, but, so far, the evidence is that the risks are small (Ross & Williams, 2005))
- psychological interventions: these are based on CBT and include assessment of the individual's readiness to change, motivational approaches and CBT.

The most effective treatment often involves nicotine-replacement combined with bupropion and CBT (Hajek *et al*, 2013; Stanton & Grimshaw, 2013). The CBT techniques used are similar to those used in alcohol cessation (Case example 12.1).

Gambling

Excessive or compulsive gambling has many similarities to drug and alcohol addiction. Indeed, functional imaging studies of reward processing and gambling-related cognitive distortions have demonstrated that in pathological gamblers there are similar changes in the core circuitry which is also implicated in drug addiction (Clark & Limbrick-Oldfield, 2013). In the UK, the rate of problematic gambling was found to increase following the introduction of the National Lottery in 1994. More worryingly, it was found that the poorest households were more likely to spend a high percentage of their income on gambling and to develop problematic gambling behaviours (Grun & McKeigue, 2000).

The increased availability of the internet led to an increase in online gambling. It was found that internet gamblers were more likely to be men, younger, single, educated and in higher-paid jobs than gamblers who did not engage in internet gambling (Griffiths *et al*, 2009). However, it was also noted that online gambling was more likely to be a contributor to problematic gambling. The widespread use of smartphones and tablets may be expected to again increase the availability of gambling opportunities and the number of problem gamblers.

Although CBT is the only treatment which has been shown to be useful for problem gamblers, it is not known which specific techniques are useful. For this reason there is currently an ongoing controlled trial comparing treatment using cognitive interventions with a more exposure-based approach (Smith *et al*, 2013). Until there is further evidence, the best approach to problem gambling is to combine cognitive approaches with exposure therapy (Case example 12.2). The assessment and treatment of gambling has been usefully reviewed by George & Murali (2005).

Case example 12.2: Uncontrollable gambling problem

Bruce had grown up in a small town in the north-east of England. He left school at 16 years and had initially intended to start an apprenticeship as an electrician. However, ill health had put an end to this ambition and Bruce had remained unemployed for several years. Eventually, through a scheme introduced to reduce youth unemployment, he was offered a job at a call centre in another part of the country. This had worked well for him and it had led to a permanent position and eventually the role of supervisor.

Although he was reasonably happy in his job, Bruce did not like living away from his family and found sharing a flat with other people difficult. He felt he was 'going nowhere' and would never be able to escape from his situation of having little money. He had occasionally joined in with colleagues at work in buying lottery tickets. However, 2 years earlier, Bruce had started online betting lured by the promises of having £30 'free cash' if you signed up with a £20 credit. On the first few trials, he won reasonable sums of money several times but always kept this to continue gambling. By the time he was referred to the clinic, Bruce was spending up to half of his income on betting and owed large sums of money to his parents and various flatmates as well as having built up a credit card debt of several thousand pounds. Bruce described how miserable and depressed he felt about his debts, but said that once he started betting, his worries seemed to lift temporarily and he convinced himself that 'this time will be different' and believed he would win.

Treatment started with a full assessment to ensure that Bruce did not have any comorbid major depression or any other impulse-control disorder. Goals were then established with Bruce:

- not to use online gaming at all
- to be able visit pubs and clubs with gaming machines without spending money on them
- to be able to go out in situations where people gamble without fearing 'loss of control', for instance to be able to accompany his father to a betting shop and join in putting a small bet on a horse winning a race without going on to spend more money; to participate in the work National Lottery syndicate.

First, the therapist and Bruce discussed the reality of gambling. Bruce realised that he was spending a large amount of money on gambling but was unaware how small the chances were of anyone making a big win. Together with the therapist, they searched the internet to find the statistics on what the percentage 'pay out' was on his favourite gambling sites. It was discovered that most of the top gambling sites pay out between 90 and 97% back to the consumer. This figure is much higher than most physical casinos and slot machines which will tend to be nearer to 80%. Initially Bruce felt that this was good news until he examined it further and realised that he was inevitably going to gradually eat away at his money if he continued. In addition, he had considerable debts which were accumulating interest. To this end, Bruce was encouraged to think about his current situation and how he would pay back his debts. He agreed to look into getting a long-term bank loan to pay off his credit cards, family and friends. It was then discussed how he would resist the temptation of getting into further debt with his credit cards. Bruce decided to destroy his credit cards immediately and to take out a card which could be pre-loaded with a certain amount of cash when needed.

During the second session, the therapist asked Bruce to relive a recent episode of gambling and to retell the story. He was asked to identify his emotions and the thoughts which came into his head. Bruce described how after a busy day at work he had returned home tired and feeling low. In addition, he received a credit card statement outlining his debts. He immediately decided to go online and try to win some of his money back. The therapist asked Bruce to look at the pros and cons of this approach and Bruce listed both.

Pros:
- 'I may win my money back and be able to pay off my debts'
- 'Gambling makes me feel excited'
- 'Gambling makes me feel happy'.

Cons:
- 'The casinos make money from every transaction'
- 'Although I feel happy initially, I inevitably end up feeling desperate'.

It was immediately apparent that Bruce was worse off gambling than not gambling. However, he lacked any other excitement and enjoyable activities in his life at present. He was asked to think of pleasurable activities that he used to enjoy and which would give him a similar thrill to gambling. Initially, Bruce could not think of anything at all. He then said that, when at home, he had had a big family and had enjoyed playing with his sister's children. He also enjoyed reading Japanese 'manga' comic books. After some discussion it was agreed that Bruce would see whether any of his work colleagues were looking for a babysitter and whether he could find any opportunities of volunteering with children's play groups or at schools. As he worked shifts, there were opportunities for him to volunteer during the day. He also agreed to explore whether there were any local manga interest groups in his area he could join. He was given the task of recording his urges to gamble during the week and to see whether any particular activity would reduce these urges.

Over the next few sessions, it became clear that Bruce had low self-esteem and found that gambling made him feel more important and in control. He realised that in fact it was making him less in control. Cognitive therapy aimed at looking at his self-esteem issues was introduced.

Towards the end of therapy, it was important to look at possible 'trigger' points which could precipitate gambling behaviour. Bruce felt that he was much happier and did have other interests but would still be at risk if he went into a betting shop. Although he had avoided these, he would go with his father when at home and put a small bet on horses to win a particular race. First, the therapist asked Bruce to try to imagine himself entering a betting shop with his father and what emotions he would feel. Then he was asked to rehearse putting a small amount of money on a particular horse and waiting for the result. At the end of this, Bruce was to imagine himself leaving the betting shop. The therapist asked Bruce to do this while sitting down and to imagine all the sensations he would feel (similar to Case example 3.1). The second time this was recorded on his mobile phone, including an ending when Bruce walks out of the betting shop feeling confident and proud that he has not spent large amounts of money. He was asked to listen to this at least twice a day before the next session. At the next session, the therapist and Bruce practised going into a betting shop, looking at the horses and not placing any money on any horse despite remaining there for 15 min. This was very difficult for Bruce but he did leave without spending any money. He was then given the task of going with a friend (who did not usually gamble) and betting just £5.

In a situation such as Bruce's, relapse prevention is particularly important. Steps that he could do to help himself included not using credit cards, going out with a small amount of cash and only the amount he would need to do what he wanted. Although total abstinence from gambling would be ideal, Bruce was keen to involve the exceptions he and the therapist came up with and so the risks of these were fully discussed with him. He knew that when he felt miserable, he was particularly at risk and had some coping strategies and alternative behaviours to implement at these times, which included telephoning his mother, putting on his favourite record track or asking his flatmate to go out to the pub with him (when he would only take sufficient money for two drinks!).

Over the past 2 years, Bruce has almost cleared his debts and is planning to move back to the north-east of England where he has found a job in retail. He has had two relapses when he has gambled £100 at a time but neither of these featured online gaming or the use of credit cards. Bruce feels he has learned from these experiences and he increasingly finds the idea of gambling less attractive.

Hypersexuality or sexual addiction

The concept of hypersexuality or sexual addiction is controversial, as is the related concept of internet sexual addiction whereby individuals constantly seek out sexual images online for sexual gratification. There was discussion about whether it should be included in DSM-5 but it was eventually omitted. Some therapists view this disorder as a form of addiction akin to substance misuse and gambling, whereas others have associated it more with other psychiatric conditions such as manic states. Although some have suggested that it should be treated in a similar way to other addictions and have attempted CBT, others have advocated the use of serotonin reuptake inhibitors (SRIs). There are no convincing trials of any treatment for this disorder.

Key learning points

- Addiction and psychoactive substance misuse is a growing problem in the UK with increasing numbers of people throughout the country consuming hazardous levels of alcohol.
- The maximum recommended limit for alcohol consumption is 14 units for women and 21 units for men per week, and half of that for those aged 65 and over.
- CBT for addictive problems should consist of motivational interviewing, coping skills training and relapse prevention strategies.
- Motivational interviewing involves expressing empathy, developing discrepancy, rolling with resistance, supporting self-efficacy.
- Coping skills training comprises managing thoughts and cravings, managing negative thinking, anger management, relaxation skills, finding new pleasurable activities, decision-making, problem-solving, planning for the unexpected, declining invitations to drink/take drugs, refusing requests.
- Relapse prevention strategies involve looking at the same areas as above but particularly at emergency planning and situations likely to cause relapse.
- Smoking is a major cause of morbidity and mortality both in the general population and, even more, in people with mental health problems.
- Treatments aimed at assessing motivation to change combined with motivational approaches and CBT can be successfully combined with pharmacological treatments to help people stop smoking.
- Gambling addiction is a growing problem in the UK and worldwide. Poorer people are more likely to spend a greater percentage of their income on gambling.
- Internet gamblers tend to be younger men, and to be better educated and in higher-paid jobs.
- Treatment is a combination of cognitive and behavioural techniques similar to those used for alcohol addiction.

Suggested measures to use with conditions covered in this chapter

- Alcohol misuse: Severity of Alcohol Dependency Questionnaire (Stockwell *et al*, 1983), Problems and targets, self-report (Chapter 2).
- Drug misuse: Semi-Structured Assessment for Drug Dependence and Alcoholism (SSADDA; Pierucci-Lagha *et al*, 2005), Problems and targets, self-report.
- Nicotine addiction: the Fagerström test for nicotine dependence: a revision of the Fagerström tolerance questionnaire (Heatherton *et al*, 1991), Brief Wisconsin Inventory of Smoking Dependence Motives (Smith *et al*, 2010), Problems and targets, self-report.
- Gambling: the South Oaks Gambling Screen (SOGS; Lesieur & Blume, 1987), the Lie/Bet Questionnaire (Johnson *et al*, 1997), Gamblers Anonymous' Twenty Questions (the GA–20; Gamblers Anonymous, 2005), Problems and targets, self-report.

References

Action on Smoking and Health (2013) *Facts at a Glance*. Available at www.ash.org.uk (accessed November 2013).

Clark L, Limbrick-Oldfield EH (2013) Disordered gambling: a behavioral addiction. *Current Opinion in Neurobiology*, **23**: 655–9.

Gamblers Anonymous (2005) *Twenty Questions*. Gamblers Anonymous.

George S, Murali V (2005) Pathological gambling: an overview of assessment and treatment. *Advances in Psychiatric Treatment*, **11**: 450–6.

Griffiths M, Wardle H, Orford J, et al (2009) Sociodemographic correlates of internet gambling: findings from the 2007 British Gambling Prevalence Survey. *CyberPsychology and Behavior*, **12**: 199–202.

Grun L, McKeigue P (2000) Prevalence of excessive gambling before and after introduction of a national lottery in the United Kingdom: another example of the single distribution theory. *Addiction*, **95**: 959–66.

Hajek P, Stead LF, West R, et al (2013) Relapse prevention interventions for smoking cessation. *Cochrane Database of Systematic Reviews*, **8**: CD003999.

Heatherton TF, Kozlowski LT, Frecker RC (1991) The Fagerström test for nicotine dependence: a revision of the Fagerström tolerance questionnaire. *British Journal of Addiction*, **86**: 1119–27.

Johnson EE, Hamer R, Nora RM, et al (1997) The Lie/Bet Questionnaire for screening pathological gamblers. *Psychological Reports*, **80**: 83–8.

Kadden RM (2001) Behavioral and cognitive–behavioral treatments for alcoholism: research opportunities. *Addictive Behaviour*, **26**: 489–507.

Lesieur HR, Blume SB (1987) The South Oaks Gambling Screen (SOGS): a new instrument for the identification of pathological gamblers. *American Journal of Psychiatry*, **144**: 1184–8.

McNeill A (2004) *Smoking and Patients with Mental Health Problems*. Health Development Agency.

Miller WR, Rollnick S (2002) *Motivational Interviewing: Preparing People to Change* (2nd edn). Guilford Press.

Pierucci-Lagha A, Gelernter J, Feinn R, *et al* (2005) Diagnostic reliability of the Semi-Structured Assessment for Drug Dependence and Alcoholism (SSADDA). *Drug and Alcohol Dependence*, **80**: 303–12.

Ross S, Williams D (2005) Bupropion: risks and benefits. *Expert Opinion on Drug Safety*, **4**: 995–1003.

Royal College of Psychiatrists (2011) *Our Invisible Addicts* (CR165). Royal College of Psychiatrists.

Smith DP, Battersby MW, Harvey PW, *et al* (2013) Two-group randomised, parallel trial of cognitive and exposure therapies for problem gambling: a research protocol. *BMJ Open*, **3**: e003244.

Smith SS, Piper ME, Bolt DM, *et al* (2010) Development of the brief Wisconsin Inventory of Smoking Dependence Motives. *Nicotine and Tobacco Research*, **12**: 489–99.

Stanton A, Grimshaw G (2013) Tobacco cessation interventions for young people. *Cochrane Database of Systematic Reviews*, **8**: CD003289.

Stockwell T, Murphy D, Hodgson R (1983) The severity of alcohol dependence questionnaire: Its use, reliability and validity. *British Journal of Addiction*, **78**: 45–156.

Recommended treatment manuals and other reading

*Linke S (2013) *Alcohol Self-Help and CBT (My Modern Health Series)*. Mercury Learning and Information.

Miller WR, Rollnick S (2002) *Motivational Interviewing: Preparing People to Change* (2nd edn). Guilford Press.

Perkins KA, Conklin CA, Levine MD (2008) *Cognitive-Behavioral Therapy for Smoking Cessation: A Practical Guidebook to the Most Effective Treatments*. Routledge.

Raylu N, Oei TP (2010) *A Cognitive-Behavioural Therapy Programme for Problem Gambling: A Therapist's Manual*. Routledge.

*Spada M (2006) *Overcoming Problem Drinking: A Self-Help Guide using Cognitive–Behavioural Techniques*. Constable & Robinson.

Spada M (2010) *Cognitive-Behavioural Therapy for Problem Drinking: A Practitioner's Guide*. Routledge.

*Williams C (2009) *Stop Smoking in Five Minutes*. Five Areas.

*Williams C (2010) *Fix Your Drinking Problem in Two Days*. Five Areas.

*Suitable to recommend to patients.

Schizophrenia and the psychoses

Overview

The concentration of psychiatric services on the effective treatment in the community of the majority of patients with severe, enduring mental illness has led to the refining of CBT techniques with these individuals. Effective medication and early treatment has meant many more people with psychoses are potentially amenable to CBT. Case examples of techniques in practice will be given. This chapter concentrates on schizophrenia but application to other conditions such as bipolar disorder is also discussed.

Schizophrenia is a very common condition affecting almost 1% of the population (McGrath *et al*, 2008). Because of the severity as well as high prevalence, treatments which improve outcome may have a considerable effect on the healthcare budget.

A review of the treatment of schizophrenia and related disorders asked the question whether or not we should be reviewing the advice that all such patients should be advised to take antipsychotic medication (Morrison *et al*, 2012*a*). The authors argue that the evidence for the effectiveness of antipsychotic drugs is less strong than previously thought and that the risk of adverse outcome and side-effects has been underestimated. The suggestion is made that patients should work collaboratively with a therapist to make an informed choice about whether or not they wish to take these drugs. Patient and therapist collaboration is a hallmark of CBT and the suggestion is that CBT and/or family therapy can be offered in lieu of dopamine-blocking drugs. However, the number of studies which examine the use of CBT without the use of psychopharmacological agents is very few (e.g. Morrison *et al*, 2012*b*). Most evidence to suggest that patients may get better without drugs relies on examination of people with poor adherence to medication. Whereas this information may be generalisable to the whole population diagnosed with schizophrenia, it may also be that some patients stop the medication because they only have mild symptoms.

In turn, this raises the question of whether a true diagnosis is always reached in these people. At the time of writing this book, therefore, the only evidence-based approach would suggest that drugs are a necessary component of the treatment of schizophrenia.

In 2009, NICE published revised guidance on the treatment of schizophrenia, recommending that all patients diagnosed with schizophrenia should be given a trial of CBT. It is suggested that most will require at least 16 hour-long sessions over a period of up to 1 year and the sessions should follow a recognised treatment manual. The aims of the CBT are described as:

1   allowing the patient to identify links between their current or recent symptoms and their thoughts, actions and emotions
2   encouraging the patient to re-evaluate their beliefs, perceptions and reasoning in respect of their target symptoms.

In addition, the CBT should include at least one of the following:

- patients monitoring their thoughts, behaviours and emotions
- therapist and patient working together and promoting alternative behaviours
- examining ways to reduce stress and emotional distress
- working towards improving functioning.

Whereas this acceptance of the importance of CBT in the treatment of schizophrenia is to be welcomed, it does also raise a number of important practical as well as academic issues.

First, there is the practical issue about the availability of specialist CBT for schizophrenia. A recent survey in the UK demonstrated that less than half of all patients with schizophrenia had received CBT (College Centre for Quality Improvement, 2012). Indeed, to be able to undertake CBT as described by NICE would mean that all trained CBT therapists would spend most of their time engaged in CBT with psychotic patients. In the 2009 update to their guidance, NICE estimated the cost of one night's in-patient care for a person with schizophrenia at approximately £256. They suggested that as CBT costs approximately £1072 per person, the average length of stay (currently 11 nights) would need to be reduced by 4 days for CBT to be cost neutral (NICE, 2009). A more recent update published in February 2014 suggested that the cost of recommended CBT was between £1750 and £1800 per person (NICE, 2014). With the average cost for an acute psychiatric bed now at over £300 (Trachtenberg *et al*, 2013), it can be seen that even more reduction in in-patient stays would be necessary to achieve cost-neutrality of CBT. Although these figures appear achievable, it would presumably require a large injection of money to train a sufficient number of CBT therapists to deliver this therapy. In addition, most of the studies have been performed in UK academic centres specialising in the technique, which poses a question about how these results might generalise to other countries with different healthcare systems and non-academic institutions.

Second, it is clear that CBT offers benefit to some patients, but which patients benefit the most from the interventions has not been fully answered. A review by Wykes *et al* (2008) examined over 30 published randomised controlled trials of CBT for schizophrenia and concluded that these demonstrated, on average, moderate benefits. Many of these studies appeared to have design flaws and Wykes and colleagues concluded that the more rigorous the study, the weaker the effect of CBT.

CBT interventions for schizophrenia

The interventions which have been used in the treatment of schizophrenia range from:

- psychoeducational models aimed at informing the patient about the symptoms of schizophrenia and what can be done to help them; in addition to psychoeducation, the experience should be 'normalised' to reduce the anxiety and stigma of the condition
- behavioural interventions, including using reinforcement models for positive symptoms as well as negative symptoms such as social withdrawal
- CBT methods aimed at looking at the links between thinking, behaviour and emotions
- third generation therapies aimed at regulating the patient's response to their emotion and not engaging in unhelpful behaviours.

Interpretation of what constitutes appropriate CBT for schizophrenia has varied among professionals and research groups. This variance may have been partially responsible for the variable outcome reported. In general, CBT should be aimed at (at least some of) the following areas: positive symptoms, negative symptoms, challenging behaviours, relapse prevention and early onset.

The cognitive model of schizophrenia is that the patient experiences a number of positive symptoms, such as hallucinations and delusions. These symptoms in turn are interpreted by the individual and it is usually the interpretations of these which result in distress. A CBT model for hallucinations can be construed (Fig 13.1).

It is understandable that hearing voices or experiencing strange and alien bodily and mental health symptoms is both alarming and distressing. All people like to have rational explanations of causation for events. In schizophrenia, the individual has such strange and unusual symptoms that the 'explanations' they devise often appear bizarre to others who have not experienced the same symptoms. These are the typical delusions seen in schizophrenia. Once the delusions have been developed, the patient may also devise ways to either try and overcome or 'get their own back' on the people/systems who they believe are causing these experiences. Thus a person with hallucinatory voices may be observed shouting or shaking their fist at the 'voices'. This behaviour, although rational given the patient's experiences and belief systems, in itself can worsen the condition by alienating and frightening others. On rare occasions, these attempts to 'get back at' the originators of the voices can result in behaviours which are violent or place the patient or others in danger.

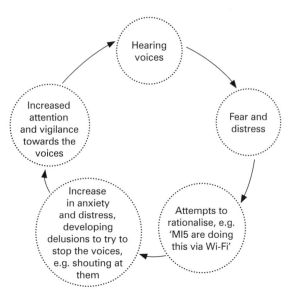

Fig. 13.1 CBT model for hallucinations.

As well as resulting in an increase in stigma and possible social rejection and ridicule, these behaviours aimed at reducing the 'cause' of the hallucination also serve to make it more prominent in the patient's thoughts. Thus, the individual is turning most of his or her attention to waiting to hear the voices. This increased attention means that hallucinations are more likely to occur and thus a vicious circle results.

Patients also often try to find other ways to reduce the frequency of their frightening hallucinations. Some may use sedative drugs such as alcohol in an attempt to try to reduce the voices or, at least, the distress generated by them. Excessive use of alcohol or other agents increases this vicious circle as many street drugs and excessive alcohol consumption can cause hallucinations as well as other potential health problems.

Education and normalisation of symptoms

One of the most useful interventions which can be made is to help the patient to understand the experiences they are having and to help them to start to challenge some of the abnormal beliefs. In fact, a high percentage of the general population experience hallucinatory-like experiences and many have abnormal beliefs which may be considered bizarre or delusionary by others. A study of third- to sixth-year students in a Spanish medical school revealed that 22% had experienced abnormal visual perceptions and 65% abnormal auditory experiences. These experiences were usually reported as being more frequent when students were anxious and hypervigilant (García-Ptacek et al, 2013). Insight that this was an abnormal perception was immediate and thus the experiences did not constitute true hallucinations but could be categorised as pseudo-hallucinations (Case example 13.1).

Case example 13.1: Psychoeducation in auditory hallucinations

George, a 25-year-old man living with his parents, had a 4-year history of hearing voices. These voices were of strangers who discussed him and made derogatory comments about his daily activities. He found these very distressing and believed that he was the victim of a plot to 'torture' him which had been hatched by the pope. He believed that, as a lapsed Catholic, the cardinals had conspired to interfere with his brain by using the neighbours' Wi-Fi system (George had thrown his parents' Wi-Fi receiver out of the window at the onset of his illness). He regularly shouted and swore at the voices and recently had made threats of violence towards his local priest.

Although George had a marked improvement of symptoms when treated with antipsychotic drugs, he was never completely symptom-free. Because he had persistent beliefs that his symptoms were a plot by the Roman Catholic church, he had poor compliance with medication. His parents were alarmed as they had recently discovered he had been trying to organise a trip to Rome, where he intended to confront the pope.

After taking a full history from George and also from his parents, the therapist started by trying to offer George an alternative explanation for his symptoms. This started with some normalisation of symptoms and the introduction of the idea of possible alternative explanations.

First, the therapist explained that many members of the general population experience the feeling of hearing noises and voices when there is no one there. It was explained that over half the population have these experiences and that these were likely to be more frequent when the individual was more stressed and vigilant. The therapist then gave the following explanation of how these experiences may arise in a situation like George's:

Therapist: 'The brain is a very complex organ and has many stored memories as well as the ability of imagining all kinds of good and bad situations and circumstances. An example of the vividness of the imagination of the brain is in our dreams. Some dreams can feel very real indeed. However, the brain is active the whole time and not just when we are asleep. Consequently the brain is constantly having vivid thoughts and 'daydreams'. We learn to distinguish these internally produced experiences from the world around us, but sometimes this barrier of distinguishing internal and external events breaks down. The tendency for this to break down increases when people are anxious as well as when they are feeling tired and sleepy. These experiences, such as hearing voices when there is no one there, are normal and very common. For some people, however, the brain 'filter' which distinguishes internal and external events is a bit more fragile or 'leaky' than in other individuals. In these cases, the person has more frequent experiences of the 'internal events' in their brain being thought to originate in the external world. This happens in schizophrenia. Because you have so frequent experiences of hearing voices when there is no one around, it is understandable that you will try and find rational explanations for your experiences. I personally do not believe that the Catholic church are interfering with your brain, but I do understand how you have come to that conclusion based on your experiences. What I would like to do is over the next few weeks examine other possible explanations of your symptoms with you. I would like us to set up some experiments to test these explanations.

One thing I mentioned was that these experiences of hearing voices are usually more common when people are stressed or tired. I wonder how that fits with your experience George?'

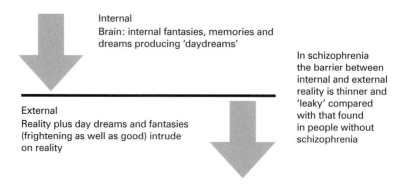

Internal
Brain: internal fantasies, memories and
dreams producing 'daydreams'

In schizophrenia
the barrier between
internal and external
reality is thinner and
'leaky' compared
with that found
in people without
schizophrenia

External
Reality plus day dreams and fantasies
(frightening as well as good) intrude
on reality

Fig 13.2   Possible model of brain function in schizophrenia.

George was far from convinced by this explanation but was happy to give the therapy a try. He was given a model of schizophrenia (Fig 13.2).

It was discussed with George how taking his dopamine-blocking medication could make the barrier between internal and external events more robust. Once again, George was unconvinced by this but did agree to have a trial where he would take his medicine regularly for a 6-week period while he embarked on some therapy. His parents agreed to supervise this and said they would discuss with the therapist if George refused his medication (they had also been ambivalent about medication in the past).

Explaining how hallucinations and delusions arise can be very useful for a patient experiencing the frightening symptoms of schizophrenia.

Cognitive reattribution for positive symptoms of schizophrenia

In the past, it used to be believed that it was counterproductive to challenge a psychotic patient's delusional beliefs or their understanding of the causation of their hallucinations. However, CBT aims to do just that. As with the cognitive techniques described in earlier chapters (for example, Chapters 8 and 9), the first principle is to establish a good rapport with the patient. Using a collaborative and empirical approach the therapist then encourages the patient to examine their belief processes and to consider other possible explanations for the symptoms that they experience. It is, however, very important to maintain a collaborative stance with the patient. If challenging thoughts is causing too much distress and anxiety in any session, then this should be terminated and an alternative approach taken. It may be that after other work the challenging can recommence at a later appointment. As with all CBT, the patient and therapist devise behavioural tests to ascertain which explanation has the most evidence and is the most likely to be correct.

Case example 13.1, continued

The first thought George wished to work on was his idea that the Roman Catholic church was causing him to hear voices making derogatory comments about his actions. The therapist had already explained to him that many people have experiences of hallucinations and that in people with schizophrenia their brains make them more likely to have these experiences. To test this out, George was asked to think of all the reasons why it may be true or untrue. This took three sessions to complete as George started with an absolute conviction that his interpretation was correct. Eventually, with the therapist's help, he produced a list.

'The voices I hear are a product of my mind and not due to intervention by the church and the pope.

Evidence for:
- This is what my therapist, the GP and my parents believe
- I have met other patients who seem to have extremely unlikely erroneous beliefs concerning their "voices"
- I cannot be the only person who is a lapsed Catholic and the pope cannot be doing this to everyone
- My aunt told me that she heard voices when lying in bed at night.

Evidence against:
- It feels as if these voices are coming from outside my brain
- The Catholic church has many "dark" secrets.'

Once George had produced this list, he was asked whether there were any ways he could think of to test these assertions. A list of activities was compiled and George was encouraged to perform them at home:
- visit Rethink's website and research their opinions about hearing voices when no one is there (www.rethink.org/diagnosis-treatment/symptoms/hearing-voices)
- ask a group of family and friends if they have ever had the experience of hearing voices when there is no one there or other unusual or unexplainable experiences of this sort
- compile a list of people who have nothing to do with the Roman Catholic church but yet believe their current problems are due to their brain rather than their lapsed religion.

By working with George in this way, he began to be more amenable to the idea that his problems may be related to his brain rather than his previous delusionary beliefs. Once he had compiled this evidence, he was encouraged to make a cue card which he was to keep in his pocket and to read whenever he experienced the 'voices' (Fig. 13.3). George did find he was able to use the cue card, but, probably more importantly, as he began to accept that his illness was due to a malfunction of his brain, he was more consistent and reliable in taking his medication. He also began to use distraction techniques (see the next section) when the hallucinations occurred.

Behavioural and other techniques used to assist coping with positive symptoms

Many patients with schizophrenia find that distraction can help with reducing hallucinations and turn their attention away from distressing delusionary ideas. Engaging with the voices or ruminating on the delusionary

> • The voices I am hearing come from inside my head even though they sound as if they are coming from outside.
>
> • My medicine does reduce these voices and so I know they are from inside my head.
>
> • If I ignore the voices they will go away.
>
> • If I distract myself they will get better.
>
> • Pay attention to what is going on around you rather than to the voices.

Fig. 13.3 George's cue card.

beliefs usually makes the symptoms increase. For example, some patients may shout back at the voices. In such cases a behavioural test could be given whereby the patient is asked to try for one day not to engage in 'answering the voices back' but to try distraction by listening to a favourite piece of music when the voices occur. They can then be asked whether the voices were more or less frequent and how distressed they felt by them when they refused to attend to them in this way. Most people will report that they feel better if they do not 'engage with' the voices.

Ruminating on delusionary beliefs also tends to make patients feel worse. Once again, this can be tested by asking the patient to try not to think about the beliefs for a set period and to see whether they feel better or worse. If this proves difficult to achieve, then a cue card can be used giving a rational response (similar to the example in Fig. 13.3).

Some patients will benefit from more structured distraction and can be taught the techniques of mindfulness (described in Chapter 8). The use of such techniques enables the patient to focus away from the distressing thoughts and symptoms on to their surroundings and external experience. In addition, it is usually found that the psychotic symptoms will be increased by stress and by sleeplessness. Mindfulness helps to reduce stress. In a similar way therapies such as ACT (described in Chapter 8) can be used to encourage the patient to accept their symptoms but to not engage with or fret over them.

Negative symptoms

The negative symptoms of schizophrenia include apathy, social withdrawal, flat affect and psychological distress, including depression (Case example 13.2). There are proven neurocognitive deficits in schizophrenia which may combine with the underlying personality so that it is easier for the individual to withdraw from many aspects of life rather than actively engage with them. In addition, the diagnosis of schizophrenia is a major traumatic life event in itself, but, in addition, schizophrenia tends to worsen at times of stress. A combination of these factors may be at least partially contributory to the apathy, social withdrawal and depression so frequently seen in chronic schizophrenia.

Cognitive–behavioural therapy aimed at addressing some of these negative beliefs and depression can be useful. The type of interventions used are similar to those in the cognitive treatment of depression (see Chapter 8). The path of this therapy can often be painfully slow. People who have paranoid delusions are often extremely anxious about social situations. Indeed, it has been noted that patients with paranoid ideation and patients with social anxiety disorder have many of the same maladaptive thought processes and attribute minor changes in expression in others as due to criticism of themselves.

Another difficult point is that too much stimulation for patients with schizophrenia can lead to an increase in positive symptoms as the stress rises. Thus therapy must be very gradual and strictly dictated by the patient's mental state and stress levels.

Case example 13.2: Treatment of social withdrawal and depression

Trilby is 28 years old and had first been diagnosed with schizophrenia at the age of 21. Her positive symptoms were well controlled on antipsychotic drugs and she generally was free of them. She had always been quiet and shy and had 'kept herself to herself', but since the diagnosis of schizophrenia her parents noticed that she spent much less time in the company of others and seemed to feel extremely anxious when in social situations of any type. Before her illness, she had been interested in art and would regularly visit local galleries as well as producing her own paintings. There was evidence that she was a competent artist and she had sold several paintings before the onset of her illness.

As the therapist started to take a history from Trilby, it became apparent that her confidence had been completely shaken by the diagnosis of schizophrenia. She believed that 'no one will want to befriend the mad woman'. In addition, she had very low self-esteem and would not engage in any artistic activities as she felt her work was of little value.

After taking a history, the principles of CBT were explained to Trilby. She admitted to feeling worthless and felt that her whole being had become tainted by her illness. It was decided with her that the first item to be examined in therapy was the view she had of herself as worthless and that she had nothing to offer other people. Initially when asked to describe herself, Trilby felt she was 'pathetic' and that she had 'no redeeming features'. Before her illness, however, she had kept in touch with two friends from school. On discussion, it was decided that for her first behavioural experiment, Trilby would ask her close family to select words which they felt best described her.

When she returned to the next session, Trilby had a list which her mother had helped prepare. Trilby had been too shy to approach her aunts, nieces and nephews to ask for their opinion of her but her mother had done so and Trilby had listened in on the telephone. Generally she was described as 'quiet, thoughtful, with an active imagination, delicate and quirky'. This was a surprise to Trilby, but she did wonder if they were just being kind. The next behavioural experiment she was given was to contact her childhood friends, to ask how they were and to monitor their response to her. This was successful and one friend was extremely excited to hear from her and asked to meet her the following week. Although she felt it would be good to meet this friend, Trilby was anxious about explaining to her what had happened over the past few years. Her friend had been doing a higher degree at university and Trilby felt embarrassed at admitting she had been ill. The therapist and Trilby discussed possible ways of tackling this, but she was adamant that she should 'tell the truth'. The therapist and Trilby therefore did some role-play practice where this subject was broached in a variety of ways.

Following on from meeting with her friend, Trilby returned to the therapy but was a little downcast. Generally the meeting had gone well, but Trilby had felt that, although she had sounded supportive, her friend had been shocked at the revelation of her recent diagnosis of schizophrenia. Trilby saw this surprise as evidence that 'no one really wants to know a mad woman'. The therapist encouraged Trilby to think of other reasons why her friend may have been shocked. Reluctantly, Trilby began to see that her story may have been a big surprise to her friend too and that she may also have felt unsure about how she should respond.

Over the next few sessions, work therapy concentrated on examining Trilby's thoughts when in the company of others and getting her to take the risk of increasingly facing up to being in more social situations.

Relapse prevention

As with the treatment of any psychiatric condition, an important component of therapy is to examine the way in which the patient can try to predict relapse and to implement coping strategies before the symptoms become a major problem. With schizophrenia it is of course important that the patient remains on medication and does not reduce or alter this without seeking medical advice and supervision. In addition, it is well recognised that certain factors may precipitate relapse. Examples of possible precipitants are stress and anxiety, being sleep deprived or tired, physical illness, hormonal changes (such as in pregnancy) and excessive alcohol or drug use.

Apart from a patient stopping their antipsychotic medication, stress, anxiety and tiredness are probably the most common identifiable precipitants for relapse.

In relapse prevention, the patient is encouraged to think of very early warning signs of relapse and then strategies can be identified to try to relieve the situation. For example, a patient may recognise that when they start to feel stressed and anxious, they tend to have difficulty sleeping and this can often herald the onset of a relapse. The patient is encouraged to write these warning signs down and then coping strategies can also be identified and written down. When tiredness and anxiety are an issue, one coping strategy may be stress-reduction techniques (as described in Chapter 9); the patient may be taught progressive muscle relaxation and techniques for sleep hygiene. Once a full relapse prevention programme has been developed with the patient, it is important to ensure that they keep this written record in a safe place so that they can consult it if or when the need arises.

Early intervention strategies

There has been increasing interest in trying to prevent chronic schizophrenia developing by intervening in the very early stage of the illness. Specialist early intervention services have been developed in a widespread manner across the UK. Although there is some evidence for the efficacy of the interventions, it is often patchy and inconclusive. Early intervention may refer to intervention either in the prodromal phase of the illness or in the first episode of frank psychosis. A Cochrane review of this subject found that there was little evidence to support CBT in isolation in either prodromal or first-episode psychosis but that in combination with drug therapy it may have a small but significant effect, as may family therapy and help with employment (Marshall & Rathbone, 2011).

The types of therapy used in early intervention are identical to those described earlier in this chapter. Identifying situations which increase the symptoms and instigating appropriate techniques to alleviate the precipitants are the keystone of the CBT treatment.

Other psychoses

Psychoses may arise in response to drug or alcohol misuse, following major trauma, or as a reaction to physical illness, to name a few. Psychotic symptoms may also form part of the spectrum of disability in patients with personality disorder. Paranoid states which appear to be different from schizophrenia can also be found and appear to be an extreme of the interpersonal sensitivity found in social anxiety disorders. There have been few high-quality, adequately powered controlled trials examining the role of CBT in the treatment of schizophrenia. In the case of other non-schizophrenic psychosis, there have been even fewer. One exception is in the emerging evidence of possible benefit of treating patients with bipolar disorder with CBT. This evidence has led NICE to recommend the limited use of CBT (mainly for depressive symptoms) in bipolar disorder (National Institute for Health and Clinical Excellence, 2006).

Bipolar disorder

The evidence base for the use of CBT in bipolar disorders is limited. A review of various meta-analyses examining the role of CBT demonstrates a small to medium effect size at the end of treatment which tends to decrease at follow-up (Hofmann et al, 2012). Similar results were found in both depressive and manic symptoms. There is little evidence to support the use of CBT without adjunctive psychopharmacological treatments. However, CBT appears to be effective in preventing or delaying relapse in individuals with bipolar disorder (Hofmann et al, 2012).

In bipolar disorder, the most important factor in treatment is psychoeducation, ensuring that the patient fully understands the condition and is fully informed of the role of medication in its treatment and prophylaxis. In the case of residual depressive symptoms, CBT for depression (as fully described in Chapter 8) should be used. For prevention of relapse of both depressive and hypomanic or manic episodes, the treatment involves identifying likely triggers or early warning factors for relapse. As with schizophrenia, the most likely triggers are stress and tiredness or lack of sleep. Interventions can then be introduced which reduce the effect of these factors, for example anxiety reduction methods and sleep hygiene.

Key learning points

- CBT appears to be a helpful adjunct to medication in the treatment of schizophreniform psychoses.
- The components of any CBT approach for psychosis should include:
  - allowing the patient to identify links between their current or recent symptoms and their thoughts, actions and emotions
  - encouraging the patient to re-evaluate their beliefs, perceptions and reasoning in respect of their target symptoms.
- In addition the CBT should include at least one of the following:
  - patients monitoring their thoughts, behaviours and emotions
  - therapist and patient working together and promoting alternative behaviours
  - examining ways to reduce stress and emotional distress
  - working towards improving functioning.
- Positive symptoms such as delusions and hallucinations can be tackled using cognitive challenging, behavioural tests and cognitive reattribution.
- Negative symptoms such as social withdrawal, apathy and depression can be tackled by examining the beliefs underpinning these behaviours and helping the patient to challenge them.
- Dealing with negative symptoms runs the risk of increasing positive symptoms and so a balance must always be struck between over-stimulation and stressing the patient and allowing them to withdraw.
- Frequent precipitants for relapse are stopping the medication, stress, anxiety and tiredness or sleep deprivation (as well as pregnancy, physical illness, alcohol or substance misuse).
- Once patients identify likely precipitants, the therapist can work collaboratively with them to identify strategies to reduce the effect of the precipitants. Frequently used techniques include anxiety reduction strategies, sleep hygiene and problem-solving techniques.
- There is some limited evidence that early intervention with CBT may help prevent some of the long-term sequelae of schizophrenia.
- There is limited evidence of the efficacy of CBT for other psychotic disorders but there is some evidence for its use in bipolar disorder.

Suggested measures to use with conditions covered in this chapter

- Schizophrenia: Positive and Negative Symptoms Questionnaire (Iancu *et al*, 2005), Brief Psychiatric Rating Scale (Overall & Gorham, 1962), Schizophrenia Quality of Life Scale Revision 4 (Wilkinson *et al*, 2000), Problems and targets and Sheehan Disability Scale (measuring impact on life), both discussed in Chapter 2.
- Bipolar disorder: Young Mania Rating Scale (Young *et al*, 1978), BDI (13-item and 21-item) (Beck *et al*, 1974; Beck, 1978), Problems and targets, Sheehan Disability Scale (measuring impact on life).

References

Beck AT (1978) *Depression Inventory*. Philadelphia Center for Cognitive Therapy.

Beck AT, Rial WY, Rickets K (1974) Short form of depression inventory: cross-validation. *Psychology Reports*, **34**: 1184–6.

College Centre for Quality Improvement (2012) *Report of the National Audit of Schizophrenia (NAS) 2012*. Royal College of Psychiatrists.

García-Ptacek S, García Azorín D, Sanchez Salmador R, *et al* (2013) Hallucinations and aberrant perceptions are prevalent among the young healthy adult population. *Neurología*, **28**: 19–23.

Hofmann SG, Asnaani A, Vonk IJJ, *et al* (2012) The efficacy of cognitive behavioral therapy: a review of meta-analyses. *Cognitive Therapy Research*, **36**: 427–40.

Iancu I, Poreh A, Lehman B, *et al* (2005) The Positive and Negative Symptoms Questionnaire: a self-report scale in schizophrenia. *Comprehensive Psychiatry*, **46**: 61–6.

Marshall M, Rathbone J (2011) Early intervention for psychosis. *Cochrane Database of Systematic Reviews*, **6**: CD004718.pub3.

McGrath J, Saha S, Chant D, et al (2008) Schizophrenia: a concise overview of incidence, prevalence, and mortality. *Epidemiological Review*, **30**: 67–76.

Morrison AP, Hutton P, Shiers D, *et al* (2012a) Antipsychotics: is it time to introduce patient choice? *British Journal of Psychiatry*, **201**: 83–4.

Morrison AP, Turkington D, Wardle M, *et al* (2012b) A preliminary exploration of predictors of outcome and cognitive mechanisms of change in cognitive behaviour therapy for psychosis in people not taking antipsychotic medication. *Behaviour Research and Therapy*, **50**: 163–7.

National Institute for Health and Clinical Excellence (2006) *The Management of Bipolar Disorder in Adults, Children and Adolescents in Primary and Secondary Care* (Clinical Guideline CG38). NICE.

National Institute for Health and Clinical Excellence (2009) *Core Interventions in the Treatment and Management of Schizophrenia in Adults in Primary and Secondary Care* (Clinical Guideline CG82). NICE.

National Institute for Health and Care Excellence (2014) *Psychosis and Schizophrenia in Adults: Treatment and Management (CG 178)*. NICE.

Overall JE, Gorham DR (1962) The brief psychiatric rating scale. *Psychological Reports*, **10**: 799–812.

Trachtenberg M, Parsonage M, Shepherd G, et al (2013) *Peer Support in Mental Health Care: Is It Good Value for Money?* Centre for Mental Health.

Wilkinson G, Hesdon B, Wild D, *et al* (2000) Self-report quality of life measure for people with schizophrenia: the SQLS. *British Journal of Psychiatry*, **177**: 42–6.

Wykes T, Steel C, Everitt B, *et al* (2008) Cognitive behavior therapy for schizophrenia: effect sizes, clinical models, and methodological rigor. *Schizophrenia Bulletin*, **34**: 523–37.

Young RC, Biggs JT, Ziegler VE, *et al* (1978) A rating scale for mania: reliability, validity and sensitivity. *British Journal of Psychiatry*, **133**: 429–35.

Recommended treatment manuals and other reading

*Freeman D, Freeman J, Garety P (2006) *Overcoming Paranoid and Suspicious Thoughts: A Self-Help Guide using Cognitive Behavioural Techniques*. Constable & Robinson.

Hagen R, Turkington D, Berge T, *et al* (2011) *CBT for Psychosis: A Symptom-Based Approach*. Routledge.

*Jones S, Hayward P, Lam D (2009) *Coping with Bipolar Disorder: A CBT-Informed Guide to Living with Manic Depression* (2nd edn). One World.

*Suitable to recommend to patients.

Personality disorder

Overview

Patients with a personality disorder use a disproportionate amount of mental health services' time. Failure to diagnose or understand a patient's personality disorder can lead to wasted trials of therapy. This chapter examines the role of faulty and unhelpful schemata in the development of these problems and how they affect long-term behaviour. Longer-term CBT interventions will be discussed. There will be a description of borderline personality disorder and the impact this has on mental health services. The application of dialectical behaviour therapy for borderline personality disorder will be demonstrated. How these treatments can be practised within mental health services will be examined. Finally, there will be a discussion about research on these approaches.

Cognitive theories relating to personality disorder

Personality disorder refers to enduring character traits and maladaptive behaviours which are egosyntonic and accepted by the patient as part of their personality. Cognitive treatments are longer-term treatments than those generally applied to conditions such as depression, anxiety and OCD and are aimed at modifying the underlying fundamental beliefs of the individual which are causing problems.

In Chapters 8 and 9, the basic principles of cognitive therapy were described. The basic triad was explored whereby our interactions with the environment and other people lead to certain beliefs about self, others and the world. These beliefs vary in accuracy and functionality and are fundamental, usually not articulated and accepted as 'absolute truths' Beck (1995). Cognitions (verbal or pictorial) are based on attitudes or assumptions (schematas), which develop from previous experiences (Beck, 1967, 1979). Another term used to describe schemata is core beliefs. The evidence of these schemata are the NATs that arise from underlying assumptions that in turn are 'rules' which are a product of these schemata.

The schemata are thus patterns of beliefs which are developed in early life in an attempt to make sense of the world and the environment. They are not logical but are held with complete conviction as absolute truths. The hierarchy of these thoughts is shown in Fig. 14.1.

Schemata are not conscious thought patterns but are the rules and patterns which an individual applies to their life and interactions with others. These core beliefs are:

- global
- rigid
- overgeneralised.

Thus a schema is a pattern of unconditional beliefs which are hard to access and are self-maintaining. These schemata are maintained by three main cognitive processes (Young *et al*, 2003):

1. *Schema surrender.* This is the way in which an individual will always seek evidence that supports their beliefs and dismiss evidence that contradicts the beliefs (e.g. a woman who believes she is ugly will focus on any minor negative comment but will ignore compliments as 'they are just saying that to make me feel better and probably would not feel the need if they did not realise that I am ugly').

2. *Schema compensation.* This refers to primary avoidance of emotional arousal by developing strategies which enforce the beliefs (e.g. a man who has core beliefs that he will be abandoned by everyone owing to his unlovable nature may be excessively self-sacrificing to his friends and family).

3. *Schema avoidance.* These are a group of blocking behaviours which help avoid emotional arousal (e.g. binge eating may temporarily reduce the emptiness and social isolation experienced by a person who had been neglected as a child. This is known as secondary avoidance of emotional arousal).

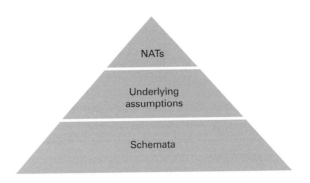

Fig. 14.1 Hierarchy of thoughts and beliefs.

Schema-focused CBT

Treatment of personality disorder using CBT was first described by Beck & Freeman (1990), who emphasised the need to focus more on the past and the relationship between the patient and the therapist and to continue therapy for at least 1–2 years. Subsequent writers have developed these ideas, for example schema-focused therapy (Young & Brown, 2003), and now consider most therapy needs to continue for 2–3 years. Given these long durations of therapy, full schema-focused treatment is unlikely to be available outside specialist centres in the NHS. Nevertheless, some of the principles can be helpful for the generalist to understand (Case example 14.1).

Case example 14.1: Schema-focused CBT for repeated self-harm and aggressive behaviour

Paula was a 22-year-old woman who had never settled at anything in life. She was referred by her local community mental health team as she regularly either cut her wrist or took a small overdose of medication whenever she was involved in an argument with her family or if she felt people were criticising her. Admission to hospital normally led to her unsettling other patients and she was unpopular with most of the staff, who felt she required excessive amounts of their time, energy and resources.

Paula had been born to parents with a drug addiction who were in an unstable relationship and who separated a few months after her birth. Thereafter followed a time when Paula had a series of 'fathers' who were in a relationship with her mother. The longest such relationship lasted 2 years. There was also a younger brother at home. Paula was sent to live with her grandmother at the age of 10 and remembered this as 'the happiest time of my life'. Unfortunately, her grandmother died suddenly 4 years later and Paula was placed in a series of foster homes and children's homes. She frequently ran away from them. At the age of 18 years, she had been placed in bed and breakfast accommodation and currently was living in a mental health hostel. The staff there found her unpredictable and often aggressive behaviour difficult to cope with and she was under threat of being evicted. Her longest period in employment was 6 months 2 years ago when she had worked as a cleaner in a hospital, but she had lost this job as a result of efficiency savings.

Paula was asked to complete a schema questionnaire. The most common is a short form of the Young & Brown's (2003) questionnaire. This asks the patient to explain how they feel about certain aspects of their life. At the end it can be analysed and a number of domains are measured. These domains are shown in Table 14.1 with the schemata that fall under each domain.

A situation such as Paula's is obviously likely to require long-term intervention to produce any change. She has a history of an abusive and difficult childhood with considerable loss and it is unlikely that long-lasting change will be produced in less than 2 years. In a case like this, the most important aspect is ensuring that there is team on hand 24 hours a day for the inevitable emergencies. In the past this would be the community mental health team with the back-up of an out-of-hours service that would have access to patient notes. In many mental health trusts this is no longer

Table 14.1 Domains and schema from Young & Brown's Schema Questionnaire

Domains	Schema
Rejection and disconnection	Mistrust/abuse Abandonment/instability Emotional deprivation Defectiveness/shame Social isolation/alienation
Impairment of autonomy and performance	Dependence/incompetence Vulnerability to harm Enmeshment Failure
Impaired limits	Entitlement Insufficient self-control/self-discipline
Other directedness	Subjugation Self-sacrifice Approval-seeking/recognition-seeking
Inhibition and over-vigilance	Negativity/pessimism Emotional inhibition Unrelenting standards/hypercritical Punitive

available to longer-term patients and other arrangements are necessary. People like Paula are at high risk of suicide, albeit accidental, as they will tend to try to demonstrate their emotional distress by self-harm or other aggressive acts. It is essential therefore that some support mechanism is available as for a person like Paula change will not be achieved overnight.

In Paula's case it can probably be predicted that she would demonstrate dominance in the schema linked with rejection and disconnection. In schema-focused therapy as described by Young & Brown, there are some differences from CBT as described earlier. The key differences are:

- more emphasis on the therapeutic relationship between the therapist and the patient, including discussing behaviours in the context of this relationship; in addition, the therapist uses 'empathic confrontation' (i.e. although being empathic to the past reasons why certain behaviours developed, the therapist still emphasises the need to change) and also limited re-parenting (i.e. the therapist provides some of the needs that the patient had as a child within the therapeutic relationship)
- encouraging the patient to 're-live' certain childhood experiences and to link these to current emotions
- rather than the term 'core beliefs', there is more emphasis on 'core emotional experiences'.

Paula's case history demonstrates how in schema-based CBT there is more emphasis on examining emotions and looking at how to deal with them as well as the underlying thoughts and beliefs. In addition, there is more emphasis on the therapeutic relationship, which in a similar way to psychodynamic psychotherapy uses the current relationship as a learning experience.

Case example 14.1, continued

The first thing the therapist did with Paula was to listen empathically to her story of neglect and the constant feeling of being 'let down' in childhood. The therapist encouraged Paula to see that her early experiences were bound to make her suspicious and wary of people but that her self-harm and aggressive behaviours were currently damaging herself rather than those who had let her down. This whole process took many sessions. Paula was initially hostile and dismissive of the therapist. She felt that in the past 'therapists and doctors would come and go, rarely sticking around for more than a few months; no one really cares'. Eventually she realised that no matter how much she poured scorn on them, the therapist still arrived for the session the following week.

After several weeks, Paula arrived and said she would like to talk about an incident which had happened during the week at her hostel. One of the other residents had walked off while Paula had been talking to her about a trip that was happening the next day. Paula had immediately reacted by shouting abuse at this woman, calling her a selection of extremely offensive names. The other woman had locked herself in her room. Paula had then gone into the main communal sitting room and had turned over the coffee table, smashed a mug and was using the broken china to try and cut her wrists before she had been contained by the staff. The first thing that happened was to try to get Paula to see that her reaction was to do with her childhood experience rather than the actual behaviour of the woman. A model of Paula's thoughts was produced (Fig. 14.2).

To obtain this model was not easy and it required an entire session to get Paula to see that her reaction was related to her past experience of being ignored and her needs not being met as a child. The therapist asked Paula to think about whether this reaction had been useful or if there were alternative, more useful ways of behaving. Using the method of collaborative empiricism, they came up with a list.

'Pros and cons for smashing a cup and cutting my wrist when I was being ignored:

Pros:
- The pain in my wrist made me feel better
- I showed Jackie she couldn't treat me that way
- The staff gave me loads of attention
- Maybe people will be afraid to ignore me in the future

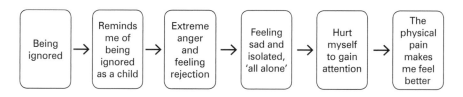

Fig. 14.2 Model of thoughts behind Paula's outburst.

Cons:
- My place in the hostel is under threat as a result of this
- I promised myself I was going to avoid such outbursts
- I have yet another scar on my arm.'

Although Paula did devise this list with the therapist, she still kept on saying that Jackie 'deserved it'. There was discussion about who suffered the most from this interaction and Paula could see it was her. She was then asked to think of the reason why Jackie may have walked off. Initially Paula came out with reasons using invectives towards Jackie, but she eventually admitted that Jackie was very anxious and that her questioning her may have caused her to panic and run away.

Finally, there was discussion about what would be an alternative behaviour in this situation. Paula felt that a 'cue card' that she could write saying 'this feeling is because I am feeling as I did as a child' would be helpful to get her to stop and think. She then agreed that if she had immediately gone and asked the staff to talk to her, they would have done so and she could have obtained attention that way. However, she said she felt very angry and would need to dissipate this. Asked for ways in which she could reduce her anger that had worked with her, she said physical activity would work but that rushing out of the hostel in a blind rage would not be a productive idea. Instead she said she could have asked one of the staff to play table tennis with her but that she was not sure if they would be happy to do so, such was the bad feeling towards her. It was agreed that the therapist would discuss this with the staff. Another way when staff were busy would be for Paula to do physical workout with her games console, which had jogging on the spot and also air boxing as options.

In the treatment there were many slip-ups and she did take overdoses and also self-harmed in other ways, but it was noted by her psychiatric team that this was far less often than previously. Initially, just having a regular appointment with a therapist seemed to help. Self-harm episodes then started to occur whenever the therapist went on holiday or was not available one week (despite Paula being given several weeks' notice of this). The therapist discussed this with her and the reason behind how this made her feel rejected as she did as a child. In reality, harming herself would not make the therapist come back from leave and so alternative strategies for dealing with her emotions were devised. Over the next 2 years, realising that the therapist did not leave was another factor, but this meant that 6 months prior to discharge she needed to be prepared for this and to look towards the other support mechanisms she had now developed. These included the people at a charity shop where she now worked part-time on a voluntary basis as well as the friends she had made at a martial arts club she attended. Despite this she needed 6 moths' warning and still had a slip-up and scratched her wrist with a kitchen knife on the day following her last weekly session with the therapist. She was then seen at 1 month, 3 months, 6 months and 1 year after discharge to check if she had maintained her gains. At the end of therapy, she had a much better understanding of how her powerful emotions of isolation and being abandoned were related to her early childhood experience. She also developed a number of 'adult' ways of dealing with these emotions and distress rather than reverting to self-harm or aggressive behaviour. In general, there had been virtually no aggressive outbursts and although there had been some self-harm attempts, these were much less frequent and much less severe than before therapy.

Borderline personality disorder

Patients with borderline personality disorder (BPD) are frequent users of both primary and secondary health services. It has been estimated that between 5 and 10% or the population have a borderline personality disorder, but the resources which are needed to deal with their problems are often extensive (Gross *et al*, 2002; Angstman & Rasmussen, 2011).

The American Psychiatric Association has defined the essential features of personality disorder as impairments in self and interpersonal functioning (American Psychiatric Association, 2013). The main features of borderline personality disorder are:

- impairment in empathy towards others (often combined with interpersonal hypersensitivity)
- difficulty with intimacy with unstable or unequal relationships
- emotional lability
- anxiety
- separation insecurity
- depression
- impulsivity
- risk-taking
- hostility.

These traits should be stable over time and not a result of an episode of illness or substance misuse. People with borderline personality disorder can frequently also have comorbid psychiatric problems, such as alcohol or drug misuse, generalised anxiety disorder, depression, bipolar disorder and eating disorder (Westphal *et al*, 2013).

Dialectical behaviour therapy for borderline personality disorder

Dialectical behaviour therapy (DBT) was pioneered by Marsha Linehan from the University of Washington. This is likely to be used in a specialist personality disorder service and does require specific training to practise but it is worthwhile considering some of the elements and how these may be useful in general psychiatric practice. The method was introduced for the treatment of borderline personality disorder. It should be noted, however, that a Cochrane Database review found only limited evidence for both psychoanalytically informed therapies (e.g. transference-focused therapy; mentalisation-based therapy; dynamic deconstructive psychotherapy and interpersonal psychotherapy) and CBT-informed therapies (e.g. Beck-style CBT; schema-focused therapy; dialectical behaviour therapy; systems training for emotional predictability and problem-solving for borderline personality disorder; manual-assisted cognitive treatment and psychoeducational methods) and concluded that 'none of the treatments has a very robust evidence base, and there are some concerns regarding the quality of individual studies. Overall, the findings support a substantial role for psychotherapy in the treatment of people with BPD but clearly indicate a need for replicatory studies' (Stoffers *et al*, 2012).

Biosocial theories of the development of personality are the underlying model for DBT (Linehan, 1993*a*,*b*). It is postulated that, as children, patients with BPD had an 'invalidating environment'. This is an environment in which appropriate attention was not focused on the child and the emotions they experienced. In addition, people who experience BPD are more emotionally vulnerable than others. Emotional vulnerability means that the individual's autonomic nervous system reacts rapidly to even low levels of stress and that these changes are extremely slow in returning to normal following stress. Thus the child experiences extreme emotions with physical symptoms but yet is not supported or helped by their environment, family or those *in loco parentis*. The child then grows into an adult with extreme physical and mental distress in response to external events. In addition, owing to the symptoms of BPD, the individual will often form unstable and unsuitable relationships and engage in unhelpful lifestyle choices, which add to the distress and symptomatology. These individuals are aware of their difficulty with coping with stress and often blame others for placing too many demands on them. But they also tend to replicate the invalidating environment internally and thus will demonstrate 'self-invalidation'. They have unrealistic goals and expectations and feel angry with themselves when they fail to achieve them. This blaming of others but also self-invalidation constitutes what Linehan called a dialectical dilemma. In addition, people with BPD tend to experience a high level of negative and traumatic external events which are related to their lifestyle and also to their extreme emotional reactions with prolonged levels of arousal. The end result is described by Linehan as a pattern of 'unrelenting crisis'.

Once the patient experiences very high levels of distress, he or she does not have the coping skills to manage this and thus many maladaptive behaviours such as self-harm, binge drinking or binge eating may be used to try and deaden the feelings.

Another feature of people with BPD is referred to as 'active passivity' and 'apparent competence'. Whereas individuals with BPD are often good at finding others who they believe will solve their problems for them, they are passive and inefficient at solving their own problems themselves. In addition, the demands placed on the people they think can solve their problems are extreme and unrelenting, and inevitably relationships mostly break down. A model for this disorder is shown in Fig. 14.3.

The term 'dialectical' refers to Greek philosophy. It is accepting that in most situations there can be no absolute truth. A thesis or belief can be challenged with an antithesis or opposite view. Using dialogue, individuals can come to a 'happy medium'.

Body dysmorphic disorder occurs more frequently in women than men and a high proportion of individuals have suffered from childhood sexual abuse. It will be seen that there are a number of similarities in treatment to that described previously using schema-focused methods.

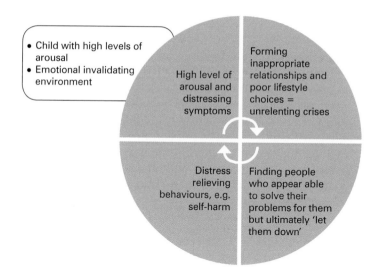

Fig. 14.3 Model of borderline personality disorder.

Before DBT commences

It is recognised that treating patients with BDD is extremely stressful for the therapist and therefore support from colleagues is always stated as an integral and essential component of DBT. The therapist is asked to accept the following about the patient:

- the patient wishes to change (despite appearances the patient is trying to achieve this change but is unable to fulfil all aspects of treatment owing to the underlying pathology)
- the behaviour is understandable when related to early life experience and current situation change will require the patient to work hard
- patients cannot fail DBT – in such cases it is the treatment that failed.

Before treatment is undertaken, the following agreement is reached with the patient:

- to work in therapy for at least 1 year and to attend (within reason) all therapy sessions
- suicidal and self-harming behaviours need urgent work to reduce them
- therapy-interfering behaviours need to be addressed
- to attend skills training.

Main treatment in DBT

Treatment has four main components:

- individual therapy
- group skills training

- telephone contact
- therapist consultation.

Most of the therapy, however, takes place in the individual therapy with the therapist and group therapy can be added in after the patient has been in therapy for a few months. The most controversial aspect of DBT is the telephone contact whereby the patient can telephone the therapist even out of hours. The idea behind this is that it is to help guide the patient through real-life situations without resorting to self-harming or other maladaptive behaviour. It should not be used after self-harm has occurred and in such situations the therapist is instructed to do nothing apart from ensuring patient safety and then the patient is allowed no further contact for 24 hours to avoid reinforcing the self-harm.

Individual therapy in DBT

The individual work with the therapist goes through several stages:

- Pre-treatment stage: this has been described earlier and concentrates on obtaining the patient's commitment to therapy and establishing the basic ground rules for the therapeutic alliance.
- Stage 1: focuses on self-harm behaviours. Included in these are any other therapy-interfering behaviours such as binge drinking and eating or sexual promiscuity as a way of self-harm. Therapy concentrates on problem-solving and developing other skills to deal with the high levels of arousal.
- Stage 2: looks at any post-traumatic stress issues. This can be done using exposure methods and also combining this with methods of reducing distress. It is important that this item is tackled *after* the work on reducing self-harming behaviours is completed or else there is likely to be an escalation of such negative behaviours.
- Stage 3: focuses on self-esteem and individual treatment goals using cognitive therapy and other problem-solving skills.

Overall, the therapist seeks to produce change using:

- problem-solving skills
- contingency management
- cognitive therapy
- exposure-based therapies
- pharmacotherapy.

There is conflicting evidence regarding antipsychotic agents as well as for SRIs.

Group skills training

There are four modules involved in this:

- core mindfulness skills
- interpersonal effectiveness skills

- distress tolerance skills
- emotion modulation skills.

Mindfulness techniques have been described in previous chapters; they are based on a technique used in Buddhism but are without any religious connotations. Using meditation, the patients are taught to concentrate on what is actually happening in the here and now rather than worrying about future or past events or concentrating on their emotional distress.

Interpersonal effectiveness skills are similar to many of the social skills described in Chapter 4.

Distress tolerance skills include using 'acceptance' of the emotion if this cannot be altered at the time (acceptance and commitment therapy is discussed in Chapter 8).

Emotional modulation skills involve:

- identifying and labelling emotions
- identifying any obstacles to changing emotions
- increasing positive emotional events
- increasing mindfulness to current emotions
- applying distress tolerance techniques.

Key learning points

- Personality disorders result from early experiences and maladaptive schemata formation.
- CBT for personality disorders is a long-term therapy taking at least 1 year and frequently 2–3 years.
- Schemata are patterns of beliefs which are generally unconscious. Schema are rigid, over-generalised and held without question.
- Three main mechanisms have been identified which maintain the schemata. These are:
  - surrender
  - compensation
  - avoidance.
- Schema-focused therapy looks more closely at the therapeutic relationship and the therapist may need to use empathic confrontation and limited re-parenting.
- In schema-focused therapy the patient may be encouraged to 're-live' certain childhood experiences and to link these to current emotions.
- Rather than the term 'core-beliefs', there is more emphasis on 'core emotional experiences'.
- Therapy thereafter involves standard CBT techniques of collaborative empiricism and Socratic questioning; challenging negative automatic thoughts and core beliefs.
- Dialectical behaviour therapy (DBT) is a treatment developed specifically for borderline personality disorders.

continued on nex page

Key learning points, *continued*

- DBT emphasises the relationship between the therapist and the patient and uses a hierarchy of modules. These start with engagement of the patient, dealing with self-harm and self-destructive behaviours, post-traumatic stress and self-esteem issues. Individual work with the therapist involves:
  - problem-solving skills
  - contingency management
  - cognitive therapy
  - exposure-based therapies
  - pharmacotherapy.
- Group therapy in DBT focuses on four main modules:
  - core mindfulness skills
  - interpersonal effectiveness skills
  - distress tolerance skills
  - emotion modulation skills.

Suggested measures to use with conditions covered in this chapter

- Measuring outcome of therapy for all personality disorders: the Personality Belief Questionnaire-Short Form (Butler *et al*, 2007), Young Schema Questionnaire (Young & Brown, 2003), Problems and targets and Sheehan Disability Scale (measuring impact on life) discussed in Chapter 2.
- For specific personality disorders: Borderline Symptom List short version (BSL-23; Bohus *et al*, 2009), Narcissistic Personality Inventory (Raskin & Terry, 1988).

References

American Psychiatric Association (2013) *Diagnostic and Statistical Manual for Psychiatric Disorders (DSM-5)*. APA.

Angstman KB, Rasmussen NH (2011) Personality disorders: review and clinical application in daily practice. *American Family Physician*, **84**: 1253–60.

Beck AR, Freeman A (1990) *Cognitive Therapy for Personality Disorders*. Guilford Press.

Beck AT (1967) *Depression: Causes and Treatment*. University of Pennsylvania Press.

Beck AT (1979) *Cognitive Therapy and the Emotional Disorders*. Penguin Books.

Beck JS (1995) *Cognitive Therapy: Basics and Beyond*. Guilford Press.

Bohus MM, Kleindienst N, Limberger MF, *et al* (2009) The short version of the Borderline Symptom List (BSL-23): development and initial data on psychometric properties. *Psychopathology*, **42**: 32–9.

Butler AC, Beck AT, Cohen LH (2007) The Personality Belief Questionnaire-Short Form: Development and Preliminary Findings. *Cognitive Therapy and Research*, **31**: 357–70.

Gross R, Olfson M, Gameroff M, *et al* (2002) Borderline personality disorder in primary care. *Archives of Internal Medicine*, **162**: 53–60.

Linehan MM (1993*a*) *Cognitive Behavioural Treatment of Borderline Personality Disorder*. Guilford Press.

Linehan MM (1993*b*) *Skills Training Manual for Treating Borderline Personality Disorder*. Guilford Press.

Raskin R, Terry H (1988) A principal-components analysis of the Narcissistic Personality Inventory and further evidence of its construct validity. *Journal of Personality and Social Psychology*, **54**: 890–902.

Stoffers JM, Vollm BA, Rucker G, *et al* (2012) Psychological therapies for people with borderline personality disorder. *Cochrane Database of Systematic Reviews*, **8**: CD005652.

Westphal M, Olfson M, Bravova M, *et al* (2013) Borderline personality disorder, exposure to interpersonal trauma, and psychiatric comorbidity in urban primary care patients. *Psychiatry*, **76**: 365–80.

Young JE, Brown G (2003) *Young Schema Questionnaire: L3a*. New York Schema Therapy Institute.

Young JE, Klosko JS, Weishaar M (2003) *Schema Therapy: A Practitioner's Guide*. Guilford Press.

Recommended treatment manuals and other reading

Beck AT, Freeman A, Davis DD (2007) *Cognitive Therapy for Personality Disorders* (2nd edn). Guilford Press.

Linehan MM (1993) *Cognitive Behavioural Treatment of Borderline Personality Disorder*. Guilford Press.

Linehan MM (1993) *Skills Training Manual for Treating Borderline Personality Disorder*. Guilford Press.

*McKay M, Wood JC, Brantley J (2007) *The Dialectical Behavior Therapy Skills Workbook: Practical DBT Exercises for Learning Mindfulness, Interpersonal Effectiveness, Emotional Regulation and Distress Tolerance*. New Harbinger Publications.

*Wood J (2010) *CBT Workbook for Personality Disorders: A Step-by-Step Program*. New Harbinger Publications.

*Suitable to recommend to patients.

CBT in combination with other therapy

Overview

Many books on CBT fail to take account of the fact that most patients with mental health problems are receiving psychotropic medication. Such medication may be unhelpful, as with long-term benzodiazepine treatment of anxiety disorders, or helpful and indeed essential, as with treatment of schizophrenia, moderate to severe depression or severe, refractory OCD. The interactive effect of medication and CBT will be discussed in this chapter. Sometimes other non-pharmacological treatments will also be necessary to effect meaningful change. Examples such as the use of EMDR for post-traumatic stress disorder (PTSD) will be described. In addition, the pitfalls of combining CBT with more analytical approaches will be evaluated as well as a brief examination of CAT and systemic family therapy.

Medication and CBT

CBT therapists have not always been accepting of the role of medication in treatment. It remains a fact, despite this, that the majority of patients who are treated by CBT in a psychiatric hospital and a significant minority treated by CBT in general practice will be on at least one psychopharmacological agent.

In 2012, an international panel of experts reported some guidelines on the psychopharmacological treatment of anxiety disorders, OCD and PTSD in primary care (Bandelow *et al*, 2012). This group of eminent psychiatrists and others concluded that selective serotonin reuptake inhibitors (SSRIs) were useful in all conditions; serotonin-noradrenaline reuptake inhibitors (SNRIs) for anxiety disorders (not OCD) and pregabalin for generalised anxiety disorder only. A combination of medication and CBT including exposure therapy was shown to be a clinically desired treatment strategy.

The benzodiazepine experience

The first benzodiazepine, chlordiazepoxide, was introduced for the treatment of anxiety in the late 1950s. Thereafter a large number of similar compounds came on the market. Unlike their predecessors, the barbiturates, these were considered to be safe and not to produce dependency and withdrawal syndromes. Throughout the 1960s and 1970s they were widely prescribed in general practice and hospitals for mild anxiety, bereavement, insomnia as well as all psychiatric disorders. In short they were considered a panacea for a whole range of human ills and emotions. However, by the 1980s it began to be clear that these drugs did in fact produce tolerance and were associated with a withdrawal syndrome in at least some people who used them for months or years. The withdrawal syndrome was even seen with gradual reduction of the drugs and was characterised by a recurrence of severe anxiety, sensory intolerance, weight loss and perceptual disturbances (Hallstrom & Lader, 1981). More extreme and potentially dangerous withdrawal symptoms were occasionally seen in patients who stopped the drug abruptly. Since that time it has generally been strongly recommended that benzodiazepines should only be prescribed for short periods of time (maximum 6 weeks), whereby the risk of withdrawal is reduced. Indeed the whole role of benzodiazepines in psychiatry has been questioned (Dell'osso & Lader, 2012).

Benzodiazepines such as chlordiazepoxide and diazepam have a long half-life, with metabolites remaining in the bloodstream for up to 3 weeks. With short-acting benzodiazepines, such as lorazepam, the clinical effect has usually diminished within 4–6 hours and it is removed completely from the body in 18–36 hours. This can be a huge problem if combined with psychological treatment, as blood levels of anxiolytic fluctuate greatly throughout the day in parallel with the levels of anxiety experienced. This is particularly a problem with exposure-based treatment methods. In such cases it is usually best to switch the patient onto the equivalent dosage of a long-acting benzodiazepine (bearing in mind that 1 mg of lorazepam is equivalent to 10 mg of diazepam) and withdraw this gradually before embarking on exposure treatment.

The other fear with benzodiazepine drugs is that they may produce state-dependent learning. State-dependent learning is when a person (or animal) learns a skill or a piece of information in a particular emotional or drugged state and then cannot recall this when the emotion has subsided or the drug level has reduced (Goodwin et al, 1969). An example of this is the belief that many darts players can only play optimally when at a specific level of intoxication. Benzodiazepines are specifically used before unpleasant medical procedures to produce anterograde amnesia (Lister, 1985). The evidence for state-dependent learning in humans is patchy, but it is probably wise to try and reduce the level of benzodiazepines to 15–20 mg diazepam equivalent a day before embarking on exposure therapy (Case example 15.1).

Case example 15.1: Multi-drug therapy for profound OCD

John was a 60-year-old man who had a severe and crippling OCD. His main fear was that he might contaminate himself or others with HIV, which he feared he could contract from anything touched by the public. His days were spent checking for anything that looked like blood or needles and avoiding public toilets and communal buildings for fear of catching the virus. Indeed, his problems were so bad that he had been a virtual recluse for the past 5 years and spent most of his days in the house, and would repeatedly wash and bathe for up to 6 hours if he stepped outside his door.

His GP had tried him on several SSRI drugs and he eventually found one which relieved his anxiety somewhat. He was still crippled by anxiety, however, and following attempts at ERP treatment from the local psychiatric services, he was started on a small dose of an antipsychotic drug as well. Although this again improved his situation, he still repeatedly telephoned the genito-urinary clinic at his local hospital to seek reassurance regarding HIV infection. His GP had first prescribed lorazepam to him 5 years earlier. At the time of referral to the clinic, he was grossly obese (BMI=40), having reduced his exercise owing to the problems. He was taking 8 mg lorazepam per day as the GP had gradually escalated the dose over the years to try to cope with his anxiety.

The first thing that was explained to John was that, although 8 mg lorazepam did not sound much, this was equivalent to 80 mg diazepam and was an extremely high dose. He was switched to 80 mg diazepam immediately and remained on this for a week. Thereafter he was reduced by 5 mg per week until he reached 20 mg diazepam. Throughout this time he was closely monitored for any withdrawal symptoms. To try and help him deal with his symptoms of anxiety, he was taught several methods of coping.

Relaxation training

John was sat in a chair and was asked to first contract and then relax his muscles starting at his feet, with the therapist modelling this and talking him through the process. This was recorded so that John could listen to it via an earpiece when he felt the need to relax.

Breathing exercises

John was asked to place his hand on his abdomen. As he breathed in, he was instructed to feel his abdomen move out as his diaphragm lowered. He should do this in-breathe for the count of 5. He should then hold his breath for the count of 5 and finally breathe out again for the count of 5, feeling his abdomen move inwards and 'collapse'.

Tension reduction exercises

Whenever John felt he was getting tense and having muscle pains, he was asked to tense and relax his muscles. Because he often felt tension in his hands, he was asked to squeeze hard on a soft tennis-sized ball and then relax.

Mindfulness techniques

John was instructed not to concentrate on his emotions but to pay attention to the external environment in the 'here and now'.

Distraction

John was asked to think of a list of things he could do to distract himself from his emotional symptoms. He listed: looking at flowers in the garden, watching TV, listening to the radio, telephoning a friend.

Once John reached 20 mg of diazepam, an ERP programme was introduced (see Chapter 7). At the same time the reduction in diazepam was commenced at a pace of 2 mg per week and then, when he reached 6 mg a day, to 1 mg a week. This rate of reduction may seem very slow but John was also undergoing therapy and so it was essential to ensure he could stick to medication reduction as well as battling with his OCD using ERP.

Selective serotonin reuptake inhibitors

In most situations, it is better to manage without medication if this does not interfere with health. There is no such thing as a 'perfect' drug and all inevitably have some potential side-effects. However, the opposite of this stance is also true as it is unethical and unreasonable not to suggest and prescribe a drug to a patient who has a condition which could be helped by medication. Selective serotonin reuptake inhibitors may be useful for a number of conditions.

Phobic disorders

People with simple phobias will rarely need any medication. The best evidence for SSRIs is with social anxiety disorder and there may also be a place for medication to treat individuals with agoraphobia (Drummond & Fineberg, 2007).

Obsessive–compulsive disorder

There is good evidence for the beneficial effects of SSRIs in patients with OCD, however, the effect is dose dependent and dosages need to be at the top end to be effective. Individuals respond differently to different SSRIs and so it is 'horses for courses'. Beneficial effects may not appear until 2 months after starting the medication and can then accrue for up to 2 years. Medication may need to be continued for life if relapse is to be prevented (Tyagi et al, 2010).

Depression

Selective serotonin reuptake inhibitors are effective antidepressants; medication should be continued for at least 6 months to prevent relapse (NICE, 2011a).

Generalised anxiety disorders and panic

Both CBT and medication can be considered for generalised anxiety and panic disorders – treatment with SSRIs, SNRIs and pregabalin has been shown to be effective (NICE, 2011b).

Health anxiety

There is a lack of good trials examining the response of health anxiety and hypochondriasis to medication. In general, it may be expected that these patients, who have similarities with OCD patients, may respond to SSRIs. Schweitzer *et al* (2011) demonstrated that patients who took long-term SSRIs were more likely to be in remission than those who did not. These drugs should thus be considered as an adjunct to CBT in patients with the more severe health anxieties.

Body dysmorphic disorder

Body dysmorphic disorder responds to SSRIs in a similar way to OCD. Thus high levels of SSRIs are necessary and this may need to be continued long term (Phillips & Hollander, 2008).

Anorexia nervosa and bulimia nervosa

In general, there is a lack of good research on the psychopharmacological interventions for anorexia nervosa but SSRIs do appear to be helpful, although occasionally low-dose antipsychotic agents are used (Herpertz *et al*, 2011). The evidence for SSRIs and bulimia nervosa is stronger (Aigner *et al*, 2011).

Personality disorder

There is conflicting evidence regarding SSRIs and antipsychotic agents. The former may be useful for comorbid depression and anxiety, and some patients, particularly those with borderline personality disorder, have reported benefit with mood stabilisers (NHS Choices, 2011).

Post-traumatic stress disorder

SSRIs should be prescribed as the first-line psychopharmacological treatment for PTSD (Bandelow *et al*, 2012).

Antipsychotic agents

Any patient undergoing CBT for schizophrenia or other psychotic illness will need to be treated with antipsychotic agents to reduce the risk of relapse.

Refractory OCD can be defined as failure to respond to ERP as well as two trials of SSRIs in maximum *British National Formulary* doses for a minimum of 3 months each. In these cases there is good evidence for the addition of antipsychotic agents to SSRI treatment. The doses of these antipsychotics are usually considerably lower than those used for psychotic disorders. For example, a patient with OCD may be prescribed 100 mg sertraline and 200 mg sulpiride daily or 5 mg aripiprazole. There is insufficient research to conclude that certain antipsychotic medications are better than others in OCD but choice may be determined by the tolerance of any sedating properties and by the ability to titrate the dose up from very small levels (Tyagi *et al*, 2010).

Antipsychotic drugs are often prescribed for patients with personality disorder but again evidence is contradictory for their specific usage. They may be useful in helping a patient cope in particularly difficult periods.

Serotonin-noradrenaline reuptake inhibitors

These drugs can be used with fairly good evidence as second-line treatment for generalised anxiety disorders, panic and some generalised phobic anxieties (Bandelow *et al*, 2012). They are effective antidepressants (Taylor *et al*, 2013), but they are not helpful for OCD and BDD, despite the fact that they are often prescribed for these disorders. In cases where SSRIs do not seem to work, it is preferable to add in an antipsychotic drug or consider supra-normal doses of SSRIs (monitoring blood levels) (Pallanti *et al*, 2002) rather than using SNRIs.

Other agents

Pregabalin

Pregabalin has been shown to be useful treatment for generalised anxiety disorder. It has been suggested for other disorders but there is scanty evidence to support recommending it as a first-line treatment (Bandelow *et al*, 2012).

Alprazolam

Alprazolam has been suggested as an alternative to antidepressants for patients with depressive disorder. A Cochrane review, however, found that most of the studies were of poor quality (van Marwijk *et al*, 2012). Alprazolam has also been advocated for generalised anxiety and panic disorders and, indeed, appears effective in these. However, it cannot be recommended for long-term use owing to the risk of developing tolerance and the abuse potential.

Tricyclic antidepressants

Tricyclic antidepressants were used in the past for depression, generalised anxiety, some phobic anxiety and panic disorders. Although effective, most of these agents have been superseded by SSRIs, which generally have fewer side-effects. Some patients cannot tolerate SSRIs, however, and in these situations tricyclics may be useful.

Similarly, the tricyclic antidepressant with particular serotinergic properties, clomipramine, was once the drug of choice for OCD. Today most patients prefer SSRIs, which have fewer side-effects (and, from the clinician's point of view, are safer in overdose). A substantial minority of OCD patients nevertheless do find the energising effects of SSRIs difficult and prefer the sedating effects of clomipramine (Tyagi *et al*, 2010).

Using other psychological therapies in combination with CBT

The original routes of behavioural psychotherapy were firmly based on pragmatism rather than theory. In other words, therapists used what works, whether or not this supported any particular theory or model of the condition. The important factor was that the patient improved. Despite multiple models and theories used in CBT, the same pragmatic approach is generally adopted. In the previous chapters, a number of 'combination' therapies have been discussed. For example, in Chapter 14 we looked at the treatment of personality disorder involving the therapist applying techniques more often associated with psychodynamic psychotherapy, such as looking closely at the relationship between the therapist and patient.

Eye movement desensitisation and reprocessing (EMDR)

One therapy that is often combined successfully with a CBT approach is EMDR. It was developed by Francine Shapiro as a treatment for PTSD (Shapiro 2001). She postulated that when an individual experiences or witnesses overwhelming or life-threatening trauma it can overwhelm their normal neurological and cognitive coping mechanisms. This leads to inadequate processing of the memories, which become 'stuck' in an isolated memory network. The results of this are the symptoms of PTSD such as flashbacks and nightmares. Treatment involves asking the patient to imagine a traumatic image and then asking them to move their eyes from side to side following the therapist's finger. According to Shapiro, this eye movement accesses both sides of the brain and allows the traumatic memories to be processed rapidly. In order to practise EMDR, a therapist is required to attend a full, several days' long course as well as to have supervision for the first few patients from a qualified EMDR specialist. The EMDR process has several phases.

- *Phase 1:* This involves full assessment and patient education. Key 'targets' for the EMDR are set. These targets may be a pictorial memory, emotion issue or event. In addition any maladaptive cognitions are identified.
- *Phase 2:* Identification of a 'safe place'. This is a memory or image which results in comfortable and positive feelings. This image can be used if the traumatic memories become overwhelming or if a session is brought to an end before resolution can occur.
- *Phase 3:* A 'snapshot' image is chosen which encompasses the negative emotions of the trauma. In addition, the negative cognition associated with this is identified as well as a positive cognition (similar to rational response in CBT; see Chapter 8).
- *Phase 4:* The therapist asks the patient to concentrate on the negative image, feeling and cognitions and a 'set' of eye movements are

performed. After each 'set' the therapists asks the patient if any other thoughts, images or emotions have arisen. At this point the therapist may need to adapt the target image and another set of eye movements is introduced. Eye movement ends when the patient reports very low levels of distress associated with the image.

- *Phase 5:* This is the 'installation phase' when the therapist asks the patient about their positive cognition and ensures this is still valid. If the positive cognition needs some adaptation, then this is done. The therapist then asks the patient to 'hold together' both the traumatic snapshot image and the positive cognition while more eye movements are performed.
- *Phase 6:* The therapist checks whether any physical symptoms have been generated. If so then the patient is asked to concentrate on the area and a further set of eye movements are performed.
- *Phase 7:* Debriefing.
- *Phase 8:* At the beginning of each new session, the therapist reviews the week's progress and any symptoms.

Eye-movement desensitisation and reprocessing has been accepted as a recognised treatment for PTSD. It often has elements of CBT involving exposure. It is recommended EMDR should be offered within weeks of a trauma in those with severe PTSD symptoms (National Institute for Health and Clinical Excellence, 2005). Medication (paroxetine, mirtazepine, amitriptyline or phenelzine) should only be used after the trial of psychological treatment. In reality, EMDR is often best delivered when combined with CBT (Case example 15.2). Care is needed, however, if the EMDR is being delivered by a different therapist to the CBT to ensure that there are no conflicts in the information the patient receives and the tasks they are set. It is often preferable to suspend the CBT and recommence after the EMDR sessions. If one therapist is delivering both therapies, then there should be few problems in combining the treatments.

Case example 15.2: Severe PTSD

Brian was a 50-year-old divorced man who had been involved in a fatal boating accident 5 years earlier. Their small craft had hit some rocks in the ocean and all four of the people on board had ended in the sea. The sea was rough. Brian had managed to save himself and his 12-year-old son, who had severely injured his arm. Another boy had been killed. Brian was plagued by flashbacks and nightmares and had avoided the coast since the accident. Immediately following the accident he had been offered some trauma-focused CBT but had declined this as he felt it would be like 'giving in'. He returned to work as a marketing manager but within 6 months was made redundant. Since that time, Brian had become increasingly isolated. He had lived alone since his divorce 8 years earlier but had previously had an active social life and also had his son staying with him every second weekend and for half of the school holidays. Over time, Brian had reduced the time spent with his son, until he now only telephoned him occasionally and hardly left the house except to buy provisions.

When referred to the clinic it was obvious that Brian was extremely depressed. He, however, did not want to take medication. Risk assessment concluded that Brian was not currently actively suicidal. A full assessment was then performed and a full description of the traumatic incident was obtained. The key traumatic image was finding his son in the water and immediately being convinced his son would die. He admitted to feeling very guilty as he wondered if he could have saved the other boy if he hadn't been so preoccupied with his son and his own safety. Throughout this discussion, it was clear that Brian was extremely distressed, and he was shaking and tearful during the interview.

Initially, it was thought that trauma-based CBT treatment would be implemented. This would involve:

- imaginal exposure to the traumatic memory, including the use of 'freeze-framing' if any memories seem to be avoided
- cognitive reattribution for the NATs which arose.

The CBT treatment of PTSD was developed on the basis that traumatic memories are avoided (in a similar way to phobic stimuli). Unfortunately, because these memories are avoided, they can emerge at other times in the form of flashbacks and nightmares. In many cases of trauma, however, there is much retelling of the story of the trauma, either for insurance purposes, to friends and relatives, or even, in high-profile events, through the television and media. Despite this, people with PTSD do not habituate because they 'gloss over' key traumatic events in the story and thus the avoidance leads to further symptoms. These avoided areas are similar to the 'key snapshot' scenes identified in EMDR and need to be explored along with the emotions and thoughts accompanying them.

Psychoanalytical therapy alongside CBT

The chapter has examined how CBT can often be usefully combined with psychopharmacological treatments and techniques such as EMDR. It is usually not helpful, however, to combine treatment approaches with an entirely different philosophy. One scenario which frequently arises is that a patient has been in long-term psychoanalytical therapy and is referred for simultaneous CBT. This is generally not a useful approach. The two approaches are greatly at variance and allowing this to occur normally means that the patient does not progress in either therapy. In such cases, it is better to ask the patient to arrange a break from the psychoanalytical therapy while the CBT takes place. If the patient is receiving short-term psychodynamically informed therapy, then it is usually possible to wait until this has finished before starting CBT. Sometimes one therapist tries to deliver a combination of CBT and a more psychodynamic approach. This is usually unhelpful because the focus and the theories are widely discordant.

Cognitive analytical therapy

One possible exception to a combination of psychoanalytical therapy and CBT is the development of cognitive analytical therapy (CAT), but in this case it is the merging of two theoretical approaches into a brief-focused but analytically based treatment. The therapy was developed by Anthony Ryle in the NHS. Trained as an analytical psychotherapist, Ryle created a time-limited talking treatment with the aim of treating more patients in the NHS (Ryle, 1990). In CAT the therapist works collaboratively with the patient and identifies goals together in a similar way to CBT. Reformulation of the problems experienced by the patient comes at the start of the therapy and the therapist looks to the patient's past and early life. There are three main pitfalls which are recognised in CAT (Denman, 2001). The first is called 'traps' and describes how individuals engage in behaviour which then confirms the negative feelings they have. For example, by not engaging in activity, a person with depression feeds into the idea that they are a failure. A second pattern is known as a 'dilemma'. In a dilemma, the individual tries to guard against unwanted emotion by trying to produce the opposite. For example, an angry controlling person may be excessively passive and accommodating. However, the continued passivity means that anger builds up and they inevitably have an outburst, which strengthens their belief that they must remain passive. Finally, there are 'snags' or subtle negative aspects of goals. An example of a snag is if an individual wanted to move away from the parental home but also believed that if they were to do so, their parents would be unable to cope alone. In therapy these patterns are examined collaboratively between the patient and therapist. The first quarter of the sessions are known as the reformulation stage of therapy, when the patient and therapist try to understand the causes and maintaining factors of the problems. At the end of this the therapist writes a letter to the patient giving the agreed reformulation of the problems. The second stage of therapy is working on the problems and looking towards change. At the end of therapy both the patient and therapist write letters outlining the advances that have been made in therapy and setting out the tasks for the patient to address in the future (Denman, 2001).

Cognitive analytical therapy was originally devised for neurotic disorders but more recently has been applied for anorexia nervosa and borderline personality disorder. There are no controlled trials which effectively test the place of cognitive analytical therapy.

Systemic family therapy and CBT groups

Systemic family therapy may be used in parallel with CBT, but again, if possible, it may be better to await the end of one before starting the other to avoid confusion and therapy conflicts.

Some patients can be attending a CBT group and also receive individual CBT. In this case there is rarely a conflict in the tasks they are set and the philosophy of the treatment. However, it is usually advisable to ensure that the individual CBT therapist and group leader are aware of the programme being set by each other to avoid any conflicting information.

Key learning points

- Most patients who receive CBT in psychiatric clinics will be on medication for their condition.
- When patients are on medication, it is important to try to ensure that the drugs will optimise the CBT.
- Benzodiazepines were considered the panacea for a number of human ills when first introduced over 50 years ago. Only over time did the problems of tolerance, dependence and potential abuse become clear. These drugs should now only be used in the short term. Despite this, many patients are still receiving long-term benzodiazepines.
- Benzodiazepine withdrawal needs to be very gradual and monitored. At high dosages, CBT intervention should be aimed at reducing acute symptoms of anxiety. Once a low dose of benzodiazepine is reached, more confrontative exposure methods can be used.
- SSRIs are the first-line psychopharmacological treatment for depression and anxiety disorders. In OCD higher doses are necessary for any effect.
- Antipsychotic drugs are essential for patients diagnosed with schizophrenia. They can also be used in combination with SSRIs for refractory OCD. The use of these drugs with personality disorders is more controversial.
- SNRIs are useful in depression and may be helpful as second-line treatments for many anxiety disorders. They are not helpful for OCD and alternative strategies should be used in refractory OCD.
- Pregabalin is a useful drug for generalised anxiety disorder.
- EMD is a technique which is best combined with a CBT approach and has been shown to be effective in the treatment of PTSD.

Suggested measures to use with conditions covered in this chapter.

- Measuring outcome of therapy for PTSD: PTSD Symptom Scale – Interview (PSS-I) (Foa et al, 1993), Problems and targets and Sheehan Disability Scale (measuring impact on life) discussed in Chapter 2.

References

Aigner M, Treasure J, Kaye W, et al (2011) World Federation of Societies of Biological Psychiatry (WF SBP) guidelines for the pharmacological treatment of eating disorders. World Journal of Biological Psychiatry, 12: 400–43.

Bandelow B, Sher L, Bunevicius R, et al (2012) Guidelines for the pharmacological treatment of anxiety disorders, obsessive-compulsive disorder and posttraumatic stress disorder in primary care. International Journal of Psychiatry in Clinical Practice, 16: 77–84.

Dell'osso B, Lader M (2012) Do benzodiazepines still deserve a major role in the treatment of psychiatric disorders? A critical reappraisal. European Psychiatry, 28: 7–20.

Denman C (2001) Cognitive–analytic therapy. Advances in Psychiatric Treatment, 7: 243–52.

Drummond LM, Fineberg NA (2007) Phobic disorders. In Seminars in Adult Psychiatry (ed G Stein): 258–69. RCPsych Publications.

Foa EB, Riggs DS, Dancu CV, *et al* (1993) Reliability and validity of a brief instrument for assessing post-traumatic stress disorder. *Journal of Traumatic Stress,* **6**: 459–73.

Goodwin DW, Powell B, Bremer D, *et al* (1969) Alcohol and recall: state-dependent effects in man. *Science,* **163**: 1358–60.

Hallstrom C, Lader M (1981) Benzodiazepine withdrawal phenomena. *International Pharmacopsychiatry,* **16**: 235–44.

Herpertz S, Hagenah U, Vocks S, *et al* (2011) The diagnosis and treatment of eating disorders. *Deutsches Ärzteblatt International,* **108**: 678–85.

Lister RG (1985) The amnesic action of benzodiazepines in man. *Neuroscience and Biobehavioral Reviews,* **9**: 87–94.

van Marwijk H, Allick G, Wegman F, *et al* (2012) Alprazolam for depression. *Cochrane Database of Systematic Reviews,* **7**: CD007139.

National Institute for Health and Clinical Excellence (2005) *The Management of PTSD in Adults and Children in Primary and Secondary Care* (Clinical Guideline CG26). NICE.

National Institute for Health and Clinical Excellence (2011*a*) *Depression in Adults (http://guidance.nice.org.uk/QS8).* NICE.

National Institute for Health and Clinical Excellence (2011*b*) *Generalised Anxiety Disorder and Panic Disorder (with or without Agoraphobia) in Adults: Management in Primary, Secondary and Community Care* (Clinical Guideline CG113). NICE.

NHS Choices (2011) *Personality disorder: treatment.* Available at: http://www.nhs.uk/Conditions/Personality-disorder/Pages/Treatment.aspx (accessed June 2014).

Pallanti S, Hollander E, Bienstock C, *et al* (2002) Treatment non-response in OCD: methodological issues and operational definitions. *International Journal of Neuropsychopharmacology,* **5**: 181–91.

Phillips KA, Hollander E (2008) Treating body dysmorphic disorder with medication: evidence, misconceptions and a suggested approach. *Body Image,* **5**: 13–27.

Ryle A (1990) *Cognitive Analytic Therapy: Active Participation in Change.* John Wiley & Sons.

Schweitzer PJ, Zafar U, Pavlicova M, *et al* (2011) Long-term follow-up of hypochondriasis after selective serotonin reuptake inhibitor treatment. *Journal of Clinical Psychopharmacology,* **31**: 365–8.

Shapiro F (2001) *Eye Movement Desensitization of Reprocessing (EMDR): Basic Principles, Protocols, and Procedures* (2nd edn): 472. Guilford Press.

Taylor D, Lenox-Smith A, Bradley A (2013) A review of the suitability of duloxetine and venlafaxine for use in patients with depression in primary care with a focus on cardiovascular safety, suicide and mortality due to antidepressant overdose. *Therapeutic Advances in Psychopharmacology,* **3**: 151–61.

Tyagi H, Drummond LM, Fineberg NA (2010) Treatment for obsessive compulsive disorder. *Current Psychiatry Reviews,* **6**: 46–55.

Recommended treatment manuals and other reading

Shapiro F, Forrest MS (1997) *EMDR: The Breakthrough Therapy for Overcoming Anxiety, Stress and Trauma.* Basic Books.

*Shapiro F (2013) *Getting Past Your Past: Take Control of Your Life with Self-help Techniques from EMDR Therapy.* Rodale.

Sudak DM (2011) *Combining CBT and Medication: An Evidence-based Approach.* John Wiley & Sons.

Taylor D, Paton C, Kapur S (2012) *The Maudsley Prescribing Guidelines in Psychiatry.* John Wiley & Sons.

*Suitable to recommend to patients.

Glossary

Activity scheduling

Working with the patient to plan daily activities, ensuring there is a balance of activities giving both a sense of mastery and pleasure.

All-or-nothing thinking

This is sometimes known as 'black and white thinking'. An example would be that someone who is on a weight-reduction diet eats a small item not on the schedule. Instead of accepting the smaller weight loss, the person may feel that they have broken their diet and that they may as well continue to eat many other items.

Anxiety-management training (stress reduction)

Treatment programmes aimed at reducing generalised anxiety and consisting of the following components:
- education
- normalisation
- identifying the maintaining factors
- coping skills such as distraction, relaxation or assertiveness
- reinforcing self-statements.

Arbitrary inference and jumping to conclusions

Conclusions are drawn without weighing up the evidence or considering alternatives.

BASIC ID

A mnemonic representing the major headings described by Lazarus for assessment (behaviour, affect, sensations, imagery, cognition, interpersonal relationships, drugs).

Behavioural activation therapy

One of the so-called third generation therapies. Behavioural activation is strongly behavioural in nature and aims to increase the activity of patients with depression, thereby improving their mood.

Behavioural exchange therapy (reciprocity negotiation training)

A behavioural form of couple therapy where each of the couple perform reciprocal behavioural tasks which are requested by the other. These tasks are performed on a 'give to get' principle.

Behavioural psychotherapy

A group of treatments with the central hypothesis that psychological distress results from maladaptive learned behaviour and can thus be unlearned.

Behavioural tests

A term used in Beck's cognitive therapy whereby the therapist works with the patient to test hypotheses. Differs from exposure as this is not repeated in a prolonged, predictable and regular fashion but tends to be a 'one off' event to disprove a hypothesis.

Classical conditioning

A basic form of learning described by Pavlov in his classic conditioning experiment with dogs. A dog will salivate (unconditioned response) when presented with food. If a bell is rung for several trials before the presentation of food, then the dog will start to salivate (conditioned response) to the sound of the bell (conditioned stimulus).

Cognitive behavioural analysis system of psychotherapy

A form of interpersonal and behavioural therapies which has been developed and patented for the treatment of chronic depression. The technique uses disciplined personal involvement with the patient rather than therapist neutrality. This interaction is used to reinforce desired behaviours in the patient.

Cognitive behavioural therapy (CBT)

A form of therapy whereby the patient's unhelpful and maladaptive thought patterns are identified and then challenged. The challenging is often using behavioural tests or experiments.

Collaborative empiricism

A term used in Beck's cognitive therapy whereby the therapist works with the patient to test hypotheses and challenge faulty thinking.

Communication skills training

A technique often used in marital therapy, though it can be applied with other relationships of groups of people. Faulty communication patterns are identified and then alternative ways of communication are introduced and practised.

Covert sensitisation

A treatment whereby a patient is asked to pair an aversive image with an image of the undesired behaviour, with a view to reducing the frequency or eliminating the behaviour.

Dialectical behaviour therapy (DBT)

A therapy devised for the treatment of borderline personality disorder. The central tenet of DBT is that the patient is taught to reconcile the inevitable contradictions in life, called the dialectical dilemma, for example the patient is asked to accept themselves for what they are but to change their behaviour.

Emotional reasoning

This describes a tendency to react to emotions despite a lack of evidence (e.g. a person who has failed their driving test may believe they will fail again despite the additional practice and thus answer questions randomly and without thought).

Eye movement desensitisation and reprocessing (EMDR)

A therapy used to process traumatic memories in patients experiencing post-traumatic stress. The patient identifies both the traumatic memories and a 'safe place' (a comforting memory which can be invoked if distress is too high). The patient is asked to induce the traumatic memories while bilateral movements are made with the eyes. The theory is that the involvement of both hemispheres of the brain encourages processing of the traumatic memories.

Faulty assumptions

These are unhelpful beliefs or rules which are held by an individual and are not questioned. They arise from early life experiences.

Functional analytic psychotherapy

This is a radically behaviourist approach which was developed from B. F. Skinner's work on avoidance. It is postulated that individuals with depression are fearful of situations and relationships. This is addressed by encouraging them to face these fears in the sessions. This approach is often combined with cognitive therapy.

Graded exposure

This is a treatment involving the patient facing up to a feared situation or object in real life until their anxiety reduces. Items are tackled in a hierarchy of fear. Once an exposure task has been devised, it should be repeated frequently (ideally three times a day), reliably (no changing to less or more frightening stimuli) and for sufficient time for the anxiety to reduce (usually approximately an hour).

Graded exposure and self-imposed response prevention (ERP)

This treatment is used for obsessive–compulsive disorder (OCD). It is the same as graded exposure except that the patient is asked not to perform the anxiety-reducing compulsions or rituals.

Guided mourning

A treatment based on the principles of graded exposure but in which the hierarchy concerns encouraging the individual to face up to their loss and to come to terms with this without denial. Often combined with cognitive therapy to ensure the patient then tries to 'move on' in their life.

Hyperventilation provocation

The therapist demonstrates hyperventilation with the patient whereby they breathe rapidly and deeply for 2 min. This should invoke physical symptoms which are usually identical to those resulting from a panic attack (where there is often unconscious hyperventilation). By being able to induce the symptoms, the patient can also learn to control them.

Integrative couple therapy

The basic tenet of this therapy is that it is the very characteristics of our partners to which we are attracted and love, but which we can also hate. The couple are taught to not only adapt their behaviour but also accept the limitations of each other and return to loving the very characteristics which were causing conflict.

Magical thinking

This is connecting unrelated items and believing them to be connected, e.g. 'it rained today because I forgot my umbrella'.

Magnification or minimalisation

Overplaying the importance of negative cues or underplaying the importance of positive cues.

Mastery and pleasure

Two components which people need in their lives to be content. In individuals who have depression both of these are at a low ebb.

Mentalisation-based therapy

A treatment based on psychodynamic principles and used in borderline personality disorder.

Mindfulness-based cognitive behavioural therapy

A form of treatment where instead of concentrating on changing the content of negative thoughts, the patient is taught to refocus and to 'distance' himself or herself from these thoughts. This is done by teaching mindfulness and focusing on the 'here and now'.

Motivational interviewing

This is a method of engaging patients who are hard to engage in therapy. The therapist avoids any conflict with the patient but tries to work with their stance to encourage them to engage with the therapy.

Negative automatic thoughts (NATs)

These are thoughts which occur spontaneously in response to situations and result in a deterioration in mood.

Negative reinforcement

This is a term from experimental psychology and of little relevance to clinical practice. It refers to learning which occurs in order to avoid negative or unpleasant consequences.

Normalisation

Refers to the education of a patient who often feels that his or her symptoms are highly unusual and worrying.

Operant conditioning

A term from animal psychology where the animal is trained to perform some instrumental response in order to gain reward. When applied to therapy with patients it involves the use of positive reinforcement.

Overgeneralisation

The belief that if one thing is wrong or bad, then everything is wrong or bad.

Positive reinforcement

Rewarding the desired behaviour, most frequently by praise and encouragement.

Premack's principle

High probability behaviours can be used to reinforce target low-probability behaviours.

Punishment

No application in clinical practice owing to ethical considerations. Refers to the application of an unpleasant negative stimulus to reduce undesired behaviours.

Rational emotive behavioural therapy (REBT)

Therapy where the therapist challenges the irrational beliefs of the patient and encourages them to engage in behaviour to counteract the irrational beliefs.

Reinforcement

An event or stimulus which when made contingent on a response, alters its probability.

Response cost

A form of reinforcement whereby the individual either loses or forteits the ability to gain a positive reinforcer.

Safety behaviours

These behaviours, most commonly seen in social anxiety and agoraphobia, are designed to reduce anxiety and can thus be seen as a form of avoidance, for instance a patient with agoraphobia may wear sunglasses when travelling outside as this reduces the stimulation of the outside world.

Schema avoidance

These are a group of blocking behaviours which help avoid emotional arousal.

Schema compensation

Primary avoidance of emotional arousal by developing strategies which enforce the beliefs.

Schema-focused CBT

The long-term type of therapy which aims to help the patient to identify deep-seated beliefs and values which have been developed in childhood. Therapy aims to examine these schemata and challenge any maladaptive and unhelpful patterns. This type of therapy is used mainly for patients with personality disorders. Therapy can continue for as long as 2 years.

Schema surrender

A model of the way in which an individual will always seek evidence that supports the beliefs and dismiss evidence that contradicts the beliefs.

Selective abstraction and disqualifying the positive

Concentrating on all the negative cues to the detriment of the positive.

Sexual skills training

Treatment developed from that devised by William H. Masters and Virginia E. Johnson in the 1960s. The aim of therapy is to remove the pressure of performance anxiety by banning sexual intercourse throughout therapy. The first stages are aimed at introducing sensual feelings into the relationship. Specific behavioural skills directed at specific problems can then be introduced.

Social skills training

Teaching how to behave in social situations by breaking down complex behaviours into the component parts and using positive reinforcement to increase these.

Socratic questioning

A form of interviewing where the patient is encouraged to work collaboratively with the therapist to discover the answers.

Squeeze technique

A technique used in sexual dysfunction therapy for premature ejaculation. The man squeezes his penis just below the corona before he reaches the stage of ejaculatory inevitability to reduce excitement levels and delay orgasm.

State anxiety

Anxiety which is induced by specific objects or situations.

Stop–start technique

A technique often used in sexual skills training where a patient has premature ejaculation. Originally described by Semans in 1956. In this technique stimulation of the man occurs until he becomes aroused to the point before ejaculatory inevitability. He then signals to his partner and all activity and stimulation stops until his arousal levels reduce.

Systematic desensitisation

An old-fashioned and now almost obsolete type of therapy where a patient with phobia was introduced to a very extensive and rigid hierarchy of fears (usually mainly in imagination) and this was paired with deep muscle relaxation. Not used since quicker and more reliable exposure methods have been developed.

Third wave (third generation)

Towards the end of the 20th century, the shortfalls of CBT for some conditions were being reported. To this end a group of therapies were developed which were often strongly behavioural in orientation. These third wave therapies had certain features in common, including empirical base, being subject to scientific evaluation or concentrating on the patient's reaction to thoughts rather than the thoughts *per se*.

Thought–action fusion

The belief that thinking about an act is tantamount to performing the act.

Trait anxiety

The inherent level of anxiety in an individual. This varies greatly from one person to another.

Waxing and waning

A technique used in sexual therapy for erectile failure. Stimulation occurs until arousal takes place but then, instead of proceeding directly to intercourse, the couple stop stimulation and allow the excitement levels to abate before recommencing. This technique is aimed at reducing performance anxiety and to reduce any catastrophising if an erection is not sustained.

Yerkes–Dodson law

There is an optimum level of anxiety for peak performance. Too high or too low levels of anxiety impede performance.

Index

Compiled by Linda English